The Preemie Parents' Companion

The Preemie Parents' Companion

The Essential Guide to Caring for Your Premature Baby
in the Hospital, at Home, and Through the First Years

SUSAN L. MADDEN, M.S.

Foreword by William Sears, M.D.
Introduction by Jane E. Stewart, M.D.

The Harvard Common Press
Boston, Massachusetts

The information and suggestions offered in this book should be used in conjunction with, but not as a replacement for, the medical care you receive from your professional healthcare providers.

The Harvard Common Press
535 Albany Street
Boston, Massachusetts 02118
www.harvardcommonpress.com

Printed in the United States of America
Printed on acid-free paper

Library of Congress Cataloging-in-Publication Data
Madden, Susan L.
    The preemie parents' companion : the essential guide to caring for your premature baby in the hospital, at home, and through the first years / Susan L. Madden ; foreword by William Sears ; introduction by Jane E. Stewart.
        p.   cm.
Includes bibliographical references and index.
ISBN 1-55832-134-9 (hc. : alk. paper). — ISBN 1-55832-135-7 (pbk. : alk. paper)
    1. Infants (Premature) 2. Infants (Premature)—Care. 3. Infants (Premature)—Development.   I. Title.
RJ250.3.M34   2000
618.92'011—dc21   99-25790
                                                                  CIP

Special bulk-order discounts are available on this and other Harvard Common Press books. Companies and organizations may purchase books for premiums or for resale, or may arrange a custom edition, by contacting the Marketing Director at the address above.

Cover photograph by Michele McDonald
Cover design by Suzanne Noli
Text design by Joyce C. Weston
Illustrations by Kathleen Gray Farthing
Any photograph not specifically credited is courtesy of the author.

10 9 8 7 6 5 4 3 2 1

To my late father, Donald B. Leach,

whose integrity and independence of mind remain an inspiration

and

To my children, Megan, Charlie, and Philip

Contents

ℰᴑ

Contents

Foreword

by William Sears, M.D.

A premature baby is deprived of the final weeks or months inside the womb. Instead, the baby—especially one with medical problems needing weeks or months of intensive care—grows in an "outside womb," where parents can watch and share in the care. While newborn intensive care units improve survival and well-being, it's easy for parents to feel displaced from the care of their baby. Care of preemies is a team approach—and parents are a valuable part of this team. *The Preemie Parents' Companion* shows parents how to be an indispensable part of the medical team.

When I was director of a premature nursery at a university hospital I would encourage mothers and fathers to sit right beside the incubator and caress their babies. I believed there was something therapeutic in a parent's touch. Recent research has validated this observation: Newborns stroked by a parent have fewer stop-breathing episodes and better weight gain. Another recent parent-care innovation in premature nurseries is the concept of "baby wearing." Babies are wrapped around the mothers in a sling-like wrap or are worn in a baby sling. Research has found that these babies gain weight faster and leave the hospital much sooner. The researchers conclude that the close proximity of mothers helps premature babies thrive. Being close to mother warms and calms the premature baby. Mother's breathing movements stimulate baby's breathing so that, in effect, mother acts as a respiratory pacemaker for her premature infant. So, parents, you can see that you are a VIP in the care of your premature baby.

A premature baby has an even greater need for mother's milk. Premature babies need more calories and protein for catch-up growth. Researchers have discovered that the breastmilk of mothers who deliver preterm babies is higher in fat, calories, and protein—just what the doctor ordered. In this book, mothers will learn the trials and rewards of breastfeeding their preterm infants.

Another way parents of premature infants can join the medical team is by an innovation dubbed *kangaroo care*, an affectionate term derived from the way the kangaroo mother carries her own preterm infant. Research by Dr. Gene Cranston Anderson in Cleveland has shown that preemies receiving kangaroo care gain weight faster, have fewer stop-breathing episodes, and experience a shorter hospital stay. With kangaroo care, mother uses a baby sling and wears her diaper-clad baby skin to skin on or between her breasts. A combination of warm milk, warm body, and warm blankets keeps a premature baby toasty, which is important because a lack of insulating body fat allows these little babies to get cold. Closeness to mother's breast stimulates baby to feed whenever he is hungry. Babies who have kangaroo care cry less, too. Crying wastes energy and oxygen, which is needed for preemies to grow.

Besides being good for babies, participating in the care of your premature infant is good for mothers, too. The closeness of baby on mother's breasts triggers her milk-producing hormones, which also help mother bond to her baby by giving her a biochemical boost in her mothering skills.

A valuable parenting concept is one we call the need-level concept. Certain babies have a high level of need, which in turn requires a high level of parenting. Premature babies are special babies that need a special kind of parenting. This book helps parents to meet the high needs of the premature baby and thereby enjoy the unique rewards of this special type of parenting.

Introduction

by Jane E. Stewart, M.D.*

ℰ

Premature births in the United States occurred at higher levels during the 1990s than they did during previous decades. In the latter part of the nineties, about 75,000 newborns each year were what doctors called *very preterm* infants, which means that they were born after a pregnancy of 31 weeks or less. An additional 361,000 babies were *preterm*—born between 32 and 36 weeks. Together, the two figures add up to about 436,000 premature births annually.

There are many reasons for the rather sharp rise in recent years in the rates of preterm and very preterm births (and in the related rates of low birthweight and very low birthweight babies). One clear reason is the rise in multiple births, which has occurred largely as a result of the increased use of assisted reproductive techniques. The number of twins has risen 52 percent and the number of triplets has quadrupled since 1980.

Fortunately, with advances in technology and in our understanding of the unique medical problems faced by premature infants, the number of babies who are able to survive despite such an early beginning continues to increase. We celebrate these successes, and yet we acknowledge that the delivery of a child so early brings tremendous challenges for parents, health-care professionals, and society as a whole. The risk of complications in extremely premature infants remains significant, and a small subset of these babies will have lifelong neurodevelopmental problems. The outcome of premature infants is a major focus of medical research that will help us to predict problems better and ultimately to prevent them. However, our inability at this point to predict health outcomes well, and

---

*Associate Director, Neonatal Intensive Care Unit, Beth Israel Deaconess Medical Center, Boston; Co-Director, Infant Follow-Up Program, Children's Hospital, Boston; Instructor, Pediatrics, Harvard Medical School

the resulting uncertainty during the first years of life, is a source of extreme frustration to parents and health-care providers alike.

The focus of *The Preemie Parents' Companion* is the family. Susan L. Madden offers important information and support for the journey—usually very unexpected—through the newborn intensive care unit (NICU) and then, at last, to home. Even among parents who have had weeks to get ready for their baby's anticipated premature birth, nothing can prepare them for the feelings of uncertainty and powerlessness they experience when they first look at their baby in the NICU. Their tiny infant, attached to machines and monitors with tubes and wires, appears so remote from their original image of a healthy full-term baby lying in their arms. One way to look at the goal of the NICU team is to say that it uses all the resources available to help parents ultimately achieve that image. That means making use of the latest medical technology and information to provide every kind of care that is needed—from managing premature lungs, to ensuring the best nutritional support to achieve the best growth and development. It also means involving parents very early in their baby's care, so that by the time their baby has grown to the stage that she is ready to go home, they feel knowledgeable and confident in their ability to provide that care at home, outside the familiar structure of the NICU. Over the past two decades, with the widespread adoption of "kangaroo care" in the NICU, parents' involvement has been starting much earlier, with even the tiniest babies still on ventilators being held by their mothers and fathers. Parents are now empowered to participate in their babies' care and to be an integral part of the care team.

The resources available to families in the NICU today have grown dramatically. The most important are the daily bedside chats with nurses, doctors, and respiratory therapists that keep parents up to date on their baby's daily progress. To supplement this, there are educational resources such as books, videotapes, and websites. For emotional help, most NICUs have family support groups run by social workers and nurses in the unit. The abundance of resources during the NICU stay provides a marked contrast to the large void most parents experience during the period of time when they first take their baby home.

Susan L. Madden's *The Preemie Parents' Companion* helps to fill that void. This much-needed and unique book is a carefully researched and up-to-date contribution to what until now has been a paucity of books for parents of premature infants. It provides parents with a wealth of practical information that is important in the NICU, but it is most valuable for parents in the period after their baby is discharged to home and in the important first years of life. During the first years of development, the importance of access to medical and other early-intervention resources in ensuring optimal long-term outcomes cannot be overemphasized. *The Preemie Parents' Companion* walks the parent through the available resources and simplifies a process that can be complicated and overwhelming. Likewise, the book shares individual parents' emotional experiences in a way that can only be done parent to parent. This book is a wonderful gift to the families of premature infants whose unique beginnings are part of their families' lives forever. I am thrilled to be able to recommend this resource to families as well as to the many health-care professionals who are involved with the care of premature infants.

Preface

༄

"Take him home and treat him like a normal baby," smiled the doctor as he discharged our eight-week-old son from the hospital's special care nursery. These were the words I had been waiting to hear since that nightmarish afternoon when Philip had been born eleven weeks early, weighing two pounds thirteen ounces.

It seemed that we were finally finished with the nightmare. Now we could try to forget the last eight weeks and pretend that our four-and-a-half pound son had just been born, a little small but healthy. Dressed in a preemie-sized outfit that was still too large, and dwarfed by the straps of his car seat, Philip was photographed by the staff of the nursery and we headed home.

Three days later my husband and I took Philip to our pediatrician for his first check-up. The pediatrician examined our son and pronounced him fine. Then he asked us if we realized that Philip was, in certain ways, still different from a typical newborn. We would probably find him to be extremely sensitive to noise, light, and handling. Unlike other newborns who can fall asleep in the middle of chaos, Philip would not yet have the ability to block out stimulation and could become easily overwhelmed. The doctor told us that Philip would need a quiet, dark place to sleep, away from the everyday noises of a home with two other growing children.

We left the pediatrician's office that day puzzled and somewhat unnerved. We had learned in the hospital that preemies are very sensitive and can become easily overwhelmed. But we naively thought that Philip, having been pronounced a "normal baby" by the expert at the hospital, had grown beyond his preemie beginnings. Now we had a pediatrician telling us otherwise—that Philip was not really a normal newborn, not yet.

Who was right? I desperately wanted it to be the neonatologist. I wanted to be finished with prematurity and all its anxiety and unknowns. But as the months went on, I was struck by many things in Philip's behavior and development that differed from what I had seen with my other two full-term children. I began to meet other parents of preemies, and discovered that they were having similar experiences. What was normal for preemies seemed to be different from what was normal for a full-term baby.

Unfortunately, there was very little information available to help us and other parents understand these differences. The books on prematurity available at the bookstore or library focused on what to expect in the neonatal intensive care unit, the possible complications of prematurity, and how to care for your baby in the hospital. None of these books told us in any detail what to expect in the months and years ahead. Books covering regular newborn behavior and development were helpful, but they lacked information specific to preemies.

This book grew out of our quest for information. Through talking with many other parents of preemies and professionals who work with preemies, and by investigating the growing body of academic research into preemie development, I have tried to put together the information for which my husband and I were searching: a detailed description of the ongoing development of children born prematurely; the special problems for which preemies tend to be at increased risk; and practical information on the common questions and concerns of preemie parents. I have tried to write the book that my husband and I needed.

When I started working on this book, I wanted to focus on what happens after you bring your baby home. But as I talked with other parents and did more research, I realized that it didn't make sense to have a book about preemies begin at the time a baby is discharged from the hospital. How early your baby was born, the types of complications he encountered, and your involvement in his care all set the groundwork for what you will be dealing with at home, so I have started with a section on the hospital period. The second section of the book focuses on the homecoming period and adjusting to home, a time that is usually filled with anxiety as well as joy. In the third section, you will find information on the longer term effects of prematurity, as well as some practical guidelines on getting the most out of early intervention and school-based programs if your child needs them. The final chapter includes stories from veteran parents on the challenges and joys of raising a preemie.

In 1998, the most current year for which data exists, almost half a million babies in the United States were born prematurely, three or more weeks before their due dates. Over half of these, almost 300,000, were born more than four weeks early. Premature births currently account for 11.6 percent of all births, and infants with low birthweights comprise 7.6 percent of the total.

These numbers have been growing over the past fifteen years, in large part because of a dramatic increase in multiple births (twins, triplets, and higher multiples). In three years, from 1995 to 1998, the numbers of triplet and higher-order multiple births increased a startling 53 percent, from 4,973 births to 7,625. Much of this growth in the numbers of multiple births appears to be the result of more widespread use of fertility-enhancing techniques. Pregnancies with twins and other multiples are more likely to result in low birthweights and premature deliveries: about half of all twins and 91% of all triplets or higher multiples are low birthweight, compared with only six percent of single births.

At the same time that the numbers of preemies are growing, the science and art of caring for these tiny babies has improved dramatically so that more and more are surviving and coming home to their parents. Most of these grow into healthy, happy children. However, babies are being discharged from the hospital earlier than ever before. This means they are smaller, more fragile, and tend to have more medical needs at discharge. For example, they may be on oxygen, special formulas, or on breathing or heart-rate monitors. Care that was once provided by professionals in the hospital is now the responsibility of parents at home. Parents need information as they face the special challenges of raising their preemies. Providing that information and sharing the hard-earned knowledge of many preemie parents was one of my desires in writing this book.

One other desire provided a driving force for this book. Periodically, books, newspaper articles, and made-for-television movies focus on prematurity, the story of a particular premature baby or babies. These stories usually present terrifying views of tiny, sick babies, and make people question the wisdom of expending so much effort and money saving tiny infants for uncertain futures. The new parents of a premature infant carry these frightening images and thoughts inside.

While not minimizing the anguish felt by parents of sick preemies or preemies who did not survive, I hope to present a more optimistic and reassuring story. Despite the different way in which these babies begin their lives, most preemies do well and develop into healthy children. This book aims to provide parents with some useful guideposts and encouragement along the way.

Like many other preemie parents, we found that our son Philip outgrew many of his early preemie differences, and by the time he started preschool I found I no longer thought very often about his prematurity. He is now a happy, healthy, physically active fourth grader. From time to time, I still find myself wondering if some learning problems will show up as he is faced with more difficult academic work, but in that I am probably no different from many other parents.

As you watch your own child grow, you may find that there is a part of you that never forgets your child's different beginning. You may feel that you take less for granted, that you appreciate more fully all that he accomplishes. You may worry more about problems or potential problems. Your child's future includes a little more uncertainty than if he had been born full-term, but you also know that he is a fighter. None of us would choose to have our children born early, but once it has happened, most parents and children show an impressive ability to cope and adjust.

PART I:
BORN EARLY

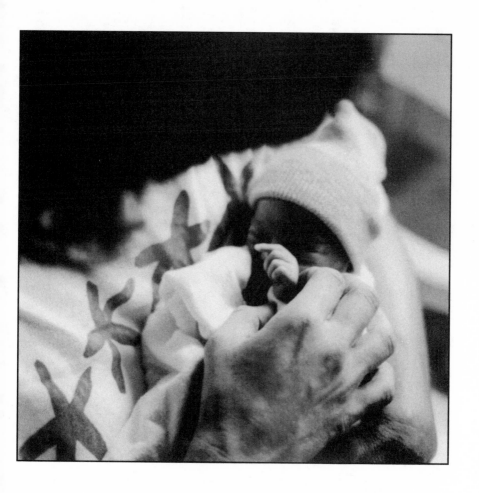

CHAPTER 1

First Questions

ᏀᎯ

FEW PARENTS ARE prepared for the premature birth of their baby. For most, the birth comes with little or no warning, cutting short an otherwise uneventful pregnancy. For others, it comes as a finale to weeks or months of complications, or even years of infertility problems. But whatever precedes it, having your baby too early is always difficult and stressful. Not only are you anxious about your child's survival and health, but you are also faced with the unfamiliar world of neonatal (newborn) intensive care, and with learning to be a parent in a hospital nursery.

Like all parents who face this situation, you will undoubtedly have many questions. The most important and immediate is: Will my baby survive and be healthy? You may wonder why this is happening, and whether something you did—or didn't do—caused your baby to be born early. In this first chapter, we will look at these and other common questions that parents ask when they find themselves facing the premature birth of their baby. This chapter also provides you with some basic information on prematurity, how you can be involved in caring for your baby in the hospital, and your rights as a parent. All of these topics will be covered in greater detail in later chapters but are offered here to help you get oriented as quickly as possible to this new world in which you find yourself.

As with all other chapters in this book, the information here should supplement, not replace, what your own medical caregivers tell you. Because they are familiar with your child's unique situation and needs, they can give you specific information and guidance.

Will My Baby Be All Right?

We all would like to have this question answered with a simple straightforward yes. But because each baby is different and the effects of prematurity are somewhat unpredictable, it is difficult to know how any individual baby will do until some time has passed. The first day or two of your child's life is particularly critical as he adjusts to life outside the womb. After this time, your baby's doctors should be able to give you much more information about how your baby is doing and any specific problems he may be facing.

In the meantime, keep in mind that advances in neonatology (the care of newborns) and neonatal intensive care over the past thirty years have resulted in dramatic improvements in the survival and health of premature babies. Babies born after 28 weeks of gestation, or weighing more than 1,000 grams (approximately 2 pounds 3 ounces), currently have a 90 to 95 percent survival rate. Even very tiny and early babies, born between 25 and 28 weeks and weighing less than 1,000 grams, have survival rates of 75 to 80 percent. As you approach the limits of viability, currently at approximately 22 1/2 weeks, the number of babies who survive begins to drop rapidly, and the survival rate is about 40 percent for those born at 24 weeks. Because your baby's chances of surviving improve so dramatically with each passing day and week, your doctors will do everything they can to help you continue your pregnancy as long as possible.

Only a small percentage of children born prematurely will suffer from serious long-term disabilities. The vast majority—at least 85 percent—will grow to be healthy children. The chances of a preemie developing a serious disability have remained steady and low even as younger and sicker babies are surviving. This means that many more babies—babies who would not even have survived in the past—are growing up with few if any serious long-term problems. As a group, preemies do seem to have an increased chance of certain types of learning disabilities, but this is an ongoing area of research in which there is still much to be learned.

Although, in general, the statistics are quite positive, the many risks and challenges inherent in premature birth should not be minimized. Nor should these statistics be used to try to predict how your own or any other individual baby will fare. Just as each child is unique, each infant's course in prematurity will be different. This means that a baby born at a gestational age of 33 weeks sometimes faces a more difficult recovery than another baby born at 28 weeks. This unpredictability is difficult for everyone—parents, doctors, and nurses. As one neonatologist put it: "We wish we had a crystal ball so we had answers for parents and could know what was going to happen, but we don't."

Like other parents before you, you will undoubtedly find that life in the neonatal intensive care unit (NICU) is an emotional roller coaster as your baby has good days interspersed with bad ones, and you have moments when you feel hopeful and others when you feel panicky. These ups and downs are a difficult but normal part of your child's recovery in the hospital. In the face of all of this uncertainty, try to take each day as it comes and remember that overall the outlook for preemies is more positive now than it has ever been.

How Early Is My Baby?

Although most people think of pregnancy in terms of months rather than weeks, a preemie's age at birth is almost always defined in terms of the number of weeks of gestation he has completed. The way that his age is calculated is explained below.

In the medical world, a pregnancy is considered to begin on the first day of a woman's last menstrual period, known as her LMP. This fairly easy-to-remember date is used as a starting point even though a baby's conception actually occurs about two weeks after this date. Using this system, a normal full-term pregnancy lasts approximately 38 to 42 weeks, with the average being 40 weeks from the beginning of the LMP. A premature birth is one that takes place before the end of the 37th week of pregnancy, also known as the 37th week of gestation, or more than three weeks early.

Your baby's age at birth—known as his gestational age—is also calculated from your LMP. So, if your baby was born 12 weeks before his due date, his gestational age is 28 weeks and you may hear him described as a 28-weeker. Your doctors will probably perform other tests to assess your baby's gestational age and level of maturity before and after his birth, but dating from the LMP is still considered an accurate measure of age, especially for women with regular monthly cycles.

Your newborn will be assessed not just in terms of his gestational age but by his birthweight as well. A full-term baby should weigh at least 2,500 grams, or 5 1/2 pounds; any infant weighing less than that is said to have a low birthweight. Babies may have low birthweights because they are premature or because certain medical problems during the pregnancy interfered with their growth, or both.

Although the definitions of birthweight are constantly evolving, the common classifications used now are the following:

Normal birthweight (NBW)	2,500 grams or more *(5¹/2 pounds or more)*
Low birthweight (LBW)	1,500 grams to 2,499 grams *(3 pounds 5 ounces to 5¹/2 pounds)*
Very low birthweight (VLBW)	1,000 grams to 1,499 grams *(2 pounds 3 ounces to 3 pounds 5 ounces)*
Extremely low birthweight (ELBW)	< 1,000 grams *(less than 2 pounds 3 ounces)*
Micro-preemies	< 750 grams *(less than 1 pound 11 ounces)*

Because of his young gestational age, it is normal for your preemie to have a low birthweight. During the last four weeks of a full-term pregnancy, most babies gain approximately half a pound a week, and develop the fat layers that give them the characteristic chubby baby look that we all expect. Since preemies miss this growth, they often have low birthweights, and are skinny and scrawny looking.

However, even though your baby is officially a low birthweight baby, he may be exactly the right size for his gestational age. This is known as being appropriate for gestational age or AGA. Sometimes preemies are born weighing less than expected because of medical or developmental problems, in which case they are small for gestational age or SGA. Less often, they may be larger than expected, or large for gestational age (LGA).

Your baby's birthweight reflects how well he has been growing in the womb. With a higher weight he starts out with some reserves of energy that will help him in the first few days of life as well. But his gestational age is a better indicator of his developmental stage and what you can expect from him in terms of behavior, appearance, and medical needs.

Why Was My Baby Born Early?

When your baby is born early, it is natural to wonder if you did something that caused it, or if you or your doctor could have caught warning signs early enough to prevent your infant's premature delivery. Unfortunately, for about 60 percent of women, premature labor and delivery occurs for no apparent reason and with little or no warning. Although the newest research indicates that some of these cases may be caused by undiagnosed genital or urinary tract infections, a great deal of mystery still surrounds the subject of why labor begins early, and how to prevent or stop it. Bed rest and certain drugs can sometimes stop or slow premature uterine contractions. Known as tocolytics, the most common drugs used are terbutaline, ritodrine, magnesium sulfate, and isoxsuprine. But for many women, nothing works, or relief is only temporary.

In about 40 percent of cases, the causes of premature delivery can be identified. The most common reasons include premature rupture of the membranes (PROM), also known as breaking your waters, and subsequent infection, and a number of obstetrical and medical problems. Structural abnormalities in the uterus that interfere with the growing fetus, an incompetent cervix in which the opening to the uterus is weak and opens too early, and bleeding behind the placenta can cause premature delivery. If a women has diabetes, kidney disease, high blood pressure or toxemia (pre-eclampsia) or her fetus has severe growth failure or serious distress, an early delivery may occur or need to be artificially induced. Mothers who have had previous premature births are at higher risk to deliver early again, as are those who have had multiple abortions. Very young (under age 16) and older mothers (over age 35) are more likely to deliver early, as are poor women. Long hours on your feet or physically demanding or stressful jobs have also been implicated in early births.

Many, if not most, mothers feel guilty or feel as if they have failed in some fundamental way when their infants are born prematurely. As a mother whose son arrived at 25 weeks said,

"When he was born, I swore it had to be something I did. I felt such guilt. That feeling was with me for a long time, but finally someone told me that it was wasted energy. You can't go back and change what happened, it's over with. You need to go on, to put your energy toward working with your baby and getting him up to being the best he can be. It didn't happen overnight, it took a year and a half for me to get beyond those first feelings. But I think it's so important to be positive."

You, too, may find yourself endlessly reviewing everything you did or didn't do that may have affected the outcome of your pregnancy. Although this is understandable, chances are that nothing you could have done would have substantially changed what happened. As time goes on, try to move beyond scrutinizing the past toward concentrating on how best to help your baby now and in the future.

Where Will My Baby Be Cared For?

Premature babies born more than four or five weeks early generally require care in a special nursery within the hospital, separate from the normal newborn nursery. Depending upon your baby's gestational age and health, he may be cared for in either a Level II nursery, sometimes known as a special or continuing care nursery, or a Level III intensive care nursery, known as a neonatal or newborn intensive care unit (NICU or NBICU).

If you are admitted to the hospital several days or more before your child is born, you may have a chance to visit the nursery where he will be cared for. Although you may worry that this will be too upsetting or scary, many parents find that seeing the nursery and learning more about what to expect actually relieves some of their anxiety. Chapter 2 provides a description of a typical NICU to help familiarize you with what you will see.

Why Was I (or My Baby) Transferred to a Different Hospital?

If you develop complications in your pregnancy or if your newborn begins to have problems after birth, you or he may be transferred to a different hospital than the one you originally planned on for your delivery. This adds another layer of stress to an already difficult situation, particularly if your baby is transferred soon after birth while you remain in the original hospital. Even though these transfers are emotionally difficult, they happen for good reasons.

As the care of preemies has improved, so have their survival rates and overall health. But caring for very premature babies is extremely complex, requiring specialized equipment and techniques, as well as medical personnel with advanced training. Because most community hospitals lack the equipment and expertise to care for these infants, a coordinated system of medical care for mothers and babies—known as regionalized perinatal care—developed in the 1970s. Currently, hospitals that provide maternity services are designated as being Level I, II, or III, based upon the complexity of obstetrical and neonatal problems they can handle. Mothers and babies may be transferred from one hospital to another within a region in order to ensure that they receive the best care possible.

Level I facilities provide care for women having uncomplicated labors and deliveries, and healthy full-term newborns. They can also usually handle large premature babies, approximately 35 weeks or older who weigh at least 4$1/2$ pounds. **Level II** hospitals usually have a neonatologist on staff in the nursery and can handle more complicated perinatal situations, including prematurity down to approximately 32 weeks. The types of cases that a Level II hospital is permitted to handle vary by region and state, but most can provide care for all but the most premature infants or those who need to be on respirators. **Level III** hospitals are equipped and staffed to provide care for all types of obstetrical and neonatal problems including extremely premature—under 32 weeks—and sick full-term infants. Level III nurseries are usually located in large, urban teaching hospitals associated with a medical school and having physician training programs.

If a transfer needs to occur, it's ideal to transfer a mother before her baby is born. Not only is it better for your baby to be born in a hospital that has the appropriate level of nursery, but you won't have to face a separation from him soon after birth.

In many cases, however, delivery happens too rapidly for the mother to be transferred. When that happens, the medical team in your hospital will provide your baby's inital care, and then transfer him in an incubator to another hospital by ambulance or helicopter. A transport team, usually consisting of a physician and nurse, will travel with and care for your baby on his trip. Most hospitals will let you see your baby before he goes and may leave a picture with you.

Having a baby transported to a different hospital is hard on everyone, but often places special burdens on fathers. When a mother is sick and must stay in the original hospital for a number of days after her baby's birth, a father feels stretched in all directions. He wants to visit his baby, but also feels a need to be with his wife. At the same time, he may face the demands of a job and of other children at home.

If your baby must be transferred, try to take comfort from the fact that your new baby is in the best place he can be and is receiving the medical care he needs. If you cannot visit him regularly during this traumatic time, regular phone calls to the nursery should help to keep you informed and involved.

On a more positive note, transfers also go in the other direction. As your baby grows and his health improves, he will be transferred from a Level III to a Level II nursery, sometimes within the same hospital or to a community hospital closer to home. Babies who have been in a Level II or III nursery are never transferred to a Level I nursery; they will continue to be cared for in a Level II nursery until they are discharged home.

Can I Help Care for My Baby in the Hospital?

When something goes wrong with your pregnancy or your baby is born early, it's hard not to feel overwhelmed with anxiety and panic. As one mother succinctly put it, "My world stopped." It's also common to feel utterly helpless in the face of a medical world which has taken over managing your life as well as your baby's. The high-tech surroundings of the intensive care unit and the number of highly skilled staff who care for your child can be intimidating at first. You may feel like an intruder in this world and unsure of your place in it.

But your importance as your baby's parent is unchanged by the circumstances surrounding his early birth. Your presence in the neonatal intensive care unit is not only welcomed but encouraged, and parents generally have 24-hour access to their child. In most units, your baby's doctors and nurses will help you to become involved in your baby's care as early as possible. Even if your baby is extremely premature or sick, you will generally be able to touch him the first time you see him. You might gently cup his head in your hand, place your hand on his back, or let him grasp your finger. Depending upon your baby's gestational age and condition, you may soon be able to hold him, change his diapers, feed and bathe him. Your baby's nurses will teach you how to help with his care.

This early involvement of parents in the care of their hospitalized infants has many benefits, both for the baby and for the parents. Hospital care, although crucial for your baby's health, has many uncomfortable aspects. In this world, your presence—the sound of your voice, your smell, your loving touch—is consistent and comforting to your baby. Babies grow and recover more quickly when they receive their parents' personal, loving care. In addition, by learning how to care for your baby, you'll gradually lose the helpless feeling that you may have had in the beginning, and you'll be better able to act as his advocate.

All parents look forward to the day of homecoming with anxiety as well as anticipation. The more involved you are during your child's hospital stay, the more confident you will be of your abilities to care for him at home, and the easier the transition will be.

Will I Be Able to Breastfeed My Baby?

If your baby is only three or four weeks early, you may be able to put him directly to your breast soon after birth. However, if he is younger than this, he will probably not have the strength or coordination to breastfeed quite yet. In this situation, you will need to use an electric breast pump to establish and maintain your milk supply so that you can supply your baby with your milk, and potentially breastfeed in the future. The postpartum floor and the nursery have breast pumps for you to use, and the nurses can show you how to operate them.

Breastmilk is particularly beneficial for preemies. It is easier to digest than formula and contains high levels of disease-fighting substances that are particularly valuable for early babies. Interestingly, the milk produced by mothers who deliver early differs from that of full-term mothers. It is uniquely suited to the needs of preemies, with higher levels of certain nutrients that preemies need. In addition, many mothers find it particularly satisfying to provide milk; it is the one thing that only you can do when so many other aspects of your baby's care are being handled by others in the nursery.

If you are undecided about breastfeeding, you might want to try pumping for a week or two. You can always change your mind, and you will have given your baby the benefit of your early milk when it is the most beneficial for him. If you decide not to provide milk, rest assured that preemies grow and thrive on formula as well.

How Long Will My Baby Need to Stay in the Hospital?

Although it is difficult to predict exactly when your baby will be ready to go home, most parents are told to expect their babies home around their original due dates. If your baby is healthy and has a relatively trouble-free time in the hospital, he may be discharged three or four weeks before his due date. If he was extremely early or has struggled with a number of complications, he may not be able to come home until a few weeks after his original birthday. Each hospital has its own set of criteria that are used to judge when a baby is ready for discharge. These are explained in Chapter 5.

How Will We Pay for All of This?

It is difficult to think about finances when your baby has just been born early and your concerns are with his health and survival. They are mentioned here because there are a number of things you should check on early in your baby's hospitalization.

In general, most insurance plans, both private and public, cover the costs of hospital care for premature babies fairly completely, although you may need to pay an initial deductible amount. Be sure to notify your insurance company about your baby's birth within a day or two, and check on your coverage. If you are uninsured or your coverage is minimal, talk to the nursery social worker or a hospital financial counselor as soon as possible.

In addition to the direct hospital costs of caring for your baby, many families incur substantial out-of-pocket expenses as a result of their baby's hospitalization. Even parking and meals begin to add up if your baby is in the hospital for several weeks or months. Ask the social worker if the hospital has any programs to help meet these costs, or can offer you discounted parking or meals. If your out-of-pocket expenses are significant, you may be able to deduct them on your income tax return. You will need to document these costs and keep a log of miles driven to visit your baby if you plan to itemize these expenses.

While they are hospitalized, many preemies also qualify for cash benefits under a federal program known as SSI (Supplemental Security Income). For some babies the benefits continue after discharge. The eligibility requirements for SSI periodically change, but currently the program covers babies born weighing less than 1,200 grams (2 pounds 10 ounces), and some babies with medical problems whose birthweights were between 1,200 and 2,000 grams (4 pounds 7 ounces). If you think your child may qualify, ask the nursery social worker for information and call the local office of the Social Security Administration (SSA) to notify them of your intent to apply. Make this phone call as soon as possible (or ask someone to make it for you) because you are eligible for benefits starting from the date you apply or notify the SSA that you intend to apply.

Talk with your nursery's social worker or a hospital financial counselor for the most complete and up-to-date information for your specific situation.

What Are My Rights as a Parent?

One of the most difficult parts of having a baby born prematurely is feeling as if you have no control over any aspect of the situation. When I went into early labor, one of my greatest fears was that the doctors would have complete control over what happened to my son and that I would be powerless to affect their decisions even though I would have to live with the consequences. As difficult as it was to ask, I wanted to know if my husband and I would be allowed to withhold or stop treatment for our son if that seemed like the kindest thing to do. I was comforted to be told that most life-and-death decisions need not be made immediately after delivery, that we would have time to see how our son was doing, and that the medical team would work with us to decide what was best for our child if he began to have serious problems.

As was true in our hospital, most hospitals in the country today consider parents to be crucial and respected participants in any decisions to be made about their own child. Despite the horror stories that you periodically hear in which the parents' wishes are ignored or parents have to go to court to have their wishes enforced, these situations are the exception rather than the rule. In most cases, difficult decisions can be made as a team, working together with your baby's doctors and nurses. Most hospitals also have a bioethicist on staff or a bioethics committee (sometimes called an Infant Care Review committee). If you find yourself facing an extremely complicated situation in which the right course of action is not at all clear, you might want to request their involvement.

Your nursery's social worker should be able to answer specific questions about your rights and provide you with the written policies of the hospital.

A Final Word

Having a baby born prematurely is one of the most stressful and frightening experiences a parent can face. But sometimes, hidden within all the negative aspects of this experience are a few positive notes. No matter how small and fragile these babies appear, most of them show an awe-inspiring resilience, strength, and will to live. And a striking number of parents describe their preemies as having a unique energy and zest for life as they grow. Despite their often rocky and uncertain beginnings, these children are fighters and they earn a special place in their parents' hearts.

CHAPTER 2

Learning Your Way Around the NICU

ℛℐ

IF YOUR BABY IS BORN more than six or eight weeks early, she will probably be cared for in a Level III neonatal intensive care nursery (NICU) right after her birth. Some babies need to spend only a few hours or days in intensive care before being transferred to a Level II special care nursery, while others remain in the NICU for several weeks or months. In this chapter you will find the basics of your baby's care explained, including the common problems faced by preemies, what the NICU looks like, the equipment used there, and an explanation of who's who in the nursery.

If your baby was born closer to her due date, she may not need the intensive care described here. Depending upon her age and condition at birth, she may need some extra support similar to that provided in the NICU, or she may adjust quickly with no problems after birth. These older preemies are often cared for in a Level II nursery or even the regular newborn nursery.

In the first few days after your child's birth, it can be difficult to absorb and understand very much of what you hear and see. Don't be surprised if it takes many visits to the NICU and repeated explanations before things begin to sink in and make sense. Throughout your child's hospitalization, but particularly in the beginning, you will have moments when you feel confused, overwhelmed, frustrated, upset, and panicky, as well as other times when you feel more positive and hopeful.

This chapter is designed to help you get oriented to the world of the NICU as quickly as possible so that you can become a more active participant in your child's care. Although your own hospital's practices may differ slightly from these descriptions, the information here should clarify much of what you see and hear.

Your First Visits to the NICU

You may have a chance to quickly see your baby in the delivery room, but your first prolonged visit will probably not occur until after she has been admitted to the NICU. This process usually takes a couple of hours. Your first visit may be postponed longer if you have undergone a cesarean birth or are ill, or if your baby must be transferred to another hospital.

Although many parents find the NICU to be alien and intimidating at first, others block out their surroundings as they focus on their baby. My husband's reaction was typical of this: "My first impression of the NICU was that it looked like a lab. But beyond that I really didn't pay much attention to it. I was much more interested in seeing my son. That's all I was looking at." Another parent had a similar memory of her early days in the NICU when she said, "I was so relieved that my daughters were alive and looked like real babies. And the NICU actually seemed kind of cozy. It was only later that I started to notice what a strange world it was."

A First Look at Your Baby

The first time you see your baby in the NICU, she will probably be lying on a small platform known as a warming bed and wearing little except perhaps a knit cap and a diaper. The warming bed keeps her from becoming chilled and also allows the NICU staff to easily watch and care for her during the critical first hours or days of her life. She may have a number of wires and tubes attached to various parts of her body and be receiving supplemental oxygen, or help with her breathing via a respirator.

If she was born more than about six weeks early, she probably won't look like any newborn you are familiar with or have seen in pictures. In fact, until you get used to their appearance, young preemies are not particularly attractive or appealing. Some parents have bluntly described them as looking more like plucked chickens or wizened old men than babies. But your baby's appearance is actually quite normal for her stage of development.

Perhaps the most obvious difference is in your baby's size. Because she didn't have time to put on the weight that babies gain in the last four to six weeks before birth, she will have little or no body fat and will look thin and scrawny. In addition, her skin may be reddish-purple and almost translucent; the small veins lying near the surface of the skin will be easily visible. Her head will seem quite large for her body, and she may be covered in downy hair called lanugo. Lanugo may be particularly noticeable on the shoulders and back and will disappear as your baby matures. Since cartilage may not have formed completely, her ears are soft and can bend over flat the wrong way. Your baby's genitals may not have matured; the scrotum in boys may be smooth and the testicles undescended, and the folds around the vaginal opening in girls may not have completely formed. Although books on preemies never mention this, my husband and I were surprised that our son had no bottom for the first few weeks of his life. His lack of fat and muscle meant that there was no rounded padding where we expected it.

If your baby is more than six to eight weeks early, she will be very weak and floppy. She will tend to lie with her arms out straight and her legs in a frog-like position when she is on her back. She'll spend most of her time sleeping, and any movements she makes will be weak and jerky. However, it doesn't take long to get used to your baby's appearance, and to see beyond all her tubes and wires. As one mother said, "Pretty soon I began to think that the full-term babies who were in the NICU looked strange. They seemed so huge next to our little one." Another parent showed pictures of his tiny, sick preemie with respirator, chest tubes, and wires to everyone he met and couldn't understand why they all fell speechless. All he saw was his beautiful baby boy.

A First Touch

One of the most important things you should do on your first or second visit to the nursery is to touch or even hold your baby, if possible. This sounds so simple, but it can seem quite daunting when you are surrounded by high tech equipment and facing a fragile or very ill baby. But most parents find that these early contacts with their baby are very powerful. Not only does it help you to connect with her and make her seem real, but touching and, later, holding her can help assuage some of your anxiety.

The Power of Touch

About two hours after Ben was born, we were taken to see him in the NICU. I don't remember much except feeling a great sense of dread and numbness. I didn't know what to expect, but whatever it was, I didn't see how it could be good. The ten days before Ben's birth had been such a nightmare; I had been in and out of the hospital in early labor. Nothing had worked and now that he had been born, twelve weeks early, I wondered what new horrible things were going to start happening. We found Ben lying spread-eagled on his back on a warming table. He was naked, with tubes coming from his bellybutton and other places. His head was no bigger than an orange and he was so scrawny, he looked like a shrunken old man. My most vivid memory of that moment is of his doctor standing beside him, grinning, and saying, "Ben is doing beautifully. I wish all my babies did this well." I remember just staring back at him. How could he say that this tiny, red, gasping baby surrounded by high tech equipment was doing beautifully? I was also struck by the fact that it was the doctor who sounded like a proud father. He seemed to be feeling the pride and excitement that my husband and I should have been feeling, while we, instead, felt numb and shell-shocked. It was all very weird.

The next day, we went back, although I don't honestly think I wanted to go very much. I felt more like running away and pretending that this whole thing had never happened. Ben had been moved into an incubator by then. As soon as we got there, Ben's nurse asked us if we wanted to hold him. He seemed so frail, I didn't think that disturbing him seemed like a very good idea. But the nurse insisted. She wrapped him up in several blankets, put a knit cap on his head, reattached his monitor wires which were peeking out of the blanket, put warming lights on over me, and handed him to me while I sat in a rocking chair.

I don't really know how to explain the effect that holding Ben that first time had on me. Maybe it was the first time he seemed real to me, as if he were something more than just a bad dream. I couldn't hold him for long—it probably wasn't more than five or ten minutes—but that short time proved to be a turning point. My numbness began to fade a bit, and even though I was still very worried about what might happen, Ben became mine in a way he hadn't been before. I was, and still am, very surprised at the impact those few minutes had on my feelings. I will always be grateful to that nurse for forcing me to hold my son.

Many parents felt they began to cope better with the situation after even briefly holding or touching their baby (see box).

Your baby's nurse can show you how best to touch your child in these early days. If your baby is too young or sick to hold, you can place a finger on her arm or leg, lay your open hand gently on her chest or back, or cup your hand around her head or legs and feet. Use a gentle but firm pressure when you touch her. Most preemies find light, feathery touches and stroking to be uncomfortable or irritating.

Many nurseries also suggest that you take several pictures of your baby to take home with you. A Polaroid camera may be available in the unit for this purpose. These pictures help you feel connected to your baby when you must be separated. And some mothers who are pumping breastmilk for their babies find that simply looking at these pictures helps to stimulate the let-down reflex and get their milk flowing.

What the NICU Looks Like

The NICU where your baby is being cared for consists of an open room or a series of rooms with designated bed sites along the walls. You'll find your baby on a warming table, in a clear plastic incubator, or in an open bassinet. Small television monitors mounted at each bed site display your baby's vital signs such as heart and respiration rates, and body temperature. There may also be one or two small isolation rooms that can be closed off from the main part of the nursery. These are used for very ill infants or infants with a contagious condition. One or more small family rooms in or near the NICU can be used for private time with your baby when she gets stronger and healthier. These rooms are usually equipped with electric breast pumps where you can express milk for your baby.

Some large NICUs consist of multiple rooms, one or more for babies needing intensive care (Level III nurseries), and others for babies in better condition (Level II nurseries). These latter rooms, which are sometimes called step-down units, feeder-grower rooms, or special or continuing care nurseries, are for babies who no longer need intensive care but are not yet ready to go home.

As your baby's health changes or as the number of babies in the NICU increases or decreases, she may be moved to a new location or to a new room in the nursery. If you haven't been told of a move in advance, it can be quite alarming when you go in to visit and discover that your baby is no longer in her normal spot. A nurse or nursery clerk should quickly be able to show you where your baby has been relocated.

The normal nursery sounds of babies crying are largely absent in the NICU; instead you will hear beeping alarms, humming incubators, and respiratory equipment. In many nurseries, efforts are made to minimize the amount of stress to which babies are subjected—lights are kept low, people speak in soft voices, and try to have conversations away from the bed sites. And in the midst of all the high tech equipment you will also find familiar items such as rocking chairs, pictures, and stuffed animals.

Typical NICU Visiting Policies

On your first visit to the NICU, the nurse caring for your baby will orient you to the nursery and explain the nursery visiting policies to you. For infection control, most nurseries require that parents wash their hands before visiting their babies. You'll find a sink with antibacterial soap just inside the nursery doors. As you wash, be sure to clean around and under your fingernails. Once you have washed your hands, try not to touch your face, blow your nose, or touch other children or babies. If you do, be sure to wash again before touching your own baby. You may also be asked to put on a hospital gown over your street clothes.

Parents are usually granted unlimited visiting privileges. But you may be asked to leave the nursery briefly during staff changes, when the staff is making rounds discussing each baby and planning care, or when your child needs certain types of medical care. Visiting policies for siblings and other family members vary by hospital. If your children are sick or have been exposed to any infectious diseases such as chicken pox, the flu, or colds, they will probably not be allowed to visit until they are well or until the incubation or contagious period has passed.

There will be times when you or your partner are unable to visit your baby. Your baby may have been transported to a distant hospital, you may be too sick to leave your own bed, you may have other children at home to care for, a job that can't be ignored, or you may not have access to transportation.

When visiting is difficult or impossible, you can stay connected to your baby through pictures and phone calls to the nursery. Your baby will spend most of her time sleeping in the first weeks of life and the staff are giving her the medical care and attention that she needs. While it is important to stay in close contact with the nursery so that you know what is going on with your baby, don't feel like you need to spend long hours sitting beside her incubator in order to be a good parent. And try not to worry about whether or not you will be able to bond properly with your baby. Bonding is a long process, not something that must take place in a few critical hours or days after birth. In the meantime, feel free to call the nursery to ask about your baby at anytime during the day or night.

Basic Medical Care for Preemies

Not simply small babies, preemies are infants who have been thrust into the world before their bodies are fully ready to take on life outside the womb. Although each preemie is different, babies born more than six weeks early usually face at least some of the following problems:

- difficulty staying warm because they have very little body fat and their muscles aren't strong enough to generate heat by shivering;
- breathing problems because their lungs are immature and/or their breathing patterns are irregular;
- difficulty being fed because their digestive systems are immature or they lack the strength and coordination to nurse from a bottle or breast; and
- jaundice (a yellowish tinting of the skin and eyes) caused by normal changes in the blood that occur with all newborns after birth but that can be more severe with preemies.

Babies born at 34 weeks or later may also have some of these same problems. But generally, their problems are milder and they recover more quickly. Most can maintain their body temperatures, but it may take them a few days to begin to feed well, they may need a bit of extra oxygen for a day or so, and some treatment for jaundice.

In this section you will find a brief description of the common equipment and procedures that are used to treat these complications. These and other potential medical problems faced by younger preemies are described in greater detail in Chapter 4. As you read this section and Chapter 4 keep in mind that not all babies will have all of these problems nor will all babies be treated in exactly the ways described below. Read the sections that are relevant to your baby, and use the information to supplement what you have seen or heard in the NICU, or to help you frame questions to ask your baby's caregivers.

Warming Tables and Incubators

Like all human beings, preemies need to have a stable body temperature, ideally around 98.6°F (37°C). A body temperature that is too low—below about 98°F—or too high—above 99.5°F—is stressful for a premature baby, and can cause her to lose weight, have an increased heart rate, or breathe irregularly. Most babies who weigh less than about four pounds have trouble staying warm because they don't have enough insulating body fat, including brown fat, a particular kind of fat that infants and young children have that is important for body heat production. In addition, their muscles are weak so they can't shiver to generate heat. Until they grow, they need to be in an incubator or on a warming table to keep from getting chilled.

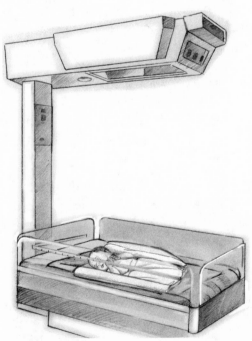

As mentioned above, when you first see your baby in the NICU, she will probably be on a **warming table,** a small open platform with heating elements above. These tables allow the staff an unobstructed view and easy access to your baby during the critical first hours or days of her life. While on a warming table, preemies are sometimes covered with clear plastic wrap. As strange as it looks, this plastic wrap acts like a transparent

A warming table keeps a preemie warm with overhead heating elements and allows staff easy access for caretaking.

blanket. It protects your baby from drafts and keeps her from becoming dehydrated while under the warming lights. This is particularly important for very young and tiny preemies whose skin is too thin to provide a good barrier to moisture loss.

After your baby's health has stabilized, which may take anywhere from an hour or two to several days or longer, she will probably be moved into an incubator. Also known as an Isolette (actually a brand of incubator), an incubator is a clear plastic box that provides a temperature-controlled environment for your baby. Porthole-like doors on the side of the incubator allow you and the staff to reach in and care for your baby. The front of the incubator also opens to allow the bed to slide out, creating a platform on which to change diapers or clothes. The air temperature within the incubator is kept just high enough to maintain your baby's body temperature in the normal range. You'll see the internal temperature displayed on the outside of the box. As your baby grows and becomes better able to regulate her own body temperature, the temperature in the incubator is slowly decreased until it equals the room temperature outside the incubator. Your baby is then ready for a regular open bassinet.

Monitors and Wires

Looking like small television screens at each bed site, monitors are ubiquitous pieces of equipment in an intensive care unit. They display ongoing information about your baby's vital signs—her heart and respiration rates, the oxygen levels in her blood, and sometimes her body temperature. If any of these readings fall outside certain preset limits, monitor alarms beep. These monitors and alarms can be unsettling at first. But the monitoring devices do not make your baby uncomfortable, and the display screen allows you to see at a glance how she is doing. Most parents find that the monitors quickly become a valuable source of information and comfort. In fact, it can be difficult to adjust to their absence when your baby no longer needs to be monitored or is discharged home. You will probably see some of the following types of information displayed on your baby's monitors.

Heart and breathing rates. Your baby's heart and respiration rates are measured using three wires attached to your baby by sticky pads. One is usually placed near the heart, another on the chest or abdomen, and a third on a leg. Your baby's heart should beat between about 110 to 160 beats per minute, and her breathing should not fall below about 30 or go above 60 breaths per minute. Until babies are about 35 weeks old, they tend to have irregular breathing patterns and will often have short periods when they pause in their breathing. If this pause continues for 10 or 15 seconds or more, and your baby's heart begins to slow down, it is known as an apnea and bradycardia spell and triggers an alarm on the monitor. In most cases, babies spontaneously begin to breathe regularly again, although some may need a slight tap to the foot or a gentle pat on the back to stimulate them. If the spells are frequent, the baby may be placed on preventive medication such as caffeine, theophylline, or aminophylline. Apnea and bradycardia will be discussed in greater detail in Chapter 4.

Oxygen Saturation Levels. Most babies are attached to monitors that measure the amount of oxygen their blood is carrying, known as the oxygen saturation level (or O_2 sat). Oxygen levels are commonly measured using one of two types of sensors. The first, a pulse oximeter, uses a small red light taped to a finger or toe to measure the amount of oxygen in the blood. The second, a transcutaneous oxygen monitor ($TCPO_2$ monitor) measures oxygen levels with a heated probe placed on an infant's skin usually on the arm or leg. Although the $TCPO_2$ probe doesn't hurt the baby, it does leave a small red dot which fades after a few days.

Blood oxygen levels ideally remain in the upper 90s, meaning that the blood is carrying close to 100 percent of the oxygen it is able to carry. If the level falls too low, an alarm will beep. This is called "de-satting" in the language of the NICU, and can occur during an apnea spell or if your baby is stressed by something—too much handling, a drop in temperature, the exertion of feeding, or a stressful medical procedure. Sometimes the baby's movement alone will trigger the alarm of the pulse oximeter, in which case the low reading is not a true one.

Body Temperature. While your baby is on the warming table, she will have her body temperature continuously monitored by a sensor attached to her abdomen in order to regulate the overhead heating elements. Usually after she has been moved into an incubator she no longer needs this continuous monitoring and her temperature will be taken periodically using a regular thermometer.

Tubes: Intravenous Lines and Gavage Tubes

In the womb babies receive all the nutrition they need for growth through the placenta and umbilical cord. With premature birth, this source of nutrition comes to an end, sometimes before a baby's digestive tract has matured to the point that it can handle food or before the baby can manage oral feedings. In the NICU, various feeding methods ensure that your baby will get all the fluid and nutrients she needs until she can begin bottle- or breastfeeding.

Intravenous (IV) Lines. During the first several days of life and often longer, almost all preemies will have an IV line (a small plastic tube) inserted into a vein just under the surface of the skin. The IV line is used to give your baby fluids so she doesn't become dehydrated; sugar and electrolytes, such as sodium and potassium; and certain medications, such as antibiotics or apnea-controlling drugs. These peripheral IVs are usually placed in the baby's hand, arm, foot, leg, or scalp, and are usually moved every day or so to prevent the area from becoming irritated. Although it can be unnerving to see an IV in your baby's scalp, this site has some advantages over the arms or legs. Scalp veins are relatively easy to find, and the baby is less likely to dislodge an IV there. Also, IVs in the arm or leg must be secured by a small padded board and a lot of tape. It can actually be more comfortable for your baby to have an IV in her head.

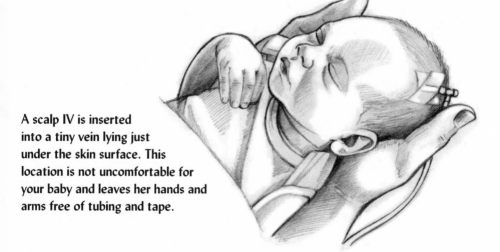

A scalp IV is inserted into a tiny vein lying just under the skin surface. This location is not uncomfortable for your baby and leaves her hands and arms free of tubing and tape.

Umbilical Catheter. The first time you see your baby, she may also have a small plastic IV tube in her bellybutton. This umbilical catheter can be painlessly inserted into either the umbilical vein or artery in order to reach the larger blood vessels in the body. Often used in the first day or two of life, umbilical catheters make it easier for your baby's caregivers to draw blood samples, monitor blood pressure, and administer blood transfusions or fluids that might be too irritating for the small veins used in peripheral IVs.

Central Lines. An alternative to the umbilical catheter is a central line. This IV is placed into one of the larger veins in the arm or leg. Central lines are used if an IV needs to stay in place for a long time or if the solution to be given might irritate the small veins near the surface of the skin. Inserting the central line may require a minor surgical procedure known as a cutdown. Using a local anesthetic, a neonatologist or pediatric surgeon inserts an IV tube into a vein through a small cut in the skin and then threads the IV up into a larger vein near the heart. Central lines do not become dislodged as easily as peripheral IVs and can stay in place for a longer time, but they do carry an increased risk of infection. If your baby is unable to take food orally for a prolonged time, she may receive nutritional solutions containing sugar, protein, vitamins, minerals, and calories through a central line. You may hear this nutritional support referred to as total parenteral nutrition (TPN) or hyperalimentation (hyperal).

Gavage or Feeding Tubes. Before they reach about 34 weeks, babies usually lack the energy to consume an entire feeding by breast or bottle or haven't yet developed the ability to coordinate the suck, swallow, and breathing sequence necessary for oral feeding. These babies are usually fed formula or breastmilk through a small soft plastic tube known as a gavage tube inserted through the nose or mouth and down the esophagus to the stomach. Gavage tubes may be left in place between feedings, or may be removed and reinserted for each feeding. Because babies don't develop a gag reflex until about 35 weeks, the insertion of the tube typically doesn't bother them. As your baby matures, she will progress through a transition phase during which she receives some feedings by gavage and some by bottle or breast, or receives part of a feeding by nipple and the remainder by gavage. Gradually, she will move to all bottle-feeding or breastfeeding.

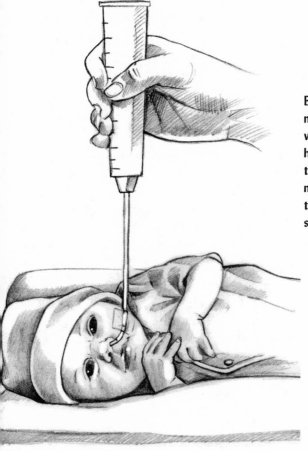

Before a baby has mastered oral feeding, she will receive part or all of her feedings through a tube inserted into her mouth or nose, down her throat, and into her stomach.

Bilirubin Lights or Phototherapy

Almost all preemies spend time under bilirubin lights or lying on a special fiber-optic bili-blanket during the first weeks of life. These blue, green, or white lights help to break down the excess bilirubin that naturally accumulates in their blood and causes a yellowish coloring of the skin and eyes known as jaundice.

While your baby is under the lights, her eyes will be protected by a small mask or goggles. She will generally wear little or no clothing so the maximum amount of skin is exposed to the lights. Her skin may take on a ruddy look which will fade once her phototherapy is finished. Some babies may seem a bit sleepy and have runny stools.

Respiratory Care and Equipment

Since the lungs mature relatively late in gestation, many preemies have breathing problems. A baby born only a few weeks early may need little or no help breathing, or may need some extra oxygen for a short time. Younger preemies may need more help, including being placed on a respirator, a machine that mechanically assists the baby's breathing through a tube in the nose or mouth.

Babies who need respiratory support may be treated in one or more of the ways described below.

Artificial Surfactant. A major advance in the treatment of respiratory problems occurred in the early 1990s with the development of artificial surfactant. Surfactant is a soap-like substance that naturally coats the inside of mature lungs and improves their function. The breathing problems that many preemies experience occur because they are born before they are producing the surfactant their lungs need. This problem can be remedied now with artificial surfactant administered directly into a baby's lungs through an endotracheal (ET) tube down the throat. In some hospitals, babies at risk of respiratory problems are given an initial dose of artificial surfactant soon after birth. In others, the first dose is not given until the baby shows signs of respiratory problems.

Supplemental Oxygen. Because their lungs are not fully mature and may not effectively absorb adequate oxygen from the air, many preemies need to breathe air with a higher than normal percentage of oxygen. Some infants need this extra support for only a short time, while others need to remain on supplemental oxygen for weeks or longer.

Room air naturally contains approximately 21 percent oxygen; with supplemental oxygen, this percentage can be raised until the air being breathed contains 100 percent oxygen, if necessary. Babies are usually given just enough oxygen to maintain their oxygen saturation levels in the acceptable range. These levels are closely monitored by sensors and through periodic blood gas measurements because too much oxygen can damage lung tissue and may be associated with the development of vision problems in preemies.

Oxygen can be delivered in a number of ways:

- Oxygen hood. Warm moist air with extra oxygen can be pumped into a plastic tent or dome placed over the baby's head. Babies who are born only a few weeks early may spend a few hours or days under an oxygen hood.
- Nasal cannula. Oxygen can also be delivered directly to the baby through plastic tubing that ends in small prongs placed in the nostrils.

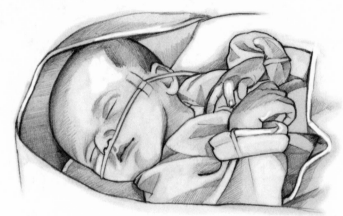

Supplemental oxygen can be supplied to your baby through a nasal cannula.

- Blow-by oxygen. As a baby gets older, she may need extra oxygen only during tiring activities like feeding. Supplemental oxygen can then be provided by blowing oxygen under her nose from a tube or small oxygen mask.
- Bag and mask. Oxygen can be manually pumped into a baby's lungs using a soft mask and attached bag. The mask is placed over the baby's mouth and nose, and the bag which is inflated with a mixture of air and extra oxygen is gently and repetitively squeezed. This is also known as bagging.

Continuous Positive Airway Pressure (CPAP). Some babies with respiratory problems may be treated with CPAP. CPAP doesn't mechanically breathe for a baby, but blows a constant stream of air into a baby's lungs at low pressure. This keeps the lungs partially inflated at all times and counteracts the tendency for the air sacs to collapse. CPAP may be delivered through nasal prongs, through a nasopharyngeal tube down the nose, through an endotracheal or ET tube down the throat, or through a small face mask. Extra oxygen can be added if needed.

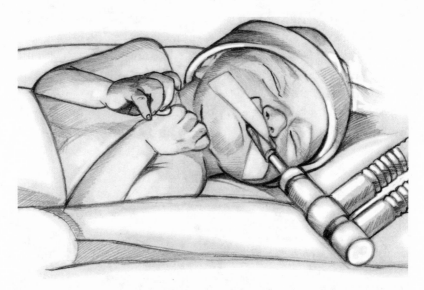

A baby with more serious respiratory problems may be placed on a ventilator which breathes for her a specified number of times per minute.

Respirator or Ventilator. If your baby is too weak to breathe well on her own or is having many severe apnea spells, she will probably be placed on a respirator, a machine which breathes for her. Your baby will be intubated while on the respirator. This means she will have a tube through her nose or mouth and down into her windpipe. The respirator will be set to breathe for her a certain number of times a minute. As babies get stronger, this rate is decreased and babies begin to breathe on their own between the breaths that the respirator takes. Often babies on respirators are given medications to keep them comfortable. Occasionally they are given muscle relaxants so that they will not fight against the machine.

High Frequency Ventilators (HFVs). These relatively new ventilators are generally used only in special situations, as when the baby is not doing well with a regular ventilator, or has developed a pneumothorax, a small hole in her lungs through which air is escaping. HFVs breathe extremely rapidly—300 to 1,500 breaths per minute—and at lower pressures than regular ventilators. Babies on HFVs often wear ear protectors to muffle the noise of the ventilator.

Your Baby's Caregivers

In most Level II and III nurseries, a specific doctor and one or two nurses are responsible for planning and overseeing your baby's care. These individuals, known as your baby's primary care team, get to know your child and her needs well, and can care for her in a consistent way. Your baby's primary nurse will oversee her care from admission to discharge. Your baby's primary physician may be a pediatric resident or neonatal fellow. Since these neonatologists-in-training are usually assigned to the nursery for four to six weeks at a time, your baby may have more than one primary doctor during her stay.

Despite this primary care approach, the staffing in NICUs can be quite confusing, and it is not uncommon to feel as if your baby is being cared for by a constantly changing parade of people. As one mother recalled,

> "I was introduced to my son's primary nurse on our first visit. I expected that I would see her every time I came in, but I'm not sure I ever saw her again before he was transferred to another hospital the next week. Every time I came in, it seemed as if someone new was taking care of him. It was hard to keep dealing with new people all the time and I wasn't quite sure what it meant that he had a primary nurse if so many other people were actually taking care of him."

In reality, your baby's care is planned and supervised by her primary doctors and nurses. But the demands of scheduling mean that a number of different individuals may care for her following the plan her primary team develops. If your baby spends more than a week or two in the nursery, you will probably get to know her primary nurse well despite these scheduling changes. This relationship can become quite intense, and for some families it continues after their baby's discharge.

While your baby is in the hospital, you should try to meet with her primary team at least once a week in order to ask questions, discuss your baby's progress or any new problems, and review the plans for her care. Request that these meetings take place in a conference or parent room outside of the NICU where it is easier to concentrate. Between meetings, write down questions as they occur to you so that you don't have to remember them all. You may also want to jot notes during the meeting to review later. It's extremely difficult to absorb, remember, and understand everything that you hear about your baby, particularly if her condition is complicated and you are upset and anxious.

You might also want to ask your baby's care team if you can audiotape these meetings. In a recent research project in Australia, parents reported that being able to listen to tapes of conferences with their babies' doctors was a tremendous help in remembering and understanding what was discussed. If one parent couldn't attend the meeting, the tapes also provided an accurate account of the discussion. Some providers may feel uncomfortable being taped, so be sure to discuss your reasons for wanting to do so ahead of time. Remember that you can always call the nurse taking care of your baby at any time of day or night for an update on your child.

Staffing in Teaching Hospitals

Most Level III intensive care nurseries are located in teaching hospitals where the staffing hierarchy is complex. Here, your baby's primary care team will consist at a minimum of a senior supervising neonatologist, a pediatric resident, and one or two primary nurses. In addition, a neonatal fellow, a neonatal nurse practitioner, a clinical nurse specialist, staff nurses, and pediatric specialists and surgeons may also be involved in your baby's care. Auxiliary staff may include respiratory therapists; nutritionists; laboratory, ultrasound, and X-ray technicians; occupational and physical therapists; and a social worker. The roles played by each of these individuals are explained below.

Physicians

Neonatologist. A neonatologist is a pediatrician who has received advanced training and has passed medical board exams (i.e., is Board certified) in the pediatric subspecialty of neonatal and perinatal medicine. This subspecialty area focuses on the care of newborns, including preemies, and in problems of pregnancy, labor, and delivery. The neonatologist who supervises your baby's primary care team is called the attending physician. There are usually several neonatologists on the staff of a teaching hospital; they share the responsiblity of acting as the attending physician in the NICU, with each typically spending a month at a time there. You may get to know more than one attending physician if your baby is in the hospital over a rotation change or for longer than a month. The medical director of the nursery, also a neonatologist, oversees the nursery and all of its staff.

Neonatal Fellow. A fellow is a pediatrician who is in a three-year training program to become a neonatologist. This physician will be more closely involved in the daily care of your baby than the attending neonatologist. Because the fellows spend more time in the unit, you will probably see more of the fellow than of your baby's attending physician.

Pediatric Residents. Residents are physicians who have finished medical school and are training to become pediatricians, although not necessarily neonatologists. Residents spend four to six weeks at a time in the intensive care unit before they rotate to a new area of the hospital. While on the unit, the resident will act as the primary physician for several babies and will report to the fellow and attending physician on your baby's progress. The residents are also referred to as house staff or house officers.

Other medical and surgical specialists. Depending upon your baby's condition, you may meet with one or more pediatric medical or surgical specialists. Discuss any questions you have about these specialists or their plans for your baby with your baby's primary care team. Because this team is most familiar with your baby, they will be able to provide you with additional information or advice.

Nurses

Neonatal nurse practitioner. A neonatal nurse practitioner (NNP) is a registered nurse who has obtained advanced training, usually through a master's degree program, in the care of full-term and premature newborns. The nurse practitioner performs a role similar to that of a neonatal fellow, and is actively involved in the daily care of your baby.

Neonatal staff nurses. Neonatal nurses are registered nurses with special training to care for preemies and sick full-term babies who require intensive care. They are with your baby night and day, and provide most of her hands-on care.

Nursing has its own hierarchy and administration although it operates under the authority of the nursery director. A head nurse is the administrative head of the nursing staff, and on each shift a charge nurse is responsible for overseeing nursing care on that shift. The charge nurse is sometimes referred to as the NIC or nurse-in-charge. If you have any concerns about the care your child is receiving, ask to speak to the charge nurse first and then to the head nurse, if necessary.

Other Important Staff

Respiratory therapists. These professionals help care for infants who are having trouble with breathing, are on a ventilator, or are receiving supplemental oxygen.

Nutritionists. Nutritionists with special training in the needs of preemies can help to assess a baby's nutritional status and needs. They may make recommendations about diet and dietary supplements and monitor your baby's weight gain and calorie intake.

Social workers. Most NICUs have one or more social workers available to work with families. These professionals can provide you with emotional support as well as information on many practical and financial issues. For example, the NICU social workers can usually answer questions about insurance coverage or eligibility for programs such as Medicaid or Supplemental Security Income. They are often involved in discharge planning and help to arrange for equipment, transportation, child care for other children, or nursing care for your baby at home. In addition, a social worker may be able to help you resolve difficulties with NICU staff members and attend primary care team meetings with you. If a social worker does not contact you in the first few days of your child's hospitalization, ask to speak to one. Because they possess a wealth of helpful information, these professionals can be a wonderful resource during a difficult time.

Physical and occupational therapists, developmental specialists, or infant educators. These professionals are specially trained to assess your baby's needs and provide feedback to you and the nursing staff on how to handle your baby to minimize stress and maximize her comfort and development.

X-ray, lab, ultrasound, and EKG technicians. These medical technicians perform many of the tests and procedures your primary care team orders. Your baby's doctors or any necessary specialists will interpret the results of these tests.

Lactation specialist. Some hospitals have trained professionals with special expertise in breastfeeding. They can help you get started pumping and storing breastmilk for your baby and in establishing breastfeeding when your baby is strong enough. Many of the NICU nurses are also quite knowledgeable about breastfeeding preemies.

Staffing in Non-Teaching Hospitals

Many special care (Level II) nurseries are located in local community hospitals. In these nurseries, the staffing is generally less complex than it is in intensive care units. In most Level II nurseries, your baby's care will be overseen by a neonatologist or pediatrician, and a primary nurse and other staff nurses. In some hospitals, your own pediatrician may become directly involved in your baby's care several weeks before discharge. In addition, you may have contact with some of the other supporting staff described above.

Adjusting to the NICU

In the first few days and weeks after the birth of your baby, you will probably experience an incredible range of emotions which may include shock, panic, anger, numbness, hope, sadness, grief, relief, confusion. Many parents report that they find it difficult, if not impossible, to concentrate; their thoughts are scattered and disorganized, they get lost or confused doing ordinary things. Some parents want to spend as much time as possible at their baby's bedside, while others distract themselves or try to counteract their feelings of helplessness by spending long hours at work. There is no way to know in advance what your reactions—or your partner's—will be, but it may help to keep several things in mind during this period.

Your feelings and the fact that they change rapidly are normal. As described earlier, parents commonly say that having a baby in the NICU is like being on a roller coaster with its dramatic ups and downs, unexpected twists and turns. The strength of your feelings and reactions will gradually decrease, but expect that the emotional impact of this experience will be long-lasting and profound.

Your partner's reactions will undoubtedly differ from yours. This can lead to misunderstandings, tension, and distance in your relationship. Although you may draw closer together during the first few panicky days in your common focus on your baby, couples often find that differences in coping styles arise as the immediate danger fades and they settle in for the long wait while their child recovers. It is important to try to keep talking with each other through this period so that you can understand what the other is feeling and thinking. Your interpretation of your partner's behavior may be quite different from his or her intention.

Your ability to understand and process what is going on will vary considerably from one moment to the next. At certain times, you may be able to absorb little of what you see or hear, while at others you may feel hypersensitive and find yourself listening not only to what is said, but also to unspoken messages. Keep asking questions in order to avoid unnecessary worry or misunderstandings. If you don't understand the first explanation, ask again. Again, it may help to write down your questions and concerns as they occur to you so that you don't have to try to remember them all during meetings with your baby's medical team. You may want to write down the answers or even tape record the meetings also so that you can review what was said. Some parents have found it useful to take along a friend, relative, or the hospital social worker to a team meeting. A less emotionally involved person may have an easier time listening and understanding what is being said and can talk it over with you later.

Most doctors and nurses taking care of your baby understand how hard this situation is and sympathize with your emotions. Experienced doctors and nurses in the NICU have seen all kinds of reactions from parents, and will not think the less of you or care less carefully for your baby if you let your emotions show. In fact, one NICU nurse said, "I worry about parents who look too good. This is such a hard time—I don't want parents to feel like they need to bottle everything up." On the other hand, most parents feel as if falling apart is not really an option—at least not in public.

Said one mother of a 28-weeker who was in the hospital for two months,

> *"I found it very annoying when people would ask me how I was able to cope so well while Sara was in the hospital. I wanted to yell at them and tell them I wasn't coping. That inside I was grouchy and angry and upset and barely functioning. But it didn't seem like it was really going to help matters very much if I let all that out. Even if you fall apart, it's not going to change things, and you just have to pick yourself up and start to cope again. Basically, you cope because you have to—there really isn't any other choice."*

Life in the NICU is usually a roller coaster of good days and bad days. You should expect that there will be days when your baby shows great progress as well as days when new complications appear, days when you feel hopeful and optimistic interspersed with days when you feel discouraged, anxious, and overwhelmed. One day, you may find that your baby feeds well, tolerates a long period of holding without showing signs of stress, and gains weight. The next day when you go in, she will do none of these things. Or she may make progress on oral feeding for a number of days, only to develop a new medical complication or problem and slip back to gavage feedings. The good news is that this uneven pattern is normal for recovering premature babies. The bad news is that the setbacks can be very discouraging and emotionally draining. Throughout this difficult period, continue to ask questions of your baby's doctors and nurses so that you understand as much as possible about your baby's health and what to expect. Look for signs of progress, no matter how small they may seem. And slowly, over time, you will notice that the ups and downs in both your baby's health and your emotions begin to level off and that the good days will begin to outnumber the bad.

The Language of the NICU: Common Terms and Abbreviations

Here are some of the common terms you may hear in the NICU. See the Glossary for more complete explanations and for terms not included here.

As & Bs Refers to apnea and bradycardia, a slow-down in breathing and heart rate.

Attending physician The neonatologist (specialist in newborn medicine, including preemies) who is responsible for overseeing the medical care in the nursery. Attending physicians usually change every four weeks.

Bagging Pumping air into a baby's lungs. A soft mask is placed over the baby's mouth and nose, and an attached bag is squeezed gently by hand.

Blood gas Blood test that measures the oxygen (O_2) and carbon dioxide (CO_2)content of the blood, and its acidity (pH).

Blow-by oxygen When a baby needs a small amount of extra oxygen during a tiring activity like feeding, it may be provided by gently blowing a stream of oxygenated air past her face through a tube or mask. This is known as blow-by oxygen.

Central line An IV line inserted into a vein, usually in the arm, and fed into a larger vein in the body. Used to deliver medicines or nutritional solutions that would irritate small veins.

CPAP Continuous positive airway pressure. A way of helping a baby breathe by blowing a constant, gentle stream of air into the lungs to keep them open.

De-satting Term used when the oxygen level (oxygen saturation) in the blood drops below a certain point.

ET tube Endotracheal tube. A soft tube placed through a baby's mouth or nose and into his windpipe (trachea). Used to give extra oxygen or to help your baby breathe.

Gavage tube A soft tube inserted through a baby's nose or mouth and into her stomach. Used to give her formula or milk if she is unable to suck or swallow.

Intubate Inserting an ET tube. When the tube is removed, the baby is extubated.

The Language of the NICU, continued

Isolette Common type of incubator. Clear plastic box used to protect preemies and keep them warm.

IV Intravenous line. Small plastic tube inserted into a vein, usually in the hand, foot, or head, and used to deliver fluids, medicines, and nutritional solutions.

Kangaroo care Holding your baby (usually wearing only a diaper) against your bare chest. Allows skin-to-skin contact, helps baby maintain her body temperature, and sleep well.

NG tube Naso-gastric tube. Another name for gavage tube.

O_2 sats Abbreviation for oxygen saturation levels, or the level of oxygen in the blood.

PICC line Abbreviation for peripherally inserted central catheter. A type of central line. Sometimes called a PVCC (percutaneous venous central catheter) line.

Spells Common term for episodes of apnea and bradycardia

Step-down unit A Level II or special care nursery. For babies who no longer need intensive care but are still recovering from prematurity.

Surfactant A soap-like substance that occurs naturally in mature lungs. Artificial forms of surfactant are given to some preemies with respiratory problems to help their lungs work better.

Umbilical line An IV line inserted through a baby's belly-button (umbilicus). Often used in the first day or two after birth.

Under the lights Refers to being under bililights—blue, green, or white lights that help a baby break down excess bilirubin in the blood that can cause jaundice (yellow coloring).

Ventilator Also known as a respirator. A machine that helps a baby breathe.

TPN Total parenteral nutrition. Also known as hyperalimentation or hyperal solution. A yellow liquid that contains all the nutritional elements a baby needs when she is unable to take food by mouth.

Vital signs Refers to heart rate, breathing rate, and body temperature.

CHAPTER 3

Parenting in the Hospital

ða

WHEN YOUR BABY IS born early, he obviously starts life differently from a full-term newborn. And you face a different beginning as a parent. Rather than being able to hold your baby at birth, to touch and examine his every finger and toe, you can only watch as he is whisked away to be cared for by a group of strangers in the corner of the delivery room. Instead of joy, wonder, and relief, you feel sadness, guilt, fear, and emptiness. You may grieve for the loss of your pregnancy, and for your expectations of a normal delivery and healthy baby. Just as this is a hard way for your baby to start life, it is a hard way for you to start being his parent.

But as the days go on, you will be able to play a more active role in your baby's life. It won't be the same as if he had been born full-term—at least not for a while—but you will be able to help care for him in simple ways even in his early days in the hospital. Even if all you can do at first is sit beside your little one, your voice and touch are consistent and comforting to him. As he grows, you will be able to assume more of his care and by the time your baby is ready to come home, you may be doing almost everything for him.

Most parents feel somewhat awkward and unsure of themselves in the beginning. But keep in mind that your presence and involvement are valued by the staff, and they are happy to teach you how to care for your child. Being directly involved also helps to build your confidence and prepares you for the day when you can bring your baby home. The more you know about your child and his needs, the better you can advocate for him when there are questions or differing opinions about his care.

In this chapter, you will find information on what to expect from your baby as he begins to recover from his early birth, as well as a description of how you can help to care for him in the hospital. This includes a detailed section on feeding your baby, which covers tube feedings, the transition to bottle-feeding or breastfeeding, and guidelines on pumping and transporting breastmilk.

Many parents find themselves pulled in many directions while their baby is hospitalized, caught between wanting to be with their baby and the competing demands of the outside world—work, family, and finances. The final sections of the chapter focus on how to care for yourself and your family during this difficult time, how to balance hospital visits and home life, and the various resources that are available to help with the financial strains of prematurity.

What to Expect from Your Baby

As you begin to work with your baby and provide some of his care, it is helpful to understand some of the common ways in which preemies behave. You can then interpret your baby's reactions more accurately and adjust the way you do things to minimize any stress to him. Your baby's nurses and doctors can give you more specific information about what to expect from your baby based on his gestational age and health. But your baby will probably show at least some of the following normal preemie behaviors.

Your baby will spend most of his time sleeping. If your baby is less than 30 to 32 weeks old, he will spend most of his time in a state of light sleep. You may notice that his arms and legs twitch while he sleeps, he may move around a bit, suck on his tongue, fingers, or pacifier, and his eyes may move under his closed eyelids. However, it is very difficult for him to come fully awake and respond to you.

As he matures, he will begin to develop a pattern to his days with noticeable periods of deep sleep, light sleep, and wakefulness. Around 32 weeks of age he will begin to have brief times when he is quietly alert. These periods are initially quite short, lasting from one to ten minutes, but lengthen as your baby matures. These are the best times to interact with your baby, but go slowly to avoid overwhelming him.

Your baby is able to see and hear you. Hearing is one of the first senses to develop and is fairly well developed by the time a baby reaches 20 weeks of gestation. Preemies dislike loud noises. They seem to prefer voices, particularly their mother's, over other sounds, and also seem to enjoy rhythmic sounds such as singing. Because a baby's eyes develop relatively late in gestation, a baby who is less than about 30 weeks old can see but has trouble focusing clearly. He is primarily able to see contrasts of dark and light. You may notice a lag in your baby's reactions, as well. For example, if you take a flash picture of a very young preemie, he will not react to the light instantaneously as a full-term baby will, but will react a second or two later. By about 35 weeks your baby's vision is nearly mature although he, like all babies, will be quite nearsighted. He can most clearly see objects that are within 8 to 12 inches of his face, and he is most interested in human faces, bright colors, and patterns in black and white.

Your baby is extremely sensitive to sounds, lights, touch, and movement. Premature babies have trouble making sense of information from the outside world, including sounds, sights, touch, and movement. Their immature brains do not yet have the ability to pay attention to some things and ignore others, so they become easily overwhelmed when exposed to too many forms of stimulation at a time. As you begin to interact with your baby it is extremely important to keep this sensitivity in mind. An activity level that a full-term baby would have no trouble with, such as being simultaneously rocked, sung to, and fed, is quite stressful or even intolerable for most preemies. Very young and sick babies and those with respiratory problems are particularly sensitive and easily overwhelmed.

Most preemies communicate primarily through physical reactions. Because crying is a tiring activity that requires energy and muscle strength, many preemies don't cry much until they are close to their due dates. Instead they show that they are stressed or upset through changes in their heart and breathing rates, by becoming limp or stiff, by becoming pale or flushed, by grimacing or hiccuping. When they are content they lie curled in your arms with their hands together, their heart and breathing rates are steady, and they have a calm, interested look (see box).

When Your Baby Is Happy...

His breathing, heart rate, and oxygen levels are steady

His skin tone is even and healthy looking

His arms and legs are relaxed and tucked up into a flexed position

His face is relaxed-looking

He looks alert and interested when awake.

His hands are clasped together

He may touch his face or mouth with his hands

He sucks on his tongue, fist, finger, or pacifier

He grasps your finger

His fingers are gently curled into fists

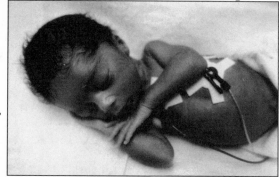

© Abraham Menashe

When Your Baby Is Upset or Stressed...

His heart and breathing rates drop or increase

He may have an apnea or bradycardia spell

His oxygen saturation levels decrease

His skin becomes mottled, pale, or dusky

He becomes suddenly stiff or limp

He may tremble or startle or move frantically

He looks worried and may grimace or look away

He may arch his back

He holds his arms out stiffly, stretching out his fingers

He holds his hands up in front of his face in a stop gesture

He cries, yawns, or hiccups

He may gag, spit up, or grunt

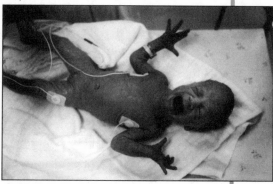

© Abraham Menashe

Your baby is a unique individual. Your baby, like any other full-term or premature infant, has a unique personality and an individual way of reacting to the world. As you spend more time with him, you will begin to recognize the ways in which he signals that he is calm and content, and ways that he indicates he is getting upset or tired. Some babies are more sensitive to certain types of stimuli than others, and each baby has particular strengths that help him cope with his environment and comfort himself. Your child's nurses can help you recognize and interpret his cues. In some nurseries, occupational and physical therapists or developmental specialists may assess your child as well and be able to give you advice on the best ways of handling and interacting with him.

Caring for Your Baby

In most NICUs, the nurses try to concentrate their care into discrete sessions and otherwise allow your baby to sleep undisturbed. If you time your visits to coincide with these activity periods, you will have more opportunities to help care for your baby. You may want to call your baby's nurse before your visit; she can tell you when she expects your baby to be awake, or she may be able to adjust his schedule so that you can provide his care when you get there.

Basic Physical Care: Taking Temperatures, Diapering, Mouth Care, Bathing

All preemies need to have the following tasks done regularly. Your baby's nurse can teach you how to do them and help you until you feel comfortable on your own.

Taking your baby's temperature

This is often one of the first tasks that parents feel comfortable performing. When you take your baby out of the incubator to hold or feed him, his nurse will want you to take his temperature to make sure he is not losing too much body heat. If you are using a traditional glass thermometer, you will probably take your baby's axillary temperature by placing the end of the thermometer in his armpit with his arm down at his side and leaving it in place for three to five minutes. If you have never used a glass thermometer before, the nurse will show you how to use and read it. Some hospitals use thermometers that give instant digital read-outs.

Changing diapers

Although diapering is not an inherently difficult task, it can be challenging to work with a tiny baby who is inside an incubator and connected to IV tubes, monitoring wires, and/or respiratory equipment. In addition, preemies who are less than about 32 weeks old are weak and floppy. If your baby is lying on his stomach or side, you must turn him over on his back to change his diaper. Unlike a full-term baby who feels like a compact, connected bundle when you handle him, your preemie is floppy and his bottom half may feel only loosely connected to his top half. You'll need to scoop both of your hands under your baby to support his whole body and head as you turn him. This can take some practice, particularly if you are a new parent.

If you are uncomfortable moving your baby, have the nurse get your baby into position first and then take over. And if working through the portholes is very difficult, ask your baby's nurse if you may open the front of the incubator and slide the bed out to give you a platform that is easier to work on. She may place warming lights above your baby so he doesn't become chilled while you work. The nurse will want to look at your baby's diaper and weigh it in order to keep track of his output of urine and feces, so leave it on top of the incubator when you are finished.

Mouth care

If your baby is on a respirator with an endotracheal tube in his mouth, you can help keep him comfortable by wiping away secretions that accumulate around the tube and applying glycerin ointment to his lips to keep them from getting chapped. This is a simple task that you can do very early in your child's hospitalization when you may be able to do little else. Some parents also learn how to suction mucous and other secretions from their baby's nose and mouth if he must remain on respiratory equipment for an extended period of time.

Bathing

At first, your baby will only be given sponge baths inside the incubator or on the warming table. Because preemies tend to have very thin and sensitive skin, they are usually just wiped with a soft wash cloth and plain warm water. As your baby gets older and bigger, you will be able to give him tub baths. In some hospitals, baths are given during the night shift when the nursery is generally less busy. If you want to start bathing your own baby, talk to the staff and try to rearrange the schedule so that you can do it yourself. Your baby's nurse will get you set up and teach you how to bathe your baby.

Holding Your Baby

As soon as your baby's health has stabilized sufficiently, you will be able to hold him. You may feel nervous about handling him at first because of his IVs and monitor wires as well as his apparent fragility, but the benefits to you and your baby far outweigh any risks. However, in the beginning, expect that you will only be able to hold him for a short time.

You can hold your preemie in one of two ways. The first is the traditional method in which your baby is wrapped in blankets to stay warm and held nestled in your arms. The second is known as "kangaroo care" and involves skin-to-skin contact between baby and parent. Many parents enjoy the skin-to-skin contact and the ability to touch and caress their baby's entire body that kangarooing allows. But others prefer the traditional approach because it allows them to look at their baby.

Traditional holding sessions

Your baby will be taken from his incubator, wrapped in blankets, have a knit cap placed on his head, and be handed to you while you sit in a rocking chair. At first, your baby's nurse will help you get set up and will transfer your baby from the incubator to your lap. However, as you gain experience and your baby grows healthier and stronger, you will be able to manage these holding sessions independently. But always check with your child's nurses first before taking him from the incubator.

To help keep your baby warm while he is out of the incubator, the nurse may place warming lights over you. These warming lights are quite bright and warm, so dress lightly or in layers for these sessions. The bright lights also make it difficult for your baby to open his eyes; shading his eyes with part of the blanket or with your hand can encourage him to open his eyes.

Kangaroo Care

During the last five years or so, the kangaroo care method of holding pree-mies has gained popularity and acceptance in NICUs around the world. In a kangarooing session, your baby will be dressed only in a diaper and knit hat, placed upright on your bare chest, and covered lightly with a blanket. The kangaroo approach was originally developed in Colombia in the late 1970s. Doctors found that when premature babies were held 24 hours a day on their mother's chests and breastfed on demand, their survival rate greatly improved.

Kangaroo care has since proven to be safe and beneficial for even very small and sick infants. Because babies are placed directly on their parent's chest, their body temperatures remain constant. In addition, babies appear to sleep more soundly, to maintain their heart and breathing rates and oxygen levels, and, in some studies, to gain weight faster.

Because kangaroo care is generally less stressful for the baby than the traditional style of holding, parents can hold their babies sooner and for

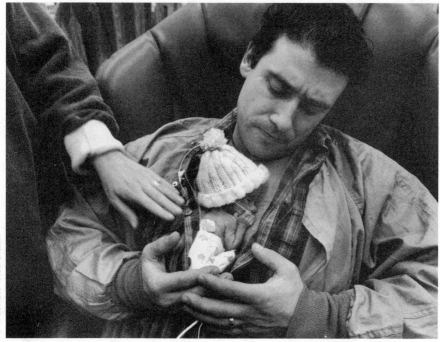

© Michele McDonald

Kangaroo care—skin-to-skin contact—is comforting to both baby and parent.

longer periods of time. Kangarooing also encourages early breastfeeding. It has even been successfully used while babies were still on respirators. Since each hospital has its own protocols governing when you can begin kangaroo or traditional holding, ask your baby's primary nurse which type of holding you should do.

Massaging Your Baby

There is some controversy over the appropriateness of massage for premature infants. Infant massage refers not to the deep muscle pressure used with adults, but to a gentle but firm stroking of a baby's body. Research conducted by Dr. Tiffany Field at the Touch Research Institute of the University of Miami School of Medicine has shown that preemies in stable health (i.e, those in Level II nurseries) who are massaged regularly gain weight faster, are discharged earlier, and show more organized behavior than babies who are not. Dr. Field's research was not conducted on very sick, young, or hypersensitive preemies who may find the stimulation overwhelming rather than comforting.

If you are interested in massaging your baby, talk with his nurse, an occupational or physical therapist, or developmental specialist for advice. Make sure your hands are warm before massaging your baby and always watch him for signs of stress while you are working. The massage used in Dr. Field's studies consisted of a series of strokes, done first while your baby lies on his tummy, and then on his back. She recommends stroking him from the top of his head to his neck, from his neck to his shoulders, from the upper back to the waist, from his thigh to his foot and back to the thigh, and from the shoulder down to the hand and back up. If your baby seems to be enjoying the experience, you can turn him over and stroke each arm and leg. Whatever you do on one side of your baby, repeat on the other side.

Even though your baby is little, be sure you use some pressure in your strokes because light feathery touches are annoying to preemies. You might want to start with just a couple of strokes to see how your baby reacts, and then gradually increase the amount of time you massage him.

Dressing Your Baby

As your baby's health improves, you may want to dress him in clothes of his own rather than hospital T-shirts. You can usually find preemie-sized clothing designed for babies under 5 pounds in stores, and there are also a number of mail-order manufacturers. Many parents feel much better when their babies are dressed in their own clothes. As one mother said, "To me, that was my way of saying this is my baby... I dressed her up, that was how I could deal with it. I found preemie clothes that fit around the leads and wires." Another mother felt it was easier to use the hospital shirts but wanted her son to have something personal. She ended up embroidering his name on one of his stocking caps. If you do bring in clothing or other personal belongings, be sure to mark them with your baby's name.

Personalizing Your Baby's Space

Some families like to place photographs of themselves or art work done by siblings on the walls of the incubator where their baby can see them. It is probably best to tape the pictures to the outside of the incubator facing in to avoid damage from the moist air in the incubator. Others make tapes of their voices singing or reading to be played while they are not there. Remember that noises can become amplified and distorted inside the closed incubator, so be careful to keep the volume low. A simple, small stuffed toy (preferably one that can be washed occasionally) can usually be placed in the incubator. Bright colors or black and white seem to attract a preemie's attention more than pastels.

However, don't feel that you need to do any or all of these things. Preemies have a tendency to become exhausted from too much stimulation, so you may want to wait until your baby is older before you decorate his surroundings. If you do want to bring in something personal, start with one thing at a time and see how your baby reacts.

Providing Comfort and Developmentally Supportive Care

Although your baby needs to be in the hospital nursery, it is not always a very comfortable or restful place to be. Lights are on 24 hours a day; machinery, alarms, people, telephones, and radios can create a lot of noise; and necessary medical procedures are often painful. Even routine caretaking activities can be tiring and disruptive.

In the last ten years, Boston psychologist Heidelise Als and others have researched and developed ways of making nurseries and neonatal care more "baby friendly." They have recommended changes in the ways nurseries operate to help lessen the negative effects of hospital care and minimize the stress babies experience. In addition, they recommend that the care each baby receives be adjusted to best fit that child's needs and coping abilities. This approach, known as individualized developmental care (or formally, NIDCAP—Neonatal Individualized Developmental Care and Assessment Program), is designed to provide an environment in which a preemie's development can continue as normally as possible despite his early birth. Research into its effects has shown that babies who are cared for using the individualized developmental care approach have fewer medical complications, shorter stays in the hospital, better weight gain, and fewer days on respirators. There may be long-term effects of this approach, as well. Some of the early research has indicated that babies cared for with the NIDCAP approach may show more organized behavior and better development in their first year of life.

As a result of this work, many nurseries have made modifications to the nursery environment and to the way in which they provide care. For example, medical and caregiving procedures are often clustered so that babies can sleep undisturbed for several hours at a time. In addition, during invasive or uncomfortable procedures, various comforting methods may be used to help babies stay calm. These include holding a baby in a curled position with hands or swaddling, giving the baby something to grasp, or a pacifier to suck on. Your nursery may have a staff member—usually a nurse—who has been trained in the NIDCAP method. She will observe your baby, help plan his care, and advise you and the staff on the best ways of handling him.

As a parent, you can provide comfort and support to your growing baby in a number of ways. These may include making modifications to your baby's surroundings to minimize stress from noise and lights, as well as learning how best to hold and interact with your baby as he grows and matures.

Observe your baby's environment and try to minimize unnecessary noise and light. There are a number of simple adjustments you can make in your baby's surroundings to help reduce the amount of disruptive stimulation that he receives.

• Make sure your baby is shielded from light either by adjusting the amount of light shining directly on him or by putting a blanket or other covering over his incubator or bassinet. If your baby is on a warming table, see if there is some way to shield his eyes from light.

- Always close the doors to his incubator quietly instead of snapping them shut. Try not to set anything down on top of the incubator, or do it quietly.
- If the nursery seems particularly noisy because of a radio playing or phones ringing, talk to the staff about your concerns. They may be able to make adjustments to lessen the noise or move your baby to a quieter location. One mother was concerned because the receiver of a wall phone hanging near her baby's incubator was constantly falling off and startling him. She finally got the nursery to replace it with a desk phone which caused much less disturbance.
- Keep voices low around your baby, particularly when he is sleeping, or move away from his bedside for conversations.
- If your baby's bed is located in an area of the nursery where there is a great deal of activity or foot traffic, ask that he be relocated to a quieter spot.
- If your baby is on a respirator, make sure that the water that accumulates in the tubing is emptied regularly.

Hold your baby in a flexed position and provide boundaries around him while he sleeps. Preemies, like all newborn babies, feel more secure when they are swaddled securely in a blanket with their legs tucked up, arms bent, and hands brought together in front of them. When they sleep, they prefer to be touching or lying up against something, and will often move in the incubator until they are up against the wall or the bottom of the enclosure. By positioning your baby in a curled position and providing boundaries for him while he sleeps, you not only help him feel calm and comfortable, but you also encourage the development of the curled position known as flexion that babies naturally assume in the womb. Preemies, with their lack of muscle strength, have a hard time maintaining this position by themselves, and, if left alone, will lie spread-eagled with straight arms and legs on the relatively hard, flat surfaces of their nursery beds.

To provide comfort to your baby and support his physical development, try the following measures.

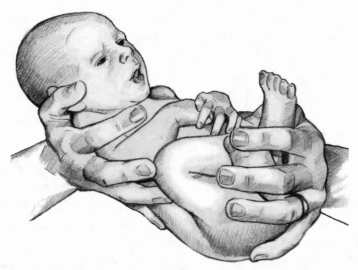

Use your hands to help your baby stay calm and comfortable.

- Swaddle your baby in a blanket with his arms and legs bent and hands brought together in front of him or to his face.
- When you hold your baby, keep him in a slightly curled position, with his legs tucked up and his hands brought forward in front of him.
- Create a nest for your baby to sleep in. Roll blankets or cloth diapers and place them around your baby to help keep his legs tucked or put them against his back and around the top of his head.
- A folded cloth diaper placed under your baby's chest when he is on his stomach can help him to feel secure and be in a flexed position.
- If your baby must sleep on his back, provide rolls along his sides to keep his arms bent and hands brought together in front of him, and another roll under his knees to keep his legs tucked up.
- In the hospital, babies sometimes sleep on artificial lamb skins or water beds to soften the surface of the bed. Artificial lamb skins and water beds are recommended for use only in the hospital where your baby is continuously monitored. They should not be used at home as they are associated with a higher risk of Sudden Infant Death Syndrome (SIDS).

Learn to read your baby's cues and pace your activities with him accordingly. As discussed earlier in this chapter, premature babies tend to express themselves through physical changes and behavior. As you spend more time with your baby and as he matures, you will begin to recognize how he signals that he is getting tired or upset, and the things he does to calm himself. The following techniques may help your child stay calm or regain his equilibrium if he has become upset.

- Provide one form of stimulation at a time: if you rock him, don't talk; if you are feeding him, try not to look him in the eye; while you are holding him, shield his eyes from strong light. Add more types of stimulation slowly, watching your baby for signs of stress.
- When your baby signals that he is getting tired and needs some time out, give him a rest period by cutting back on some of the stimulation he is receiving. For example, if you are rocking and looking at him, look away and just hold him quietly, perhaps shading his eyes from light until he relaxes again. Or decrease the intensity of the stimulation by talking more softly, or rocking more slowly. If these approaches don't work, your baby may simply need to be placed back in his incubator or bassinet to rest and sleep.
- Help your child bring his hands to his face or mouth, or offer him your little finger or a pacifier to suck on.
- Handle and move him slowly and gently.
- If your baby must be unwrapped from his blankets during certain procedures, use your hands to keep his arms and legs tucked and to create boundaries around him. This will comfort him and help him feel more secure.
- Apply gentle but firm pressure on your baby's back or chest with your open hand. This helps him to block out other stimuli, calm down, and organize himself.

Bonding with Your Baby

The sensitivity of premature babies to handling and external stimuli and the brevity of their wakeful periods can be frustrating at times. You may find yourself yearning to hold and talk to your baby but worrying that any action you take will cause him stress or harm. Or if your child is unable to noticeably respond to you or is so overly sensitive to stimulation that you are very limited in what you can do, you may feel cut off or even rejected.

You may worry that all of the obstacles that come between you and your baby in the NICU will affect your feelings and that you will never feel very connected to your child.

It is important to remember that the process of bonding is not one that takes place in the first few hours or days of your child's life as was once thought. For the parent of any baby, the growth of affection and of feelings of connection is a gradual one. It is not surprising that the process takes longer in the NICU for some parents and babies. However, this period when your baby feels very inaccessible and your role as his parent feels limited is a relatively short one. As your baby grows and matures and his health improves, the opportunities for interaction and involvement with him will increase, and your feelings will grow as well.

Caring for Twins and Other Multiples

Parents who have had twins, triplets, or higher multiples in the NICU offer several pieces of advice on how to handle the additional challenges involved.

- Ask to have your babies' schedules staggered, if possible, so that their feeding and care take place at different times. If your babies are on different schedules you will be able to participate in caring for both (or all).
- Take what you have learned caring for one baby and apply it to the other(s). If your babies are cared for by different nurses, you may learn different skills or techniques from each. You can apply this knowledge to all of your babies and feel confident and competent more quickly.
- Do not feel that you must spend all day every day in the hospital. Your children are being well taken care of in the NICU, and it will help you both physically and emotionally to take a break periodically.
- If one baby is sicker than the other(s), spend more time with that baby. If the worst happens and that child does not survive, the memories of the time you spent with him will be incredibly precious. Parents who have lost a baby stress how important this is to your later peace of mind.

Feeding Your Baby

Perhaps no other single activity of preemie parenthood absorbs as much time and emotional energy as feeding your baby. Not only is feeding a tiny infant challenging and time-consuming, but concerns about weight gain are universal. Almost every phone call or visit to the NICU includes a report on how much weight your baby has gained or lost in the previous 24 hours.

In fact, your baby, like all newborns, will lose approximately 10 percent of his body weight in the first days after birth. If your baby weighed about 3 pounds at birth, he will lose about 5 ounces or 140 grams. This weight loss is normal and to be expected. It usually takes between one and three weeks for most preemies to get back to their original birth weight; the younger and sicker the baby, the longer it can take. Unfortunately, when your child is tiny to begin with, waiting through this period is particularly stressful. As one parent recalled, "Our son was so little to start with, I hated to see him lose any weight. It didn't seem like it was possible for him to lose very much and still be okay."

Your baby will begin oral feeding, either from bottles or the breast, when he is approximately 32 to 34 weeks old. If he was born at that gestational age or older, you may be able to bottle- or breastfeed him soon after birth. If he is younger, or too sick to feed orally, he will probably be fed first intravenously, and then by gavage tube directly into his stomach, as explained in Chapter 2.

In this section, you will find general information on what to expect as your baby begins to feed orally, and some of the common feeding challenges presented by preemies. Many mothers want to provide breastmilk for their babies and potentially breastfeed in the future; information on the advantages of breastmilk for preemies, how to pump and store breastmilk, and how to begin to nurse your baby are also included here.

Tube Feedings

Even before your baby can take bottles or nurse at the breast, you can participate in his feedings. During gavage feedings, you can hold the tube of milk and measure how much he takes. At first your baby may be fed in the incubator, but later you may be able to hold him during these feedings.

You may also be able to give him a pacifier or your finger to suck on while he is being fed. This helps to develop the muscles in his mouth and cheeks that he will need for bottle-feeding or breastfeeding. It also helps him associate sucking with getting a full tummy.

Early Bottle-Feeding Sessions

Although feeding practices in many nurseries are changing to encourage earlier breastfeeding, most preemies still have their first oral feeding experiences with a bottle. Preemies are usually fed from small plastic bottles marked in cubic centimeters (cc) or milliliters (ml) and topped with a soft red preemie nipple. These nipples require less sucking strength and make it easier for your baby to feed.

It takes most babies a few weeks to master the suck-swallow-breathe sequence involved in feeding and to develop the muscle strength and energy to take all of their feedings by mouth. As your baby is learning, he will receive some feedings by mouth, some by tube, and some as a combination. Young preemies are generally slow, erratic nursers. During his early bottle-feeding sessions, your baby will probably take only small amounts of milk or formula at first, and may doze between short bursts of sucking. As your baby develops the coordination necessary for bottle-feeding, he may also experience short episodes of apnea when he forgets to breathe as he concentrates on sucking. These apnea spells are unnerving, but are usually easily corrected by pulling the nipple from your baby's mouth to give him a chance to catch his breath. Babies with respiratory problems tend to tire easily and may need extra oxygen while feeding, while those who have been on respirators for an extensive period may have developed a strong aversion to having anything placed in their mouths or a poor suck reflex which can make feeding even more problematic. Your baby's nurse will help as you and your baby learn the skills involved in oral feeding.

Helping Your Baby Feed Well

Oral feeding is a very demanding activity to a preemie. As your baby is learning, help him focus his energies on feeding by limiting other forms of stimulation. In particular, avoid making eye contact with him, rocking him, talking or singing while you are feeding him. Hold your baby in a gently flexed (curled) position, with his arms brought forward and legs

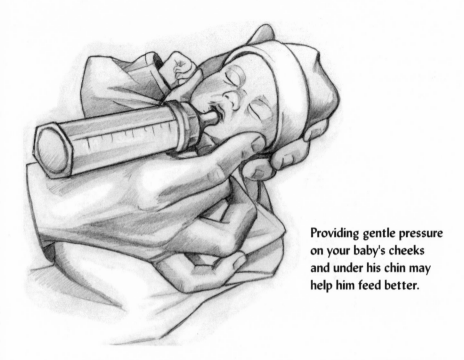

Providing gentle pressure on your baby's cheeks and under his chin may help him feed better.

bent. Be careful not to let your baby slump too much because this can make it hard for him to breathe properly as he feeds. It may help to have a nurse take a Polaroid picture of you with your baby positioned correctly so that you can refer to it later at home.

The traditional way of holding a baby by nestling him close to your body in the crook of your arm may not provide the support that your baby needs. You may find it easier to sit him in your lap, supporting his back and head with one hand as you hold the bottle with the other, or you can lean him back against your thighs (raise your feet on a support and bend your knees) so that he is facing you. Both of these positions allow you to see your baby more clearly as you feed him and to provide him with more support. Some babies also feed better if you provide some support to their jaws and cheeks. You can give gentle pressure or support by placing a finger under your baby's jaw or chin, or by pressing very gently on both cheeks. You might also try placing a finger in the palm of your baby's hand; this can help to stimulate the sucking reflex.

You may find it easier to burp your baby by sitting him up in your lap rather than up against your shoulder. Support him with a hand on his

You may find it easier to burp your tiny baby by sitting him in your lap and supporting his chin with one hand while you rub or gently pat his back.

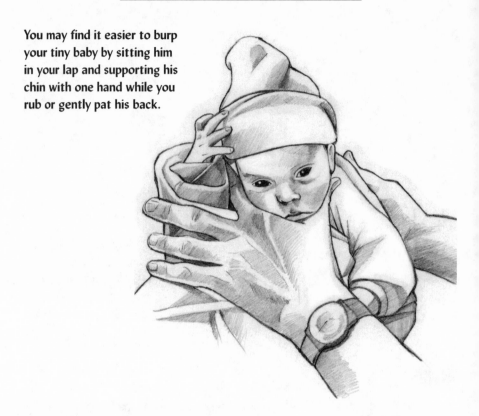

chest, and your thumb and forefinger under his jaw to keep his head from sagging forward too much. With your other hand, rub or pat his back. Babies can also be burped lying across your knees.

Do You Want to Breastfeed?

If your baby has been born very early, you may not have had time before his birth to think about whether or not you want to breastfeed. Even if you had already decided you wanted to nurse your newborn, you may wonder if it is still possible. Physically, it is possible since your breasts will have developed the capability of producing milk by the fifth or sixth month of pregnancy, but your baby may not have the ability to nurse quite yet. Until he can, you will need to express your milk, preferably with an electric pump, and store it for his later use.

There are many factors that may affect your decision to pump breastmilk for your baby or use formula. On one side there is evidence that breastmilk is particularly beneficial for preemies (see below). In addition, many mothers find it comforting to pump and supply milk for their babies. In the face of all the high tech care your baby may be receiving and all the strangers who are caring for him, it is nice to know that there is one important element of your baby's care that only you can provide. The routine of pumping also provides many mothers with a structure and focus during a chaotic time.

However, pumping breastmilk can be tiring and time-consuming, and not all mothers are willing or able to make this commitment. The need to return to work, the demands of other children, time spent traveling, conflicting advice or lack of support, stress, and exhaustion can all interfere with your ability and desire to develop and maintain a milk supply. If your baby is fed formula instead, there is no reason to worry or feel guilty. Special infant formulas are available for preemies and babies thrive on these as well.

If you are undecided about pumping milk, it is probably worth giving it a try. Electric breast pumps are relatively easy to use, and you can change your mind at any point knowing that you've given your baby your milk when it was most important to him.

The Benefits of Breastmilk for Premature Babies

Breastmilk is the best food for all newborns but has particular benefits for preemies.

- Breastmilk is easier to digest than formula. The nutrients are easier to absorb, an important advantage for preemies whose digestive systems are still immature and inefficient.
- Milk produced by mothers whose babies are born prematurely differs in composition from that produced by mothers who deliver at term, and is uniquely suited to the early nutritional needs of preemies. It contains the higher concentrations of protein, sodium, chloride, and lipids (fats) that these babies need. The reasons for the differences in preterm milk are not yet understood. One theory suggests that it is an adaptive reaction by the mother to match the needs of the baby. A second theory proposes that the differences are caused by the relative immaturity of the mother's milk glands themselves. By about a month

postpartum, these differences have disappeared and the breastmilk produced is similar to term breastmilk. At that point, your baby's nurse will probably mix certain additives to your milk to provide the additional calories and protein needed by a growing preemie.

- Breastmilk contains numerous anti-infective substances, including antibodies and white blood cells that help fight infections and provide immunity to certain diseases for as long as nursing continues.
- Colostrum, the first milk produced postpartum, is particularly loaded with antibodies and white cells. It is easy to digest, and stimulates the digestive system to mature. Colostrum also helps your baby eliminate excess bilirubin from his system.
- A number of recent studies have suggested that breastmilk helps to protect premature babies from necrotizing enterocolitis (a serious intestinal infection), other infections, and allergies.
- Breastmilk contains special types of fats that aid in the maturation and development of the brain and the retina of the eyes.

How to Get Started Pumping

The sooner you are able to begin pumping your breasts after your baby is born, the easier it is to stimulate a good milk production. Ideally your first pumping session should occur within two to six hours of delivery. However, if you are unable to pump that quickly, simply try to get started as soon as you can. As long as pumping begins within about five days, it is usually possible to successfully establish an adequate milk supply.

You will need to pump at least six to eight times a day for the first week or two in order to stimulate your breasts just as a newborn would. You may want to pump more frequently during the day so that you can get a decent interval of five to six hours of uninterrupted sleep at night. After your milk supply is well-established, you may be able to cut back a bit on the number of times you pump.

Electric Breast Pumps. If you will be pumping milk for more than a few days, you will need to use an electric breast pump in order to develop and maintain an adequate milk supply. Most nurseries and maternity floors have electric breast pumps available for your use. Before you leave the hospital, you will need to arrange for one to use at home. As these pumps are quite expensive, most mothers rent pumps (the cost of rental is usually between $1.00 and $2.00 a day). The nursing staff can give you a list of rental agencies which can usually deliver a pump to you in less than 24 hours. In some hospitals, the staff will make the calls and arrangements for you. Save your receipts for rental charges since some insurance companies will cover the costs of the pump rental if you have a doctor's prescription.

Double-collecting kits. Many pumps have double-collecting kits that allow you to pump milk from both breasts at the same time. Not only does this decrease pumping time but it also stimulates higher levels of prolactin, the hormone which activates the milk-producing cells in the breasts. Double-collecting kits are particularly useful if your baby weighs less than 1,500 grams, if you will be pumping for more than two weeks, and if you have had twins or higher multiples.

What to expect. Don't be discouraged if you seem to be producing very little milk in the early days of pumping. Most mothers produce only drops of colostrum and very little milk (approximately 1/2 ounce) in each session in the first few days. Luckily, your baby doesn't need much milk initially. Your production will increase as your real milk comes in on about the third day postpartum, and you become accustomed to using the pump and settle into a routine. Many mothers find that they have an easier time getting their milk to start flowing if they look at a picture of their baby or have something of their baby's with them (a piece of clothing, a burp rag, etc., that smells of the baby) while they pump. You may be particularly successful if you pump right after visiting your baby.

The steps involved in pumping milk are outlined in the box below.

Storing and Transporting Breastmilk

The nursery will have a refrigerator and freezer available for you to use to store your breastmilk. Be sure to label your milk with your baby's name, and the date and time the milk was expressed. Milk is usually given to babies in the order in which it was pumped, with the oldest milk used first. This way your baby will receive your colostrum in his first feedings.

Be sure to ask your baby's nurse for the storage guidelines used in your nursery. Some nurseries prefer that you use glass bottles for storage while others prefer plastic bottles or bags. If your baby is sick or will be receiving

Guidelines for Pumping

1. Discuss your desire to provide breastmilk for your baby with his nurses and physicians, and review your hospital's guidelines for pumping and storing breastmilk. Also inform them of any medications you are taking.

2. Wash your hands thoroughly before beginning. Your hands should be clean before you handle any of the parts of the breast pump and collecting containers that will come in contact with the breastmilk. Try to pump in a quiet location where you can relax.

3. Make sure all tubing and overflow bottles are connected correctly.

4. Before you begin pumping, roll your nipple gently between your fingers, or run your fingertips very lightly over your breast to stimulate milk let-down. Massage your breasts for about 3 minutes before pumping and during pumping to improve and speed milk extraction. Having something that reminds you of your baby, such as a picture or piece of clothing, can stimulate your let-down reflex.

5. Center the flange of the collecting cup over your nipple and aureola (the dark area surrounding the nipple). Pumps usually come with two sizes of flange—experiment to see which is the most comfortable. If you have trouble maintaining suction, the inside of the flange can be moistened with warm water or a few drops of breastmilk.

milk through a continuous feeding pump, you may need to use extra precautions to keep your milk as clean and germ-free as possible.

Unless your hospital nursery instructs you differently, use the following guidelines for storing your milk.

- If your baby will be using your fresh milk soon after you pump it, store it in a plastic container. The white (disease-fighting) cells in milk tend to stick more to glass surfaces than to plastic ones, decreasing the number your baby receives. Since freezing destroys many of the white cells, you can use either glass or plastic to store frozen milk.

- When freezing milk in plastic bags, use the type of bags that are specifically designed for breastmilk storage. If these are not available, use the plastic bags designed for regular nursers. Leave extra room at the top of the bag to allow for expansion as the milk freezes. Place the bag

Guidelines for Pumping, continued

6. Set the pump on the lowest suction setting and increase slowly until your milk is flowing freely and you are comfortable (pressure that is too high and/or painful will not increase the amount of milk you will express).

7. If you are using a single set-up, plan to pump each breast for approximately 5 minutes at first. Then return to each breast for a few minutes more. As production increases, you will pump each breast until milk flow slows down (approximately 10 minutes), and then return to each breast one or more times for a few minutes more. Always turn the pump off before removing the flange from your breast.

8. If you are using a double set-up, pump for approximately 10 minutes until milk flow has slowed. Check frequently to make sure the flanges are positioned properly and good suction is maintained.

9. Transfer milk to clean storage container, label with your name and your baby's name, the date and time collected, and place in refrigerator or freezer.

10. Wash flanges, tubing, and containers (anything that came in contact with your milk) in hot soapy water and rinse well. In the hospital, you will probably use a new sterile set-up for each pumping session. These supplies should be thrown away after each use.

inside a paper cup in your freezer to keep it from spilling. You may want to double bag or place several small bags into a larger ziplock bag or airtight container to protect against punctures.

• Freeze milk in small quantities (2 to 3 ounces) to avoid wasting it. You can add more milk to some that was previously frozen, but cool the new milk first in the refrigerator before adding it.

• Transport your milk to the hospital in a small cooler with cold packs or styrofoam pellets. Regular ice is warmer than frozen breastmilk and will tend to melt it.

Early Breastfeeding Sessions

Recent research has found that preemies actually have an easier time at the breast and experience fewer spells of apnea and bradycardia during breastfeeding sessions than when feeding from a bottle. In many nurseries, feeding protocols are changing and mothers who want to nurse are encouraged to put their babies to breast earlier and earlier.

Your first breastfeeding sessions with your baby should be thought of as opportunities to get acquainted with one another rather than as real feeding sessions. The first few times you try to nurse your preemie, do not expect him to be able to latch on to your breast like many full-term babies can. If he simply nuzzles your nipple and perhaps get a drop or two of milk on his lips or in his mouth you should consider it to be a successful session. As you progress, you may want to try to stimulate your milk let-down reflex before you put your baby to your breast. With your milk already flowing, your baby will have an easier time suckling. Remember that breastfeeding is a learned skill on the part of both mother and baby; with preemies the transition to successful breastfeeding is a slow process. Many babies do not really catch on until they get closer to their due dates, and some never make the transition to full breastfeeding.

Where to Get Help and Information

Surveys have found that only about a third of mothers with low birthweight babies begin breastfeeding, and only about half of these continue until their babies are discharged from the hospital. Lack of support and information are cited as the biggest barriers to successful breastfeeding.

However, as the benefits of breastfeeding preemies have become more widely known, support services for nursing mothers are beginning to improve in many NICUs. Find out if your NICU has a lactation specialist on staff who can work closely with you, or if any of the staff nurses are particularly knowledgeable about the problems and challenges of nursing preemies. The LaLeche League in your area may be able to give you the names of volunteers who have experience in working with mothers of preemies, and there may be other organizations in your area that provide lactation education and support. There are a number of good books available on breastfeeding, most of which have sections on feeding preemies (see Appendix E). Chapter 8 also contains detailed information on the special challenges of breastfeeding preemies.

Caring for Yourself and Your Family

Although your primary focus will be on your baby in the hospital, it is also important to take care of yourself and your family during this period. Finding the right balance can be very difficult. Some of the common issues that parents face during this time are discussed below.

The Postpartum Period

Even though your pregnancy has come to an unexpectedly early end, during the first six weeks after your baby's birth you are a postpartum mother whose body is going through all the normal adjustments and changes that occur at the end of every pregnancy. Most women find that they tire easily and are quite emotional during this period. If you had a cesarean birth, you are also recovering from major abdominal surgery.

Although your primary concern is for your baby, you need to take care of yourself as well, making sure that you eat well and get adequate rest. You will be in better shape to care for your baby when he comes home if you allow yourself time to recover from your pregnancy and delivery. One of the few benefits of having a baby born prematurely is that some or all of the postpartum period of recovery can occur before you are responsible for physically caring for your child 24 hours a day. The following suggestions may help you during this period.

Eat nutritious meals. Many women find that their appetites decrease for a few weeks after giving birth. Distraction, anxiety, and fatigue also make it difficult to think about cooking or shopping, but eating well is an important part of the recovery process. If you don't have any interest in fixing meals, try eating smaller meals or snacks throughout the day instead. Keep nutritious foods handy such as yogurt, lunch meats, cheese, cottage cheese, tuna, soups, peanut butter, whole grain bread or crackers, fruits, and vegetables. Friends and relatives can help during these early weeks by doing your grocery shopping for you or by delivering prepared meals.

If you are pumping milk or nursing, make sure that you drink at least six to eight glasses of water or other fluids (such as juices and non-

caffeinated beverages) a day. One easy way to remember to drink enough is to always have a glass of water or juice at hand when you sit down to nurse or pump. A nursing mother also needs approximately 500 more calories a day than when she is not pregnant, including at least 65 grams of protein. If you are nursing twins, increase your caloric intake by 1,000 calories to approximately 3,000 calories a day.

Getting extra rest should be a priority for the first few weeks after giving birth. This can be particularly difficult if you must go back to work, have other young children at home, or spend long hours commuting to and from the hospital. If at all possible, try to take one nap a day or at least lie down for half an hour. If you are pumping milk, you may want to pump more often during the day so that you can sleep uninterrupted through the night.

Minimize the number of household chores you try to do or arrange for help from friends, relatives, or others. It can be difficult to ask for and to accept help, but your friends and family certainly want to help you in some way; they just may not be sure what to do. Aid with the basic chores of life—laundry, grocery shopping, preparing meals, caring for children—can be enormously helpful to you and gives people something concrete to do. One mother was lucky enough to have a friend who offered to act as a central clearinghouse for such offers of help. "It was so much easier just to refer people to her when they offered to help out. She knew what we needed and when—I didn't have to think about it or try to organize people."

You may want to limit the number of phone calls and/or visits you receive. Telling and retelling the story of your child's birth and current condition can be extremely taxing, even though you appreciate people's concern. You may want to use an answering machine to screen calls or ask a friend to be the primary source of information for you.

Periodically, take a day off from visiting your baby in the hospital. He is being well cared for and your spirits could probably use a lift from a break in your routine. Try to get out for an evening with your spouse; see a movie, go out to eat, or just take a walk. Even treating yourself to something simple like a long soaking bath or shower can be a refreshing mini-vacation. A brisk twenty-minute walk or some other form of mild exercise every day can help you feel better physically and emotionally.

Expect that you will experience dramatic ups and downs in your energy levels and emotions. Most postpartum mothers experience these fluctuations during the first few weeks after their baby's birth. For preemie parents the ups and downs tend to be more intense and longer lasting.

Balancing Hospital Visits and Outside Life

Most parents are shocked and panicky during the days surrounding their baby's early birth and find it hard to cope with the normal demands of life. Unfortunately, responsibilities at work and at home generally do not come to a halt. Although you may be able to arrange for time off or flexible hours at work for a while, there comes a time when you must return to your job. The needs of other children or relatives may have never diminished. One way of coping with the competing demands of a hospitalized baby and your other responsibilities is to try to arrange your visits around times when your baby tends to be awake and alert. In this way, you can maximize the satisfaction and pleasure of the time you spend with your baby while minimizing the actual amount of time you need to spend in the hospital.

If your baby was born ten or more weeks early, he will spend most of his time sleeping. Although it is important to visit and begin to help with his care, it is not really necessary to sit beside him all day long. Most nurseries cluster their caregiving at certain times of the day, usually around feeding time. Find out when those times are because your baby will most likely be awake, and you may be able to help in his care. As your baby grows and matures, he will begin to develop his own sleep and wakefulness patterns. Ask the nurses to note if there are certain times of the day or evening when your baby tends to be awake so you can coordinate your visits with these periods. In addition, it may be useful to call the nursery before your visit to let them know when you are planning to come. If your baby's nurse knows when to expect you, she may be able to plan a feeding or some other caretaking activity around your visit.

Another way of balancing your desire to spend time with your baby with other demands is for parents to take turns visiting their baby.

Although you may find support and comfort in visiting together, there are also benefits to visiting separately. Separate visiting is particularly valuable for a new parent when his or her partner has older children and is more experienced. The inexperienced parent may be tempted to defer to the more experienced partner when they are together. Confidence and skill in handling your baby come from practice; although you will probably be nervous trying things on your own at first, it is the best way to gain confidence. The nurses will always be close by to help you. Being by yourself gives you a chance to have some precious one-on-one time with your baby and simplifies some of your family's need for child care if there are other children at home.

Sibling Reactions

The trauma of premature birth is felt not only by parents but by other children in the family as well. They will be aware of your upset and the disruption of their routines and react to it, often by acting up themselves. Although it can be difficult, it is important to dredge up extra patience for them during this period and to explain to them in a simple, straightforward way what is happening with their baby brother or sister. Try to spend time with each of your other children during the week, even if it is just for a few minutes, so that they know they are still important to you also. You might want to read an extra story one night, play a short game, or talk for a few extra minutes at bedtime.

There are a number of good books written for young children that explain prematurity and what is happening with their baby brother or sister. Some of these are listed in Appendix E.

Sibling Visits

Your children's involvement with their preemie brother or sister should be geared to their age level. A mature eight-year-old can probably actively participate in his sibling's care, learning to do things like change diapers and hold the baby. Younger children can be brought in for short visits periodically, but don't expect a young child to be able to sit quietly and patiently for very long. It may help to bring along a bag of quiet activities that your child can play with. Some nurseries have sibling corners where younger children can play under supervision while you visit.

Your children's attachment to the new baby will take time to grow, as is true with any addition to the family. Short periodic visits to see the baby usually work better than long ones, which can be boring for older children and stressful for you.

Other Family Members and Friends

Hospitals have different policies regarding visits in the nursery by grandparents and other relatives. Most require the presence of one of the parents or their permission before they will allow anyone else to visit the baby.

Many grandparents face a double load of anxiety, worrying about their grandchild as well as their child. Their expectations may be quite pessimistic, since in their experience there was little that could be done for babies born prematurely. A visit to the nursery to see, and possibly touch or hold, the baby may be beneficial for grandparents or other relatives.

But if relatives cannot visit, they can still help support the family through this crisis. If they live far away, they should call. If they live nearby, they can take care of some everyday tasks such as babysitting your other children, meal preparation, laundry, and grocery shopping.

Most people have little or no experience with prematurity and have no idea what to say to a couple whose child has been born early. Let your friends and family know that you want and need to talk about your baby. If they ask if there is anything they can do to help, try to give them a concrete task such as a specific household chore.

Financial Issues

As difficult as it is to think about, when you are anxious and preoccupied with your baby's survival and health, issues of health insurance and the costs of having a preemie rear their heads rapidly. Most government and private insurance plans include fairly complete coverage for a baby needing intensive care, although you may need to pay an initial deductible amount. Be sure to call your insurance company to notify them and check your coverage early in your infant's hospitalization. Your hospital may help with such incidental expenses as parking or meals. Ask the nursery social worker for information about these and other sources of financial aid.

You should also know about several government programs.

Supplemental Security Income (SSI)

The Supplemental Security Income (SSI) program, administered by the federal government through the Social Security Administration (SSA), provides income to the elderly and to those who are blind or disabled at any age. Many premature and low birthweight babies qualify for this benefit; if your baby weighs less than 1,200 grams (1 pound 10 ounces) at birth, or if he weighs between 1,200 and 2,000 grams (4 pounds 6 1/2 ounces) and is 4 weeks small for gestational age, he is considered to be disabled and is automatically eligible to receive SSI payments.

As long as a premature baby is hospitalized, the parent's income and resources are not considered in determining eligibility. After discharge, the parent's economic situation is taken into account to determine whether eligibility will continue. SSI benefits start the day you file, or notify your local SSA office that you intend to file, an application. A phone call to the local SSA office will establish intent; be sure to note the date and time of your call and with whom you spoke. If the parents are not able to make the phone call, another person (the hospital social worker, a friend, relative, or legal guardian) may do so on behalf of the infant.

Because the SSI program is primarily a program that provides income assistance for the elderly and disabled, various SSA offices may be less aware that certain premature infants also qualify for SSI payments. The SSA acknowledges this problem and is working to correct it but recommends that you be "patient, persistent, and firm" in your request.

Medicaid

Medicaid is a federal program (Title XIX of the Social Security Act) which provides health insurance for certain eligible groups, including families with incomes below a certain level, individuals with disabilities, or some working families with high medical costs. The Medicaid program is jointly administered and funded by each state and the federal government. In many states, Medicaid eligibility is automatically established with SSI eligibility. In other states, a separate application is required. The eligibility criteria for Medicaid as well as the benefits included vary from state to state. Your hospital social worker can provide you with detailed information on your state's program and eligibility requirements.

State Child Health Insurance Programs (CHIP)

In 1997, the federal government established a new children's health insurance program under Title XXI of the Social Security Act. Under this new program, states can expand health insurance coverage for currently uninsured children and receive matching funds from the federal government. As with Medicaid, the eligibility requirements and services covered vary from state to state. Your hospital social worker should have details on your state's program.

Federal Income Tax Deductions

If you itemize deductions on your federal income tax return using Schedule A of Form 1040, some of the out-of-pocket (i.e., unreimbursed) costs you incur related to your child's medical care can be counted toward the deduction for medical and dental expenses. Unfortunately, this benefit is rarely useful since your out-of-pocket expenses must exceed 7.5 percent of your adjusted gross income before you can begin to deduct them. However, if you pay your own health insurance premiums or have high deductible or co-payment amounts, you may be able to take advantage of this deduction.

The types of expenses that can be deducted as medical expenses include premiums for health insurance that you pay yourself, out-of-pocket expenses for medical and laboratory services and prescription drugs (including deductibles and co-payments), lodging (up to $50 per person per night), the costs of transportation (bus, taxi, train, or plane fares), parking fees and tolls, and car expenses (actual expenses such as gas and oil, or $.10/mile). You must keep a log book to account for mileage and save receipts for other expenses in order to substantiate your claim.

For more detailed information on the medical expense deduction, order Publication 502, "Medical and Dental Expenses," from the IRS at 1-800-TAX-Form (1-800-829-3676). Or for answers to specific questions, call the IRS at 1-800-829-1040.

CHAPTER 4

Coping with Medical Complications

ℰᕽ

PREMATURE INFANTS MAY develop a number of medical problems as a result of their early arrival in the world. Some of these are unavoidable and occur because a preemie's organ systems—her lungs, her digestive system, her eyes—are being asked to function before they are fully mature and ready. Other complications happen, unfortunately, as a side effect of the medical care that is so crucial to a preemie's survival. And still others occur for reasons not yet fully understood. Some problems are temporary and are so common in the world of the NICU as to be almost routine—although they never feel that way to parents. Others occur less often or are potentially more serious.

This chapter gives you an overview of the most common problems that preemies face. It is important to keep in mind that no baby will experience everything described here. You may want to concentrate on those parts of the chapter that pertain to your baby's situation, and use the information to supplement what your own doctors and nurses tell you. Since explanations in the NICU can be rushed and confusing, it can be helpful to have something to refer to later in the quiet of your home.

In the first part of this chapter, you will find information on the medical problems that most preemies experience. These include apnea and bradycardia, newborn jaundice, and anemia. Difficulties with temperature regulation, and nutrition and fluid intake were discussed earlier in Chapter 2. The second part of the chapter covers more serious medical problems. These include respiratory distress syndrome, chronic lung disease, brain bleeds, vision problems, and others. For further details on these and other less common problems, see the Bibliographical References at the end of this book for a listing of additional sources of information.

Common Complications

The following complications are extremely common among premature infants, are generally short-lived, and do not usually cause any long-term problems.

Anemia

Anemia occurs when the number of red blood cells, the component of the blood that carries oxygen, falls below normal. This can affect the amount of energy that a baby has, causing her to tire quickly, gain weight slowly, have more apnea spells, or have trouble coping with other medical complications.

Almost all premature babies will develop anemia over the first few weeks and months of life. For most, it causes no problems and gradually goes away on its own. However, some very premature or sick babies may begin to show the symptoms described above and need a blood transfusion to boost quickly the number of red blood cells in their bodies.

What causes anemia? Anemia can occur for a number of reasons. Among premature babies, the primary cause is a series of changes that naturally occur in the composition of the blood during the first weeks of life. Before birth, a baby's blood supply carries extra red blood cells in order to help her pick up oxygen from her mother's blood stream through the placenta. Once a baby is breathing on her own, she no longer needs as many red blood cells. The body temporarily stops producing them, and the number of red blood cells in her blood stream slowly decreases. When the level gets too low—that is, when the baby becomes anemic—her body responds by beginning to produce red blood cells again and the anemia gradually goes away.

Although both full-term and premature babies go through this transition, premature babies usually become anemic faster and their levels of red blood cells drop lower. A full-term baby usually hits her lowest point at about six to twelve weeks of age compared to a preemie who becomes most anemic between four and ten weeks after birth.

Preemies can also become anemic because of the number of blood tests (including tests for anemia) they undergo. Even though these tests can now be run on tiny volumes of blood, the blood loss caused by repeated testing becomes a significant factor for some babies. Premature babies may lose blood during or soon after birth, or due to hemorrhage as well.

How it is treated. Many healthy premature infants are able to tolerate fairly severe levels of anemia without showing any ill effects, and your baby may simply be monitored by periodic blood tests known as hematocrit or hemoglobin tests. The hematocrit measures the proportion of red blood cells, and the hemoglobin test measures how much hemoglobin— the oxygen-carrying component of the red blood cell—there is in the blood. Another test known as a reticulocyte count is usually performed as well. Reticulocytes are new, immature red blood cells. Their presence in the blood indicates that your baby's body is beginning to produce red blood cells again.

A blood transfusion may become necessary if a baby develops anemia-related problems, such as poor weight gain, apnea, increased heart rate, or poor feeding. If a baby has respiratory or other medical problems, her doctors will probably want to keep her hemoglobin levels fairly high and she may need multiple transfusions. Transfusions are usually done using packed red blood cells which contain a high number of cells in a low volume of blood. Further information about transfusions can be found later in this chapter.

And finally, in some hospitals, anemia is treated with a substance known as erythropoietin (EPO) which stimulates the production of red blood cells. This is a fairly new approach that may help avoid transfusions, but it is not in common use yet.

The need for iron as your baby grows. Anemia of prematurity is further complicated by the fact that preemies are born with lower reserves of iron in their bodies than full-term babies. Iron is a necessary part of the hemoglobin in red blood cells. As preemies begin to grow and produce red blood cells again, they can quickly run out of the iron they have stored for this purpose. To avoid this, they need to have iron supplements added to their diet. Most babies receive iron supplementation in the form of liquid drops or iron-fortified formula when they begin taking food orally. You may want to ask your baby's doctor about this. With iron supplementation, your baby's anemia should have disappeared by the time she is about three months old.

Apnea of Prematurity

Apnea is defined as a pause in breathing that lasts for more than 15 to 20 seconds, or a pause of any length when a baby's heart rate drops to less than 100 beats per minute (known as bradycardia). During an apnea episode, a baby's skin color usually changes as well. Babies with light skin turn dusky—bluish or purplish—and babies with dark skin become pale. This change in color can be seen most clearly around the mouth, and in the beds of fingernails and toenails. In the NICU, these episodes may be called spells, or As and Bs, for apnea and bradycardia.

Apnea episodes are extremely common among premature babies, and the younger the baby the more likely it is that she will experience apnea spells. About one fourth of all preemies, and four out of five of those born before 30 weeks, will have apnea spells. The first episode generally occurs sometime within the first two days of life; if your baby does not have a spell during the first week after her birth, there is a good chance she will not experience any apnea.

What causes it? The most common type of apnea seen among premature babies—known as apnea of prematurity—occurs because the respiratory and nervous systems are immature. The centers that control breathing are not fully developed and are still somewhat unreliable. Because this is a developmental problem, most babies outgrow it by the time they reach about 37 weeks of age, although for some it may take a few weeks longer.

Apnea spells can also indicate that a baby is getting sick or developing other problems, particularly if the spells begin suddenly or become more frequent. Apnea spells can be triggered by infections, low blood sugar, a body temperature that is too low or too high, brain injury, or respiratory problems. If your baby begins to have more apnea spells or they continue beyond her due date, her doctors will run tests to determine what is causing them.

How it is treated. Almost all babies in intensive or special care nurseries are routinely placed on heart and breathing monitors which will sound an alarm if an apnea or bradycardia spell occurs. Most of these spells are short; babies quickly begin to breathe again on their own, or need only a gentle pat or rub on their foot or back to remind them to breathe. These short pauses aren't harmful for your baby. But if they occur regularly, she will probably be placed on apnea-controlling medication, such as theophylline, aminophylline, or caffeine, until she outgrows her tendency to have apnea. Some babies need a little extra oxygen to help them recover from a spell. Still others will be placed on CPAP or a ventilator until their apnea improves.

Are apnea and Sudden Infant Death Syndrome (SIDS) related? Once your child has experienced apnea spells in the hospital, it is natural to worry that she might stop breathing again at home, or be at higher risk for SIDS. But apnea of prematurity is a developmental problem that most preemies outgrow by 37 weeks gestational age. It is not the same as SIDS. Although it is true that premature and low birthweight babies are at higher risk for SIDS, that risk is not increased if your child experienced apnea of prematurity.

Bradycardia

Bradycardia or a slowdown in the heart rate usually occurs during an apnea spell but can occur for other reasons as well. Preemies' hearts usually beat between 110 and 160 times per minute. If the heart slows down below about 100 beats per minute, it is considered a bradycardia spell and your baby's monitor will beep. As you begin to handle your baby more, you may notice that her heart rate changes in different situations. When a baby is feeling stressed, her heart rate may speed up or slow down. It also may slow down periodically when she is learning to feed from a bottle. The heart rate usually comes back up by itself, although sometimes a baby may need a gentle pat or rub, or some blow-by oxygen.

Jaundice or Hyperbilirubinemia

During the first weeks of their lives, almost all premature babies will need to be treated for jaundice, also known as hyperbilirubinemia. Jaundice is a yellowish coloration of the skin and whites of the eyes that occurs when the level of bilirubin in the blood rises above normal.

What causes it? Like anemia, jaundice occurs as a result of normal changes in the blood of newborns. It does not indicate liver problems as it does in adults. As the excess red blood cells in a baby's circulation begin to break down in the weeks after birth, they release a yellowish substance known as bilirubin. All newborns show increases in the levels of bilirubin in the blood over the first weeks of life, but with premature infants this build up occurs faster and bilirubin levels can go higher.

Bilirubin is normally processed by the liver and excreted in the stool. Because their livers are still immature, premature babies don't process bilirubin efficiently. In addition, they are eating little and so producing few stools (which normally help eliminate bilirubin from the body). Bruising that occurs during birth can also contribute to high bilirubin levels.

How it is treated. Jaundice is primarily treated by phototherapy or by being "under the lights." During phototherapy, a baby is exposed to special lights which may be blue, white, or green. These lights may be placed above your baby or they may be embedded in a fiber-optic blanket. Sometimes both methods are used together. Babies usually wear nothing or only a diaper so that as much of their skin as possible is exposed to the lights.

Bilirubin is very sensitive to light waves, and the light exposure breaks down the bilirubin in your baby's body into products that can be elimi-

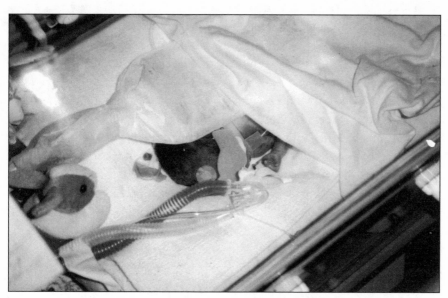

A 6-day-old baby on a respirator, eyes protected by eyepatches, receives phototherapy from a biliblanket.

nated in the urine and stools. Your baby may have more frequent or loose stools during phototherapy. She will also wear a shield to protect her eyes from the bright lights.

Rarely, bilirubin levels rise to such high levels that a baby will need an exchange transfusion to lower the level quickly. During an exchange transfusion, a specific amount of blood is withdrawn from a baby and replaced with an equal amount of donor blood from a carefully matched donor (see information on transfusions below).

Slight or moderate increases in bilirubin levels are not harmful to your child. But because high levels can cause permanent brain damage, a condition known as kernicterus, your baby's bilirubin levels are monitored closely. Younger, sicker, and smaller babies are most sensitive to excess bilirubin. To keep your baby safe, treatment with bililights usually begins at fairly low levels of bilirubin and often starts within the first few days of birth for very premature babies. Through this aggressive management, the occurrence of permanent damage has become extremely rare.

Breastmilk Jaundice. A few breastfed infants develop a condition known as breastmilk jaundice, in which breastmilk itself appears to contribute to high levels of bilirubin. True breastmilk jaundice occurs in only 1 or 2 percent of breastfed babies for reasons that are not yet clearly understood. If your baby is nursing or being given your breastmilk and her bilirubin levels remain high despite treatment with lights, your doctor may recommend temporarily switching her to formula. Bilirubin levels usually fall quickly, and your baby will be able to resume breast milk again within a couple of days. Once bilirubin levels have been brought down by the short break in nursing, they never again rise as high.

If your baby develops breastmilk jaundice, it does not mean that there is anything wrong with your milk or that it is harmful for your baby. The benefits of breastmilk far outweigh this temporary problem. It is not a reason to avoid or stop breastfeeding, or to stop supplying your baby with your pumped milk.

If Your Child Needs a Blood Transfusion

Blood transfusions can help babies recover quickly from a number of complications and even save lives. But in this era of HIV and other blood-born diseases, it is hard not to worry about the risks to your child of receiving donor blood. A combination of factors has made it much safer for your child to receive blood if she needs it. First, most neonatologists use blood transfusions sparingly. They will only recommend one if your child absolutely needs it, or if they feel that the benefits to your child are considerable. In addition, the blood supply is safer now than it has ever been. Potential blood donors are carefully screened for health history and risk factors, and the blood itself is tested extensively, including tests for HIV and hepatitis A, B, and C. New and more sensitive tests have significantly lowered the risk of transmission of disease. Currently, the risk of HIV is estimated as being 1 in 420,000 units; hepatitis A is 1 in 1,000,000 units; hepatitis B is 1 in 200,000; and hepatitis C is in the range of 1 in 2,000 to 1 in 6,000.

Additional processing. Blood used for preemies usually receives extra processing as well to further minimize the risks to your child. Two common practices are irradiation and leukocyte (white cell) depletion. These procedures kill or remove certain viruses that may be carried in the white cells of the blood. Removing the white cells also lowers the chances of your baby having a reaction to the transfused blood.

Using a single donor. Babies receive tiny amounts of blood in a transfusion. For example, a 4 1/2 pound baby has a total of about 3 ounces of blood circulating in her body. A baby that size would typically receive about 1/3 to 1/2 teaspoon of blood in a transfusion. Because babies need so little blood, many hospitals will break down a single unit of blood into eight smaller portions. If this service is available at your hospital, your baby can potentially receive up to eight tranfusions using blood from a single donor. This minimizes her risks even more since she is not exposed to blood from many different people.

Directed donors. Many hospitals also offer directed donor programs in which you, a relative, or friend with the same blood type as your baby can donate blood for her. Directed donor blood is tested and processed like that from any other donor, and it usually takes 48 to 72 hours before it can be used. Studies have not shown that directed donor blood is any safer than regular blood-bank blood. However, if you donate your own blood or limit requests to people whose health and lack of risk factors you feel confident of, it is reasonable to feel less anxious. If you are considering asking relatives or friends to donate, it is important to be sensitive to the fact that some people are afraid to donate blood and may feel uncomfortably pressured by your request. Others may be pleased to be asked.

More Serious Complications

The following section covers the most common serious medical problems that some babies face in the NICU. These include problems with the lungs and heart, the brain and senses, the digestive system, and, finally, infection. Again, no baby will experience all of these complications, and the understanding of and treatment methods are constantly improving. If your baby experiences any of these problems, your baby's doctors and nurses can provide you with the most current information about relevant treatment options.

Respiratory Distress Syndrome (RDS)

Because a baby's lungs mature relatively late in gestation, many preemies develop breathing difficulties known as respiratory distress syndrome (RDS). In the past, this condition was also known as hyaline membrane disease (HMD). Advances in the treatment of RDS have allowed many more preemies to survive, and have lessened the severity of the disease for many.

In general, the younger the baby, the greater the risk of her developing RDS. However, when babies have been been under some stress before delivery—including babies with intrauterine growth retardation, those whose mothers have been in early labor, whose membranes have broken early, or who have high blood pressure—their lungs often develop more quickly, lessening their chances of RDS. If a premature delivery can be postponed for a day or two, this natural process can be duplicated by giving the mother one or two injections of corticosteroids such as betamethasone or dexamethasone before delivery. These medications, different from the type of steroids sometimes abused by athletes, accelerate the development of a baby's lungs. They reach maximum effectiveness in about 24 to 48 hours.

What causes it? RDS occurs when a baby's lungs are immature and do not produce enough surfactant, a soaplike substance that coats the inside of the breathing sacs (alveoli) of the lung. Without surfactant, the air sacs collapse as the baby exhales and the sides of the sacs stick together like deflated balloons. With each breath, the baby must work hard to re-inflate the sacs. Soon she grows tired and has more and more trouble breathing.

A baby with RDS looks as if she is working hard at breathing: she grunts with each breath, the skin is drawn in between and below her ribs (retractions), she may breathe quickly, her nostrils may widen as she inhales (flaring), and her skin may be bluish or pale. As she grows tired, her breathing becomes irregular and she may pause periodically. A baby with RDS usually gets worse for three or four days and then gradually gets better as her lungs begin to produce surfactant.

How it is treated. Babies with RDS usually receive a number of doses of artificial surfactant until their own lungs begin to produce sufficient amounts of natural surfactant, usually within about two weeks. Artificial surfactant cannot prevent babies from developing RDS, but its use has made a significant improvement in the survival and recovery of babies with the disease.

Babies with RDS usually need supplemental oxygen, and some will be put on CPAP or a respirator. If the disease is fairly mild, a baby may only need some extra oxygen for a few days. In more severe cases, babies usually show improvement after a few days, but progress is slower. Some babies with RDS develop chronic lung disease, which is explained below.

Air Leaks

Some babies with respiratory problems develop a complication known as an air leak. An air leak occurs when one or more of the air sacs in the lungs tears and air escapes from the lung into surrounding tissues. Air can enter the spaces within the lung itself (pulmonary interstitial emphysema or PIE), between the lung and the chest wall (a pneumothorax), or into the space in the center of the chest where the heart lies (a pneumomedi-astinum). Although leaks may be small and not cause serious problems, they can become dangerous if enough air escapes to press on the lung or heart, making breathing or circulation difficult. Fortunately, the number of babies who develop air leaks has been decreasing with the use of artificial surfactant.

What causes them? Air leaks can develop spontaneously, but they often occur when a baby with severe lung disease must be on a ventilator set to high pressures. Sometimes air leaks develop when babies on ventilators try to breathe out of rhythm with the ventilator.

How they are treated. If an air leak is small, the baby's body may be able to reabsorb the air by itself with no treatment necessary. When an air leak is more serious, a baby may show signs of increasing respiratory distress and need some help. In some cases, a pocket of air can be drawn out using a needle and syringe. If the air is between the lung and chest wall, the doctors will often place a small plastic chest tube into the space. This tube is connected to a suction device that prevents air from accumulating in the chest space. Chest tubes are usually left in place for a few days while the baby's lung heals. Babies may also need to be temporarily placed on higher concentrations of oxygen, or have the pressures on a respirator or CPAP increased. Some babies are placed on high frequency ventilators which operate at lower pressures in order to avoid injuring the lung further.

Chronic Lung Disease (Bronchopulmonary Dysplasia)

Unfortunately, some babies who are treated successfully for RDS develop a condition known as chronic lung disease (CLD), or bronchopulmonary dysplasia (BPD). Chronic lung disease develops when babies' lungs are damaged by the ventilators and oxygen that must be used to treat their RDS. Areas of bleeding and scarring occur in the injured lungs, causing the airways to become narrower and more rigid. In addition, some areas of the lung may collapse while others overexpand, and increased mucous secretions may clog the air spaces. In mild cases, only small areas of the lung are involved; in more severe cases a large proportion of the lung may be affected.

Doctors begin to suspect CLD when a baby with respiratory distress syndrome does not progress as well as expected. She may need to be on a ventilator longer than usual and may continue needing supplemental oxygen. Infants are diagnosed with CLD if they are still receiving supplemental oxygen past 36 weeks of age (gestational age), and if certain changes are seen in their lungs on X-ray.

The use of artificial surfactant has significantly improved the outcome of babies with CLD. Although preemies, particularly very young ones, still develop the disease, it is usually less severe than in the past. Most babies recover from CLD by the time they are two or three years old as new lung tissue grows and damaged tissue is repaired.

What causes it? Chronic lung disease develops when a baby's lungs are damaged by the oxygen and ventilators used to treat their RDS. The longer a baby must be on oxygen and a respirator, the greater the risk of developing CLD. However, not all babies with RDS develop chronic lung disease. The reasons that some babies do and some don't are not clearly understood at this point. Babies from families with asthma seem to be at higher risk, as are babies with a patent ductus arteriosus (explained below).

How it is treated. Babies with chronic lung disease are treated with a number of medications that help the lungs work better and make breathing easier. These include steroids such as dexamethasone to reduce inflammation of the lungs; theophylline, aminophylline, and albuterol (Ventolin) to help expand the breathing tubes in the lungs; and diuretics such as Lasix, Diuril, or Aldactazide to get rid of excess fluid in the body. Excess fluid can accumulate in the lungs of babies with CLD making breathing more difficult. Many babies remain on supplemental oxygen throughout their stay in the hospital and are discharged home on oxygen. Some infants with CLD outgrow their need for extra oxygen within a few months of discharge. Others continue to need it, or need it periodically during growth spurts or with new levels of activity for two or three years while they recover from CLD.

Recovery from CLD can be long and frustratingly slow. As infants, these babies are often very sensitive and irritable. They need extra calories to help them grow and recover but can be very difficult to feed. They may become seriously ill with colds or respiratory infections and may develop asthma-like symptoms.

However, throughout the first years of life, a baby's lungs continue to grow and develop. And as new tissue grows, the damaged part becomes an ever smaller portion of the lung. Most children recover from CLD by the age of two or three, and are subsequently able to participate in vigorous activities like any other child without showing any ill-effects of their earlier problems.

Patent Ductus Arteriosus (PDA)

Before birth, a baby receives oxygen from her mother through the placenta. Because she does not need her lungs, a special structure known as the ductus arteriosus allows blood being pumped from the heart to by-pass the lungs and go directly out to the body. At birth, as a baby begins to breathe on her own, the ductus arteriosus closes, and the pattern of blood flow changes. Now, blood begins to travel from the right side of the heart through the lungs to pick up oxygen. It then leaves the lungs and returns to the left side of the heart, and is pumped from there out to the body.

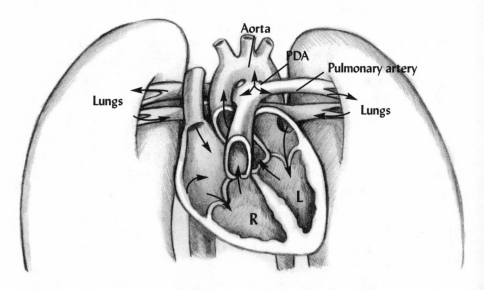

PDA: The ductus arteriosus connects the pulmonary artery (which carries blood from the heart to the lungs) with the aorta (which carries blood from the heart out to the body). If the ductus remains open (patent), it allows some non-oxygenated blood to be pumped directly out to the body, or allows extra blood to be pumped through the lungs, causing strain on the heart and lungs.

However, sometimes the ductus does not close, or reopens in the weeks after birth, leading to a condition known as a patent (open) ductus arteriosus (PDA).

What problems does it cause? A patent ductus arteriosus is a fairly common condition among preemies. Approximately 20 percent of babies born weighing less than 1,500 grams (3 pounds 5 ounces) and 40 percent of all babies weighing less than 1,000 grams (2 pounds 3 ounces) have a PDA. It is particularly common among babies with RDS.

Although there is nothing wrong with the heart itself, the continuation of the fetal circulatory pattern is problematic for several reasons. In the early days of a baby's life, a PDA allows blood to by-pass the lungs so that the heart is pumping blood that is not fully oxygenated out to the body. This may continue during the first phase of RDS while the baby's lungs are not functioning well, and is known as a right-to-left shunt. As the lungs improve and circulation through them increases, the effect of the PDA changes. It now allows some of the oxygenated blood being pumped out to the body from the left side of the heart to be diverted back into the lungs. Known as a left-to-right shunt, this blood flow pattern puts an extra strain on the heart and lungs. If a large volume of blood is diverted in this way, it can cause congestive heart failure (CHF), a condition in which the heart is unable to keep up with the demands being placed upon it, and/or pulmonary edema, in which fluid leaks into the lung tissue itself, making it more difficult for a baby to breathe.

How it is treated. The effects of a PDA depend upon how large the opening is and how much blood is flowing through it. A small PDA may cause few, if any, problems. Your baby's doctors may simply wait to see if it closes on its own. A larger or more serious PDA may cause increasing respiratory problems. For example, your baby may need more oxygen or higher respiratory settings; she may have more apnea spells or appear to be working harder at breathing; or she may develop a heart murmur, an enlarged heart, or an increased heart rate. If your baby appears to have a PDA, the diagnosis will be confirmed by a test known as an echocardiogram. Like an ultrasound, this test uses sound waves to produce a picture of the heart and to estimate how much blood is flowing through the PDA. An echocardiogram is done at your baby's bedside in the nursery and should not disturb her.

Most PDAs can be treated with medication that helps the ductus to close off. The most common drug used is indomethacin (Indocin). In addition, your baby's fluid intake may be reduced or she may be given a diuretic to get rid of extra fluid while the ductus is open. This lessens her chances of developing pulmonary edema or congestive heart failure. Your baby may need several doses of indomethacin before the ductus finally closes.

If the medication is not effective or can't be used because of other medical problems, the ductus may need to be closed surgically. The surgeon will make an incision in your baby's chest and tie off the ductus in an operation that takes about an hour. Your baby will have a chest tube for a couple of days after the surgery to drain air out of the chest as the incision heals. Although a scary prospect for any parent, PDA surgery has become fairly routine and babies usually do very well.

Intraventricular Hemorrhage (IVH)

Intraventricular hemorrhages, also known as brain bleeds, are among the scariest problems that your baby may face. However, bleeding in the brain as it occurs with a premature infant is vastly different from a stroke or brain bleed in an adult. Most brain bleeds in premature infants are small and cause no short- or long-term problems. More serious brain bleeds can but don't always cause permanent damage or developmental problems.

Historically, brain bleeds were categorized using a grading system from I to IV, with I being the mildest and IV being the most serious. As more becomes known about brain bleeds, new ways of describing and classifying them give more detailed information about the location, size, and characteristics of the bleed. Your hospital may use the traditional grading system or may describe brain bleeds in a more detailed fashion.

In the mildest form of IVH (known as a Grade I), a small amount of bleeding occurs in the germinal matrix, the tissues around the ventricles. This blood is gradually absorbed by the body over two to three weeks and appears to cause no lasting damage. If the IVH is more extensive (a Grade II), a small amount of blood is also found in the ventricles. This type of bleed usually resolves on its own as well and causes few if any problems. At the next level (Grade III), there is more bleeding into the ventricles, which may fill with blood and become enlarged. In the most serious type of bleed (a Grade IV), the ventricles fill with blood and there is additional bleeding in the surrounding area of the brain. These two more serious types of bleeds may resolve on their own or may cause a number of short- and long-term problems including hydrocephalus (described below) and developmental problems. But many infants who have suffered the most severe types of brain bleeds have gone on to develop perfectly normally.

What causes it? Brain bleeds typically occur in a rapidly developing area of the brain laced with tiny, fragile blood vessels that break easily when blood pressure or oxygen levels fluctuate. This area, known as the germinal matrix, lies around the ventricles of the brain. The ventricles are interior fluid-filled spaces which act as shock-absorbers or cushions for the brain.

The incidence of brain bleeds has been decreasing over the last decade, and most hospitals report that between 17 to 25 percent of babies born at less than 34 weeks have an IVH. Like many other complications of prematurity, the risk of IVH is greatest for the youngest babies; for babies weighing less than 1,000 grams (2 pounds 3 ounces) at birth, the rate may be as high as 60 percent. However, the majority of these are small bleeds (Grades I and II), and usually cause no serious problems.

How it is treated. Since brain bleeds typically occur in the first few days after birth, preemies under the age of 34 weeks are routinely given a head ultrasound on about the third day of life. This is usually followed up a week later with a repeat ultrasound, either to monitor an existing bleed or to check for late occurring bleeds. The ultrasound test for brain bleeds is done in the nursery at your baby's bedside. An ultrasound scanner or trans- ducer, which looks like a fat wand, is placed on your baby's fontanel, the soft spot on the top of her head. Using sound waves, the scanner produces clear pictures of the brain and ventricles. Most babies sleep right through this painless test.

Most brain bleeds stop quickly, produce no symptoms, and need no treatment. In more serious cases when there is more extensive bleeding or the ventricles become swollen, a baby may show symptoms such as anemia, apnea and bradycardia, a bulging fontanel, limpness, or even seizures. As the bleeding stops, the swelling of the ventricles may slowly disappear as the body reabsorbs the fluid. In other cases, medication or a spinal tap (also known as a lumbar puncture) may be used to control or reduce the swelling in the ventricles. A spinal tap is a procedure in which a needle is inserted into the space between two vertebrae (back bones) in the small of a baby's back and used to withdraw a small amount of cerebrospinal fluid.

Hydrocephalus

Hydrocephalus, a term which means literally water on the brain, is one of the most serious complications of a severe brain bleed. Hydrocephalus occurs when the bleeding causes a blockage in the circulation of cerebrospinal fluid in the ventricles, or scarring which slows the absorption of fluid in the ventricles. As fluid accumulates, the ventricles swell and press on surrounding brain tissue. Hydrocephalus generally occurs slowly, and can often be controlled with medication or a series of spinal taps which draw off the excess fluid, as explained above. However, if the swelling becomes too great, or cannot be relieved quickly enough, it can cause permanent damage to the brain. If your baby has had a severe brain bleed, she will be closely monitored for signs of hydrocephalus. The circumference of her head will be measured daily to look for signs of unusual swelling, and she will have repeat ultrasounds on a regular basis.

If your baby develops hydrocephalus, she may need to have a shunt surgically implanted. A shunt is a thin plastic tube that is inserted into the baby's ventricle in the brain and then passed under the skin (usually behind the ear) and into the abdomen. The shunt allows excess cerebrospinal fluid to drain harmlessly into the abdomen, where it is reabsorbed. You will find more information about shunts and hydrocephalus in Chapter 11.

Periventricular Leukomalacia (PVL)

Periventricular leukomalacia (PVL), meaning damage to the white matter of the brain, is not a disease, but is a diagnosis based on an ultrasound examination of a baby's brain. When signs of PVL are seen, it indicates that something has happened to cause an injury to a particular part of a baby's brain. The injury occurs early in a child's life, possibly even before birth, but is usually not visible on ultrasound until a baby is three or four weeks old. PVL may appear as scattered tiny holes or cysts in the brain tissue but can sometimes involve larger areas. In order to make a more precise diagnosis, the newer forms of imaging are sometimes used. These include MRI (magnetic resonance imaging) and NMR (nuclear magnetic resonance) spectroscopy.

What causes it? The causes of PVL are still unknown and are the focus of a great deal of research at this time. However, infections that occur right before or after birth have been implicated, as have periods of insufficient blood flow to the brain. The brain's blood flow can be disrupted when a baby's blood pressure drops suddenly or is unstable because of other conditions such as a patent ductus arteriosus. PVL occurs more often—but not always—in infants who have had brain bleeds. Approximately 7 percent of infants born weighing less than 1,500 grams (3 pounds 5 ounces) develop PVL.

What problems does it cause? White matter, which lies deep inside the brain, contains nerve fibers that connect the cells in the gray matter at the surface of the brain to other parts of the brain and the spinal cord. Damage to the white matter can disrupt the way signals are transmitted along the affected nerves. Not all children who are diagnosed with PVL will develop later problems. But one common area affected is motor development, including delayed development and cerebral palsy (CP). The type of cerebral palsy that occurs most often with PVL, known as spastic diplegia, affects the legs more than the arms and hands. Chapter 11 has more information on CP. Other children with PVL may have problems with vision or visual-motor coordination, or learning disabilities.

There is still a great deal to be learned about PVL, its causes, and prevention. In the meantime, if your baby is diagnosed with PVL, her development should be closely monitored. You may not be able to prevent some of the problems that may show up, but through early identification and therapy, you will be able to ensure that she has the best possible chance to overcome or adapt to any developmental difficulties that may arise.

Retinopathy of Prematurity (ROP)

Retinopathy of prematurity (ROP) occurs when the normal development of the retina, the inner light-sensitive lining of the eye, is disturbed. Normally, tiny blood vessels begin to grow in the retina beginning at about the sixteenth week of gestation. This growth starts at the back of the eye, where the optic nerve enters the eye from the brain, and moves toward the front until the entire retina has a sufficient blood supply. Although the process is nearly complete by the thirty-second week of gestation, it continues until the second or third month after birth. When a baby is born prematurely, the growth of these retinal blood vessels can stop temporarily. When the capillaries begin to grow again, they may grow rapidly and irregularly. The abnormal growth can cause scarring and damage to the retina. In most cases of ROP, the disease progresses to a certain point and then gradually improves without treatment. However, in a certain number of cases, ROP leads to severe damage to the eye, with detachment of the retina and blindness a possibility.

The disease itself is described by a classification system called the International Classification of Retinopathy of Prematurity or ICROP. ICROP defines the disease in terms of its location relative to the optic nerve, how much of the retina is involved, and by stages of disease. The closer to the optic nerve disruption of blood vessel growth is seen and the more of the retina that is involved, the more serious is the disease.

What causes it? The causes of ROP are still not completely understood, but prematurity and changes in blood oxygen levels appear to play important roles. The earlier in gestation a baby is born, the greater her chances of developing ROP because the blood vessels in the retina will not have grown very far before they are disrupted. Of babies born at less than 28 weeks, 85 percent have some ROP; between 28 and 31 weeks, 57 percent will have ROP; after 31 weeks, the percentage drops to 30 percent. Most of these cases are mild and improve without treatment.

Several decades ago, experts thought that ROP occurred when premature babies were treated with high concentrations of oxygen. Further research has shown that a high level of oxygen is only one of the factors involved. Careful regulation and monitoring of oxygen levels has helped to decrease the incidence of ROP. Other treatments, such as the use of vitamin E and protecting babies' eyes from bright lights, have had mixed results. Research is continuing into the causes and treatment of ROP.

How it is treated. All babies at risk of ROP—which includes any baby born at less than 32 to 34 weeks—should be examined by a pediatric ophthalmologist at approximately four to six weeks of age. During these exams, the eye doctor places drops in your baby's eyes to dilate the pupil and examines the retina. The exams are usually repeated every two weeks until the blood vessels have completed their growth.

In most cases, ROP improves without treatment. Unfortunately, when this doesn't happen and the ROP progresses to the point that it needs to be treated, it usually occurs between the ages of 34 to 42 weeks of gestational age, no matter when the baby was born. For many parents this is a time when things are going well for their baby in other ways, and discharge home seems imminent. The diagnosis of severe ROP at this point is extremely difficult and discouraging.

However, there are some treatment options which may prevent further deterioration of your baby's vision. ROP may be treated with cryotherapy, in which a small probe is used to freeze and destroy sections of the retina in order to prevent the disease from progressing. Unfortunately, cryotherapy is painful. It is usually performed using local or general anesthetic, but many babies have a difficult time during the treatment and for several days afterward. They may have an increased number of apnea spells or need to have oxygen levels increased. A newer approach using laser treatments appears to be just as effective and less traumatic. Ask your baby's doctor about this approach.

If laser or cryotherapy treatments are unsuccessful and the retina begins to detach, there are some surgical options. A scleral buckle may be used to help prevent further retinal detachment. A scleral buckle is a tiny belt which is placed around the eye and tightened in order to bring the retina close to the wall of the eye so that it can re-attach, or to prevent further detachments. In very severe cases, the eye may be opened, the retina repaired and repositioned against the back of the eye. Known as a vitrectomy, this surgery is usually used only in extreme cases as an attempt to preserve some vision.

Hearing Problems

Although the chances of your child having a problem with her hearing are still very low, premature babies as a group do have a much higher incidence of sensorineural hearing loss than full-term infants. Sensorineural hearing loss occurs because of damage in the inner ear or with the nerve that carries sound from the ear to the brain. It affects between 1 and 15 percent of premature babies, compared with 1 out of 1,000 full-term babies.

What causes it? All of the reasons for this increased risk are not well understood. Prematurity itself plays a role, as does exposure to certain types of drugs, including some antibiotics and diuretics. Brain bleeds, levels of bilirubin high enough to require an exchange transfusion, chronic lung disease, and infections such as meningitis can all affect hearing. The noise from incubators and respirators has also been implicated.

How it is treated. Preemies who are at increased risk of hearing loss, including those born weighing less than 1,500 grams and those experiencing certain medical complications and treatments, usually have their hearing tested before they are discharged from the hospital. Interestingly, a panel of the National Institutes of Health has recently recommended that all newborns, not just preemies, be screened for hearing loss before they come home from the hospital. Hearing problems are rarely diagnosed before children reach the age of 2 to 21/2 years of age, by which time they have experienced significant delays in their speech and language development.

At this point, because preemies fall into a high risk category, they are more likely to be diagnosed early enough to avoid some of the problems that can develop when hearing loss goes undetected. A description of hearing tests given to preemies before discharge and follow-up recommendations can be found in Chapter 5.

Necrotizing Enterocolitis (NEC)

Necrotizing enterocolitis is a very serious disorder of the bowel in which a portion of the bowel wall is damaged or dies. Bacteria that are normally present in the intestine may attack and further injure the weakened section of the bowel, and the wall may rupture, releasing infection into the abdomen.

The number of cases varies from hospital to hospital, but NEC generally occurs in about 5 percent of all NICU admissions. It occurs more frequently among the smallest and youngest babies. As treatment methods have improved, the mortality rates for babies with NEC have improved over the last five years. Currently, between 72 and 91 percent of babies with NEC will survive. Among the smallest babies—those under 1,500 grams (3 pounds 5 ounces)—the mortality rate can still reach as high as 45 percent, however.

What causes it? The causes of NEC are not well understood, nor does there appear to be any way to prevent its occurrence. Prematurity is the primary risk factor, and NEC almost always starts after a baby has begun oral feedings. Infection, damage to the intestinal lining, and disruption of the blood supply to the intestines may all play a role, causing damage or death to the cells involved. Babies fed breastmilk appear to be somewhat protected from NEC, but breastmilk alone does not prevent NEC. In one study, babies whose mothers were treated with steroids before the baby's birth had a significantly lower incidence of NEC compared with a control group.

Premature babies are watched carefully for signs of NEC as they begin to take feedings by mouth. Symptoms include feeding difficulties, such as a swollen or tender abdomen, increasing amounts of milk left in their stomachs between feedings (known as residuals), the presence of bile (greenish liquid) in the residuals, vomiting, apnea spells, and general signs of illness.

How it is treated. At the first sign of NEC, all oral feedings are stopped. This is known as being NPO, nothing by mouth. Your baby will be fed intravenously while she is being watched or treated for NEC so that her bowel can rest and heal. A tube may be passed down your baby's throat into her stomach to drain air and fluids from her stomach and intestine. She may receive antibiotics for infection in the intestine, oxygen or ventilation for support, and X-rays to check the progress of the disease and look for evidence of rupture of the intestine. It can take two or more weeks for a baby to recover from NEC. She may need to have a central line inserted so that she can be given complete nutritional support during that time.

In serious cases of NEC, surgery may be necessary to remove the injured part of the intestinal wall. When this happens, the healthy bowel above the injured portion is often brought to the surface of the abdomen to allow the remaining part of the bowel to rest and heal. This opening is known as a stoma; the baby's stools will empty into a plastic bag attached to the stoma on the skin of the abdomen rather than traveling through the rest of the intestine. If the surgery is on the small intestine, the opening is known as an ileostomy; if it is on the large intestine, it is a colostomy. When your baby is larger and healthier, she can usually undergo a second operation in which the two ends of the intestine are reconnected so that she will no longer have a stoma.

Most babies recover from NEC with no lasting problems. However, some babies with serious cases of NEC will need special nutritional support in the first year or two of life. These and other potential complications are discussed in Chapter 11.

Infection

Premature infants are particularly vulnerable to infections for several reasons. First, they are born without all of the disease-fighting antibodies that full-term babies have. Because antibodies are transferred from the mother's body in late pregnancy, most preemies arrive before they have received the full measure of these protective agents. In addition, preemies' immature immune systems cannot respond as quickly to infection. What might be a small infection in a full-term baby or adult can more easily become a serious widespread one in a preemie. Finally, IV lines, endotracheal tubes, and blood tests—all of which are necessary in caring for preemies—can introduce germs into the body.

Some of the common types of infections that preemies develop are:
- an infection in the lungs, known as pneumonia;
- a generalized infection of the body or blood stream, known as sepsis;
- an infection of the lining of the brain and spinal cord called meningitis;
- a bladder or kidney infection, also known as a urinary tract infection.

Infections can also occur in the skin, especially around the umbilical cord stump.

What causes it? Infections occur when germs—bacteria, viruses, or fungi—attack certain parts of the body, causing inflammation and illness. Many infections are caused by germs that are normally present around our bodies. When these germs enter an area where they should not be, or when a baby's immune system is not able to respond quickly, an infection develops.

How it is treated. If the doctors suspect that your baby is developing an infection, samples will be taken of your baby's blood, urine, spinal fluid, or secretions from wounds. These samples are sent to the laboratory for testing and analysis. Until the results of these tests are known, your baby may be placed on a broad-spectrum antibiotic that is effective against a wide range of germs. This antibiotic may be changed to a more specific one when more information is available. Most infections respond fairly quickly to antibiotics and the babies recover without lasting complications.

Facing Difficult Situations

One of the many challenges facing you as a parent in the NICU is to understand what is happening with your baby, to know what questions to ask, to understand the answers, and, sometimes, to make difficult decisions about your baby's care. When your baby is experiencing a setback or is seriously ill, the situation is complicated in a number of ways: it is inherently stressful, the language you are hearing is foreign and confusing, and it is rare that you have the knowledge to know how to balance your options. In addition, you may be faced with situations in which the right course of action is not very clear to you or to your baby's medical team. And you may be asked to help make a decision about your child's care when you are upset and not thinking clearly.

This chapter can help by providing you with some basic information, but it cannot replace what you learn directly from your baby's caregivers as you wrestle with difficult decisions. Your baby's doctors and nurses have experience and training in neonatology that is an important source of information for you. But you are your baby's parent, and what is in your heart is another important part of any decision. Luckily, most hospitals increasingly recognize the crucial role that parents play in making difficult decisions for their babies.

Making Sense of Things

Whether you are talking about routine care or difficult situations, the first step in understanding and participating in your child's care is to get information. But what is useful information for one person is not always helpful for another. Some parents want explanations that use numbers, statistics, and probabilities. Others want a general summary, the doctor's opinion or advice, or explanations in simple, non-medical language. While most caregivers in the NICU try to provide parents with the kind of information and support they need, some are better at this than others, as this mother of a 29-weeker explained.

"When our son was two or three days old, he was started on an antibiotic, gentamicin, because the doctors were worried that he might have meningitis. We were told that at high levels gentamicin could damage Dan's hearing, but that the levels in his blood would be monitored closely. Perhaps this should have been reassuring, but it wasn't. No one seemed to be able to tell us how much risk there was. Was hearing damage a rare problem, a common one, or an unpredictable kind of thing?

"We kept hearing vague reassurances until a few days later when a new doctor told us that the level of gentamicin in Dan's blood would have to be about ten times higher than it was before it could harm his hearing. Knowing that was a great relief; finally we could understand exactly how much risk he was running, and how the risk was being monitored.

Getting the Information You Need

- Meet with your baby's medical team at least once a week or more often if your baby's condition is serious, complicated, or changing rapidly.
- Ask that the meeting take place out of the NICU in a quiet room where you can concentrate and take your time asking questions.
- Write down your questions and concerns in advance and bring them to the meeting.
- Write down the answers and explanations you are given during the meeting.
- Consider audiotaping the meetings.
- Consider taking a friend or the nursery social worker with you to medical team meetings. A less emotionally involved person may be able to remember more clearly what is said. This person can then help you understand and interpret the information later.
- If you don't understand an answer, ask your question again. Someone else on the care team may be able to explain it in a different way.
- If you don't think you can handle any more information, take a break. You may be able to cope or understand better in a day or two.

"My husband and I knew the other doctors were trying their best to reas-sure us, but vague explanations didn't help. Unfortunately, when there are so many unknowns, it can be hard to even figure out what kind of question to ask. And a lot of times you get an answer to your question, but you still don't really know what the answer means for your child. There are just too many unknowns."

Another parent talked about a different type of barrier to getting information: "Everybody always tells you to ask questions if you don't understand something. And I think you do have to do that. But sometimes you don't want to ask because you're afraid of what you might hear."

If you have trouble understanding the explanations given to you by one doctor or nurse, or if someone you are dealing with is not very helpful, ask if you can talk to another member of your baby's care team. And if you know what sort of information is most useful to you—statistics and num-bers, or non-medical-language explanations—try to let your baby's med-ical team know. They deal with many different parents, all of whom cope in different ways, and they may not know at first how they can best help you. Unfortunately, there are also many situations in the NICU for which there aren't good explanations and no one will be able to supply you with all of the information or answers that you want.

Making Difficult Choices

There may come a time when you need to make a difficult decision about your child's care. It may be a situation in which it isn't clear what the best course of action is. There may be several choices, or the benefits of a par-ticular approach may also carry substantial risks of complications. Or, most agonizing of all, you may need to make a decision about whether or not to continue your child's care.

In situations like these, your child's medical team should work closely with you to try to reach the best decision possible. In the case of life and death decisions, everyone's focus should be on determining what is in the best long-term interests of your baby. If she seems to have no chance for survival or a decent life, or if continuing her treatment would only prolong her suffering, you and your baby's medical team might decide to stop actively treating her. You would focus instead on helping your baby die comfortably and peacefully. Sometimes this decision is clear, although it is never simple.

However, in many other cases, the right decision is not at all clear. In these latter situations, your baby's team will probably call in other senior members of the staff to give them another assessment of the situation. You can also ask that the hospital ethics or Infant Care Review committee become involved in your child's case. Usually, the medical team and you can reach a decision together about what to do. And you will usually, although not always, have time to make your decision without feeling rushed.

But even then, when you have done everything you can do to make the right decision, you will probably find that you continue to have doubts or regrets. This is particularly true when you made a decision to help your baby die peacefully, or when you opted for aggressive medical treatment but your child was left with long-term problems. You may rehash the decision in your mind, wondering whether you left something out, were not thinking clearly enough, or simply didn't understand enough about what you were facing to make the right decision.

Although simpler said than done, it is important to try not to be too hard on yourself. Keep in mind that in many of these situations there is no one right decision. There is only a decision that seems to be the best at the time, given what you and your doctors know, and what you feel in your heart. There may be times when you wonder if you would have made a different decision if you knew then what you know now. Remember, hindsight is always clearer. You did the best you could under the circumstances, and that is all anyone—including your baby—asks of you.

Saying Good-bye

The grief borne by parents whose babies do not survive their premature births is a subject that cannot adequately be covered in this book. Rather than gloss quickly over its many facets, I have put together a list of books and resources in Appendix E that offer a more complete source of information and support. I want to include here just a few things that were mentioned by a number of parents. These are things that they felt particularly unprepared for, things that meant a lot to them, or things they wished they had done.

Stay with and preferably hold your baby while she is dying. You may not feel like you want to watch your baby die, or you may not feel like you can handle it, but parents who have been through this ordeal continually stress how important it is to stay with your baby. Your grief is real and tremendous, and you do not shield yourself from it by not being with your baby. In fact, you may be giving yourself reason to criticize yourself later. If you are there, holding and comforting your baby, you know you have done everything you possibly could to make her brief life as good and full of love as possible. And you will probably find that touching her gives you a sense of peace and comfort as well. Ask to spend as much time as you need with your baby after she has passed away.

Should you consent to an autopsy? Your baby's doctor will probably ask you to sign a consent form for an autopsy to help determine the reasons for your baby's death. You do not have to agree to this, but there are a number of issues that you may want to consider. First, an autopsy can provide you with information about exactly what happened and why your baby died. This may not seem important to you now, but you may begin to have more questions in the future. The autopsy findings can provide you with more precise answers. In addition, the knowledge that has been gained from these examinations has expanded doctors' understanding of the problems of prematurity and led to improved care for preemies. Some parents feel that they are contributing to the future of other babies and parents by allowing their baby to be examined. However, many parents do not want their baby to go through anything else and prefer to let their baby rest in peace. And some religions put restrictions on the practice of autopsy.

Before you make your decision, talk with your doctor about the pros and cons of having your baby autopsied, and of what you can expect in either case. If you do decide to go ahead, the autopsy can usually be done quickly so that it doesn't interfere with the timing of your funeral arrangements. You will be able to have an open casket if you prefer, even if your baby has had an autopsy. You may request that your baby's head remain undisturbed, or she can wear a bonnet or knit cap to hide the incision on the upper part of her head.

Parents are often asked to make a decision about an autopsy soon after their baby has passed away. If you don't feel able to decide right away, ask to be given some time to think about it. Don't be rushed or pressured into making a decision that you are not comfortable with.

Keep some mementos of your baby. Again, you may be too grief-stricken right now to think of keeping anything of your baby's. But many parents commented on how important it was later to have a picture, a hat, a footprint, a lock of hair—something tangible with which to remember their baby. If you don't want to take anything home with you right now, ask your baby's nurse to put something away in her medical record that you can retrieve later if you want it. Your baby's life may have been brief, but her impact on yours will be lasting. Having something concrete to remember her by may be very important to you in the future.

Make sure you invite at least a few friends and family members to the funeral. You may not realize in advance how comforting it is to have friends with you during such a time. And a funeral is also a public recognition that your child did exist. As one mother said,

> *"We had so much else going on at the time since we still had one child in the NICU. And Leah was with us for such a short time. No one else had known her, so I didn't really think of inviting anyone to the funeral. This was something my husband and I had been through together, so I thought we would just go through the funeral together too. But when we got there it seemed very strange and lonely. Thank God one of our good friends showed up anyway. It helped a lot to have him there to share this with."*

Your close friends and family will be honored to be asked to attend your baby's funeral, and your shared memories will be a link with your baby through the years.

PART II:
COMING HOME

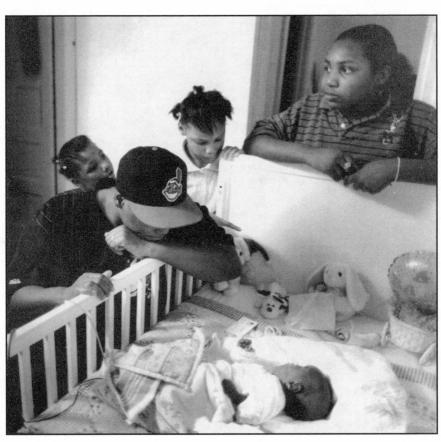

CHAPTER 5

Making Progress
Toward Home

ℐᴥ

I F   Y O U R   B A B Y   W A S
born more than a few weeks early, he has probably spent several weeks or
even months in the hospital intensive or special care nursery and has been
cared for by a small army of highly trained professionals. It will soon be up
to you to take over that care. Many parents approach this transition appre-
hensively, while others are ready and eager. My husband was anxious: "I
knew they were taking good care of him in the hospital, and he was doing
well. I wasn't sure we could do as well, so I was in no hurry to get him
home." Another parent voiced the opposite view: "I'd been caring for my
daughter for weeks—changing her diapers, feeding her, giving her baths. I
felt prepared for anything and everything. I was ready to have her home."

Most parents are told to expect that their babies will be discharged
near their original due dates, but this date can move forward and backward
dramatically depending upon your child's progress or setbacks. If your baby
is healthy and has a relatively smooth course in the hospital, he may be
discharged three or four weeks before his due date. If he arrived extremely
early or struggled with a number of complications, he may not be able to
come home until a few weeks after his original due date.

The following scenario described by one couple whose baby had been
in the hospital for three months is typical of how unpredictable your
baby's discharge can be.

*"We were told on Tuesday that Katie would be coming home at the end of
the following week. Then on Thursday, they told us she would be coming
home on Saturday—in other words, in two days. We had almost no time to*

prepare. We both were supposed to be working on Saturday, I needed to notify my boss that I would be starting my leave, and the hospital wanted us to spend the night with Katie in the hospital on Friday night. After all the time she'd been in the hospital, the end felt very rushed and chaotic, and we were totally exhausted by the time we got her home that first day."

Other parents have the opposite experience. They are told to expect that their baby will be ready to go home on a certain date only to have a new problem—an apnea spell, difficulty feeding, an infection—arise to postpone the discharge. When this happens repeatedly, it can be enormously discouraging, and the waiting can seem endless.

Although there is no way to take all of the uncertainty out of your baby's recovery—including when he will come home—it will feel less mysterious if you can recognize the signs of progress that your baby will show. This chapter describes what typically happens in the hospital as your baby recovers, and how the nursery staff decides when he is ready to come home. It also includes information on specific things that you can do to prepare for your baby's homecoming.

As Your Baby Grows: The Feeder-Grower Period

At some point in your baby's hospitalization, he will become what is commonly called a feeder-grower—a baby whose health has improved enough that he no longer needs intensive care, but who still needs time and special support as he grows and matures. When your baby becomes a feeder-grower, he will usually be shifted out of the intensive care (Level III) nursery to a Level II nursery. Depending upon your baby's gestational age and medical needs, this transfer may take place after only a few hours or days, or it may take many weeks. Your baby may be moved to a different room or location in his current nursery. Or you may be offered the option of having him transferred to a nursery in a community hospital closer to your home.

Even though your baby's transfer out of intensive care represents significant progress, the feeder-grower period is not always smooth and problem free. Your baby will still have good and bad days, days of good weight gains and energetic feeding alternating with days when he is tired, has apnea spells, needs more oxygen, and gains little or no weight. He may even need to go back to the Level III nursery for a few days. But generally, your baby is making progress, the problems that arise are less intense or serious, and life settles into some type of routine.

Transfer to a Level II Nursery in a Community Hospital

When your baby is transferred to a Level II nursery it is a clear indication that his health is improving, and is a reason to feel encouraged and excited. However, when it involves a change of hospitals, the transfer can also be quite anxiety producing. Not only must you become familiar with a new hospital and its rules and procedures, but you must shift your trust and faith from one set of providers to another. If your baby has had a rocky course or you have already spent a significant amount of time at one hospital, making this change may be particularly difficult.

But a nursery in a community hospital may offer you and your baby a number of advantages. These nurseries are generally smaller and quieter with fewer alarms and monitors beeping. Because the pace is less hectic, they can be less stressful for babies as well as parents. Medically, they are closely linked with the referring Level III nursery, which helps to ensure continuity in your baby's care. There are fewer staff members to get to know, your pediatrician may be able to help care for your baby, and the nursery may provide more flexible and individualized care.

On a practical level, travel time to the hospital may be shorter, and parking easier and cheaper. If the nursery is in the hospital where you were originally planning to deliver, returning there may help you feel like life is beginning to return to normal.

However, some community hospitals have lagged behind the larger teaching hospitals in instituting family-centered care. Some have stricter policies regarding siblings and family visits, and may not encourage the same level of parent participation. Your baby will not be transferred without your permission, so before you agree, you may want to call or visit the new nursery to ask about their policies.

On the day of the transfer, your baby will be transported by ambulance in a special incubator and accompanied by one of the nurses from the NICU. In some cases, your child's primary nurse will be able to travel with him.

The following suggestions may help to ease the transition to the new nursery.

Call and, if at all possible, visit the nursery to which your baby is being transferred a day or two before the actual transfer. It is a good idea to have a tour of the facility, and to review some of the following issues: visiting policies, nursery rules and procedures, what to expect on the day of the transfer, attitudes toward parent involvement, support for breastfeeding, and any other concerns or questions.

Give your baby time to adjust to the new nursery. Many babies seem unaware of their transfer. However, the extra movement and activity involved in the transfer process is tiring for others. You may notice that your child seems tired or sleepy for a day or two after the move, and may drink less or gain less weight. Don't be overly concerned about this; within a couple of days, your baby will have settled into his new surroundings and be making consistent progress again.

Be prepared to find that some of the ways in which your baby is cared for will be different in the new hospital. For example, in some hospitals gavage tubes are typically inserted through the nose and left in place taped

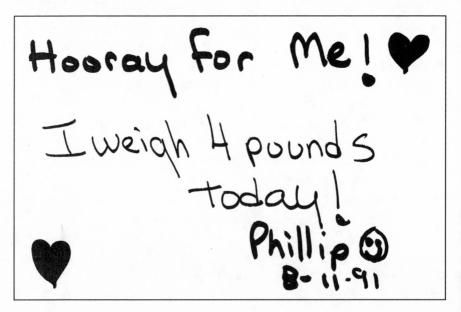

to the cheek between feedings, while in others they are inserted through the mouth for each feeding and then removed. The fact that things are done differently does not mean that one hospital is doing them correctly and the other isn't. In most cases, they are just different approaches, and you may find that the new approach actually works better. In other cases, they may reflect your baby's changing needs as he grows and matures.

Give yourself time to adjust also. Although most transfers occur smoothly, it is natural to be more anxious at first, and to worry about whether your baby will be cared for as well by the new staff. Give yourself a day or two to become accustomed to the new nursery, and to get to know your baby's new nurses and doctors. Be sure to ask about anything that concerns you.

Signs of Progress

As you are waiting through the feeder-grower period, it may seem as though your baby, like most preemies, is making little if any progress; his weight gain is slow and erratic, he feeds well one day and not the next, his need for oxygen goes up and down, his hematocrit continues to drop slowly.

But finally, he will turn a corner. It may happen when you least expect it and when you are most discouraged, but it will happen. Your baby will finally begin to make steady, consistent progress and you will see concrete signs that he is getting better.

For example,

- he will begin to take more and more of his feedings by mouth and need fewer tube feedings;
- he will begin to gag and grimace as the feeding tube is passed down his throat;
- he will begin to gain weight more consistently, usually between 15 and 45 grams a day;
- his need for oxygen will first stabilize and then begin to decrease;
- his hematocrit (red blood count) will stabilize and begin to increase;
- he may begin to develop short periods when he is awake and can gaze at you quietly;

- he may begin to have periods of crying or fussing, a sign of increased strength and energy;
- his body will start filling out as he gains weight, his skin will lose its translucence, the veins will no longer be as clearly visible under the skin, and the lanugo (hair) that once covered his shoulders fades and disappears;
- his muscle tone will improve and he won't feel as floppy and fragile as he once did.

The medical equipment used to care for your baby will also change. He may move from CPAP to a nasal cannula to periodic blow-by oxygen, or he may outgrow his need for extra oxygen altogether. He will no longer need to be under the bilirubin lights, and his heart and apnea monitors may be disconnected—although most hospitals today continue to monitor preemies until discharge.

Your baby's ability to feed by bottle or breast will slowly improve during this period. You can expect that by the time he has reached 34 or 35 weeks gestational age, he will generally have the muscle strength and energy to take most of his feedings by mouth. Some breastfed babies can handle feedings even earlier than this.

However, expect that his progress will be erratic. He will take some feedings by mouth and others by tube, or parts of feedings by mouth with the remainder given by tube. Feedings are usually slow, and many babies continue to have trouble coordinating the suck-swallow-breathe sequence for quite a while. For some babies, the transition from tube feedings to oral feedings goes agonizingly slowly, but all babies have better and worse days as they learn this skill.

Most dramatically, your baby will graduate from his incubator to an open bassinet. As your baby matures and gains weight, he is able to maintain his own body temperature more easily. The heat in his incubator is slowly decreased until it equals the room temperature of the nursery. At this point, the incubator doors are left open and your baby is monitored to see if he can maintain his body temperature. If he can, he will be moved to an open bassinet. During this transition period, his weight will be watched carefully. If he is having a hard time keeping himself warm, he will use up too many calories, and the rate at which he is gaining weight will slow down or even stop. If this happens to your baby, it means he was not quite ready to leave the incubator. He will be moved back for a few more days, and then tested again. This is discouraging but will be only a short set-back. Ask your baby's nurse to point out other ways in which your baby is showing progress.

Your Changing Feelings: Gratitude and Impatience

The feeder-grower period can seem endless for parents. At times, many parents find themselves feeling impatient with and even resentful of their baby's caretakers. As one mother recalled,

> *"I loved Sharon [her son's primary nurse]. She did such a wonderful job caring for Justin, but I got so tired of her being the expert, of her saying try this, hold him this way... After a while, I just wanted my baby to be mine. I wanted to be in charge."*

These mixed emotions of gratitude and impatience are common to most parents whose babies must spend an extended time in the hospital. Dealing with a long hospitalization is exhausting and frustrating. There are days when you feel only admiration and appreciation for your baby's doctors and nurses. And other days when you doubt their abilities, feel critical of how they are handling your baby, and annoyed by their comments.

If possible, try to keep a perspective on your shifting feelings. If you are particularly down or upset, it may signal that you need to take a break from the nursery for a day or two to recharge your batteries. Your short fuse probably signals more about your own state of mind than about the actual care your baby is receiving. And if you have some real concerns, you will be able to talk them over more productively with the staff when you are rested and in a better frame of mind.

How the Hospital Decides When to Discharge Your Baby

Hospital nurseries use a number of criteria to determine when a baby is medically able to be discharged. A decade or so ago, babies needed to weigh at least five pounds before they could go home. Today, as long as a baby can maintain a normal body temperature, he can go home at any weight. Some go home weighing four pounds or even less.

Although your nursery has its own set of discharge guidelines that you should ask about, they will probably include at least some of the following:

- **Your baby is no longer having apnea spells.** He no longer needs apnea-controlling medication and has completed a certain number of days—usually five to seven—with no apnea or bradycardia spells. These apnea-free days must be consecutive. In other words, if after three days, your baby has a spell, the counting starts over and he must pass another five to seven spell-free days.
- **He can maintain a normal body temperature of 98.6°F in a regular open crib or bassinet.** He no longer needs to be in an incubator to stay warm.
- **He is able to take all of his feedings by mouth,** either by bottle, breast, cup, or a combination.
- **He is gaining weight consistently.**

Most babies reach this stage in their development somewhere between 36 and 40 weeks of gestational age, although for some it may take a little longer. These criteria are sometimes adjusted for individual babies as well. For example, some babies get to a point where they meet most of the discharge requirements but continue to have a problem in one area. They may have apnea spells or continue to need tube feedings, oxygen, special formulas, or medications. Your baby's medical team may decide to discharge him even with ongoing medical needs as long as the necessary equipment, medication, and/or nursing care can be arranged at home.

Final Tests and Procedures

Before he is discharged from the hospital, your baby may receive several common tests and procedures. Not all babies will need all of these tests, and your baby's nurse or doctor can explain to you which ones they recommend for your baby and why.

Vision and Hearing Tests

Although the risks are still quite small, some preemies have problems with vision and hearing as a result of their early birth or complications that occur after birth. If your baby meets certain criteria described below, he will be given an eye exam, a hearing test, or both before he is discharged.

Depending upon the results, he may need to have a follow-up test at a specified time after he has gone home.

Eye Exam. According to guidelines from the American Academy of Pediatrics, all infants with birthweights of less than 1,500 grams (3 pounds 5 ounces) and any infant who receives supplemental oxygen during the newborn period should have an eye exam. During this exam, the pupil of the eye is dilated (enlarged) so that the ophthalmologist can examine the retina or back wall of the eye to make sure it is developing properly (see the explanation of retinopathy of prematurity [ROP] in Chapter 4).

If your baby meets the criteria that put him at higher risk for vision problems, his first eye exam is usually conducted between five to seven weeks after birth. If he has some signs of ROP, your baby will be examined weekly to monitor his progress, and may need to have follow-up exams or continuing treatment with a pediatric ophthalmologist after he has gone home.

Hearing Test. As described in Chapter 4, many preemies are at higher risk for hearing loss than full-term newborns and are routinely tested before discharge. Babies routinely tested before discharge include those who

- were born weighing less than 1,500 grams (3 pounds 5 ounces),
- had brain bleeds or infections such as meningitis,
- were exposed to certain antibiotics or diuretics,
- needed an exchange transfusion for hyperbilirubinemia (jaundice), or
- have a family history of hearing loss.

A number of tests can be used with infants, but the most reliable is called the Auditory Brainstem Responses (ABRs). In this test, monitoring wires are placed behind your baby's ears and on his forehead to record his brain's response to clicking noises coming from earphones placed over his ears. The test is painless and is conducted while your baby dozes.

Since test results are affected by the immaturity of the hearing system, an abnormal test result in the hospital does not necessarily indicate a hearing problem. However, if this happens, your baby should be re-tested between one and three months after his original due date.

Head Ultrasound and Chest X-rays

Babies are usually given head ultrasounds early in their hospitalizations, and again at about three weeks of life or before discharge. These later tests are used to diagnose any problems such as PVL (periventricular leukomalacia) that may not have been visible in the earlier ultrasounds. Ultrasound tests are done at your baby's bedside and are not bothersome to him.

If your baby had or continues to have respiratory trouble, he will also have a final chest X-ray. You should request a copy of this X-ray to take with you. Your baby may have scarring in his lungs, which can be mistaken for pneumonia on future X-rays. If the radiologist has his old films for comparison, he will have an easier time correctly interpreting what he sees on any future X-rays.

Blood Tests

Final blood tests include a hematocrit or hemoglobin test to assess your baby's level of anemia. A reticulocyte (immature red blood cell) count will probably be included, as well, to make sure he is beginning to produce red blood cells again. If your baby is being discharged home on medications, the blood levels of these drugs will also be measured.

Car Seat Test

Research shows that some preemies and low birthweight babies have trouble breathing adequately in the semi-upright position of a regular car seat. For this reason, the American Academy of Pediatrics (AAP) now recommends that all babies born before 37 weeks of gestation be placed in their car seats and monitored for apnea, bradycardia and/or oxygen desaturation before they are discharged home. This test should be performed a day or two before your baby is discharged.

For the test, your baby is properly positioned in his car seat, connected to the monitors, and observed for episodes of apnea, bradycardia and oxygen desaturation. The AAP does not specify how long the observation period should last, so hospitals test for varying amounts of time. You may want to make sure that your baby's test lasts at least as long as you expect to spend in the car with him getting home from the hospital, or the amount of time it will take you to get from home to the pediatrician's office.

If your baby has trouble during this test, he should ride lying flat in a car bed until he has grown bigger and stronger. Your baby will probably be ready for a car seat within a month or two, when he has gained enough strength in his neck and back that he doesn't slump forward as much as he does now. Check with your pediatrician to see how long your baby should use a car bed. The AAP also recommends that you not use infant seats, swings, or carriers if your baby has difficulty during the car seat test.

Pneumogram (Sleep Study)

If your baby continues to have apnea and bradycardia spells as he nears discharge, he may be given a test called a pneumogram, or sleep study, to try to determine the cause. The test is sometimes known as a pneumocardiogram. During this test, your baby will be attached for several hours to a monitor that records his heart and breathing rate, oxygen saturation level, the air flow through his nose, and, for some babies, the occurrence of gastro-esophageal reflux, or spitting up. This information helps to pinpoint why your baby is continuing to have apnea spells, and how to best treat them. Depending upon the results, your baby's medical team may recommend that he either continue apnea-controlling medication, or that he remain on an apnea monitor at home, or possibly both.

Immunizations

Premature babies are immunized on the same schedule recommended for full-term infants. In other words, your baby will begin to receive his shots two months after birth, regardless of how early he was born.

If your baby is in the hospital nursery at two months, he will be given his first diphtheria, pertussis, and tetanus immunization (DPT shot) there. He will probably not receive the oral polio vaccine (OPV) until discharge since there is some risk of transmission of the virus between babies. The hepatitis-B vaccine is usually postponed until babies weigh at least 2,000 grams (4 pounds 7 ounces) or until two months after birth.

Babies who come home close to their two-month birthdays are usually immunized in the hospital nursery before discharge. Detailed information about immunizations can be found in Chapter 7 and Appendix D.

RSV Protection

If your baby is discharged in the winter months (November through April), was less than 32 weeks gestational age at birth, or has ongoing respiratory problems, he may be given an initial dose of Synagis (an injection) or Respigam (an IV solution) a few days before he comes home. These medications help to protect your baby from a common type of cold germ, RSV (respiratory syncytial virus), which is particularly prevalent during the winter. Although RSV generally causes only simple colds in older children and adults, it can cause serious respiratory illness in young babies. For more information on RSV, Synagis, and Respigam, see Chapter 7.

Common Surgical Procedures Before Discharge

Two common surgical procedures—inguinal hernia repairs and circumcisions—are usually performed in the hospital a few days to a week before discharge.

Hernia Repair

If your baby has an inguinal hernia, a weak spot in his groin where a bit of intestines pushes through the muscles, it will probably be repaired before he is discharged (see Chapter 9 for an explanation of hernias). This prevents your baby from developing any complications from the hernia at home. It also means that he can continue to be cared for in the NICU before and after his surgery. Although the surgery to repair a hernia is quick and routine, it does require that your baby be given general anesthesia. If your baby has had or continues to have respiratory problems, it is particularly comforting to know that he is being cared for by people who know him well.

However, some hospitals prefer to send a baby home and perform the operation later when he is older and stronger. In this case, the surgery will probably be done on an outpatient basis and your baby should be able to come home the same day.

Circumcision

Circumcision is a simple surgical procedure in which the foreskin, a piece of skin that covers the tip of the penis, is removed. In a new policy statement released in March, 1999, the American Academy of Pediatrics stated that although there were some medical benefits to circumcision, these were not significant enough for the Academy to recommend that infant boys be routinely circumcised. According to the research analyzed, circumcised boys have fewer urinary tract infections. Circumcision can also prevent some later complications, and decrease a man's chances of developing cancer of the penis (a rare form of cancer). However, the rates of these problems are so low to begin with, that the benefits of lowering them further are not compelling.

Circumcision is quick and complications are very rare and usually minor, occurring in approximately 2 to 5 of every 1000 procedures. The main problems that can occur are slight bleeding and infection. However, circumcision is painful, and the AAP now recommends that pain relief always be provided. There are several choices: a cream, called EMLA, which is applied to the penis about an hour before the procedure; and local anesthetics that can be injected into the penis (either a dorsal penile nerve block or subcutaneous ring block). In addition, babies can be comforted by swaddling or positioning, by being offered a sugar-coated pacifier on which to suck, and with acetaminophen (Tylenol). Be sure to talk with the doctor who would perform the circumcision about pain relief and other comfort measures.

If you do opt to have your baby circumcised, the procedure is usually performed a few days before your baby is discharged so that he can be watched by the nursery staff for any signs of complications. If your baby requires a hernia repair or other surgery in the near future, you might want to postpone the circumcision. It can be performed while your baby is under anesthesia for the other surgery. Be sure to check with your insurance company to make sure they will pay for a circumcision done later.

Deciding whether or not to circumcise a son is often a complicated one for parents. In some cases, there are specific health or religious reasons that make the decision clear. But in most cases, as long as your baby is healthy, your decision is a personal one in which you must balance religious preferences, your doctor's advice, what has been done in the past in your family, and your own opinions. When your baby has already been through a long hospitalization and has had a number of painful experiences, it can be even more difficult to decide what to do. But most babies, including preemies, have few if any problems with the procedure.

Talk with your baby's doctors and take some time to make your decision. Although circumcision was almost universal in the past, this is no longer true. Whatever decision you make, your son will be among boys who are circumcised and boys who are not as he grows up.

Preparing for Your Baby's Homecoming

One of the few benefits of having your baby spend so much time in the hospital is that you have the opportunity to practice many aspects of his care before you take him home. This can help assuage some of the anxiety you may feel about being on your own soon. But even if you haven't been able to spend as much time as you wished with your baby in the nursery, there are a number of things you can do in the last week or so that will help make the transition home easier.

For the most part, the preparations you make to bring your baby home are the same as those made by all parents. However, your baby's extended hospitalization makes some aspects of homecoming quite different. These additional needs are the focus of this section.

Preparations in the Hospital

Practice As Much of Your Baby's Daily Care As Possible

Before you bring your baby home, make sure you have done the following at least once, and preferably more often:

- give him a tub bath;
- change his diaper and clothes;
- prepare his bottle and feed him—or breastfeed him—as often as possible. Do some of these feeding sessions in the family room away from the nursery;
- take and read his temperature.

If your baby will come home with special medical needs—oxygen, medications, special formula, a monitor—be sure to practice his care under the supervision of the nurses until you feel confident about taking over on your own (see Special Situations at the end of this chapter).

If at all possible, practice these basics over several days and weeks. Try not to pack a lot of new activities into the final days. One couple recalled,

"We spent the last two days of our baby's hospital stay doing all kinds of things we hadn't done before: giving him a bath, learning CPR, fixing his bottle. The hospital hadn't really encouraged us to be very involved up until

then. The last few days felt very rushed and I'm afraid a lot of what we learned went in one ear and out the other."

Break the Habit of Watching Your Baby's Monitor

Monitors serve an important role in safeguarding your baby's health. But for many parents, they play an additional role, by providing you with an easy way of judging your baby's condition from one moment to the next. The monitors can give you instant feedback on how your baby is reacting to handling, feeding, or other activities. As one mother said,

"For three months I depended on the monitors. I could tell when Joey was contented, when he was stressed, when it was all right to pick him up, and when he needed to be put down to rest. I was so used to watching his heart rate and his oxygen levels that when the monitors were first disconnected I was a nervous wreck. I actually turned my chair around and watched the baby's monitor across the room the first time I fed Joey after he had been disconnected. It seems totally crazy now, but at the time it made me feel better."

In the past, it was common for hospitals to discontinue monitoring babies as soon as they had passed a certain number of apnea-free days. This gave you a chance to become accustomed to your baby being off the monitor before you took him home. However, most hospitals now monitor babies until the moment of discharge. If you are accustomed to watching your baby's monitor, it is a good idea to break this habit as much as possible before you take him home.

You might first try turning your chair around so that your back is to the monitor. If your baby tends to hold his breath while feeding, ask a nurse to stay close by for support and advice the first few times you feed him without a monitor. With practice, you will find that you can accurately judge your baby's condition by watching him rather than the monitor.

Use the Parent or Family Visiting Room

As often as possible, take your baby to a parent or family room separated from the nursery but within calling distance. This gives you an opportunity to finally spend private time with your baby, and to be on your own with him just as you will be at home. If your nursery continues to monitor babies up until discharge, the family room can provide an opportunity for you to be with your baby without the monitors.

Siblings and other family members can usually visit with the baby in the family room as well. One mother with older children felt this was extremely useful.

"The nursery was very small, and didn't allow siblings to visit. If we took the kids to the hospital with us, they had to wait in the hallway, and they were bored and irritated by the whole thing. It helped a lot when we could finally take Annie to the family room where the kids could hold her and even feed her. It made it much more interesting for them, obviously, and they started to feel like they were a part of things too."

Stay Overnight with Your Baby

Some hospitals offer parents the opportunity to spend the night with their baby in a family room close to the nursery but away from the direct supervision of the nursery staff. This dry run can be very helpful particularly if you haven't been able to spend a lot of time in the nursery, if your baby will come home needing ongoing medical care, or simply to assuage your anxiety a bit. A night alone can help you learn more about your baby's habits and boost your confidence. And you have the added security of knowing that the nursery staff is close by if you need them. Because you will probably get very little sleep, do this several days before discharge rather than the night before your baby is released. Try to get a good night's sleep before your baby comes home. As is the case with any newborn, it will undoubtedly be a while before you get another!

Learn Infant CPR (Cardiopulmonary Resuscitation)

Most special care nurseries will not allow you to take your baby home until you have learned infant CPR. Knowing CPR skills will help you know what to do in the unlikely event that your baby should stop breathing, or, when he is older, if he should choke on something.

CPR is an important skill for all parents to know. As one neonatal nurse explained, "We wish we could teach all parents CPR before they take their babies home, but we don't have the time or personnel to reach everyone with babies in the regular nursery. So we concentrate on the parents with babies in the special care nursery who are usually with us for a longer time."

The elements of infant CPR are reviewed in Appendix C. Refresher courses as well as courses in first aid can usually be found at a Red Cross center in your area.

Preparations at Home

Stock Up on Basic Infant Supplies

Despite their unusual start, preemies have the same basic needs as all other newborns. One of your first purchases should probably be a good book on baby care. These books can answer many of the questions that will come up in the first weeks at home, and also provide lists of clothing and equipment that you will want for your baby. The following items are suggested in addition to those you find on any layette list.

Preemie-sized diapers. If your baby weighs less than five pounds, preemie-sized diapers are easier to use than the regular newborn size. Your baby will probably go through at least 10 to 12 diapers per day. If you have trouble finding preemie-sized disposable diapers you can usually order what you need from your local pharmacy, but it may take several days for the order to arrive. See Appendix E for phone numbers to order diapers directly from the manufacturers.

Preemie-sized clothing. Your baby will probably be able to wear regular newborn-sized clothing soon after getting home, but you may want to have a few smaller pieces to use at first. Most stores that sell baby clothes now carry sizes for babies weighing less than five pounds. There are also a number of mail-order companies listed in Appendix E.

Bottles, formula, nipples, and pacifiers. While your baby is still in the hospital, ask the nurses if you can take home some of the small plastic bottles, nipples, and pacifiers that your baby is accustomed to using since they are usually unavailable in retail drugstores. The small feeding bottles used in the hospital are particularly useful in the early weeks at home. It is also a good idea to come home with several days worth of infant formula, especially if your baby is on a special diet. If you will be switching formulas after you get home, have enough of the hospital formula on hand to make the switch gradually or to use while you experiment with other formulas. If you need to order a special formula, give your drugstore enough time to order it for you. If your pharmacy is unable to supply you, you may be able to order directly from the manufacturers by phone (see Appendix E for phone numbers). Again, be sure to leave enough time for the order to be delivered.

Cloth diapers and soft receiving blankets. Try to have a number of these on hand as they are particularly useful for many purposes beyond their primary ones. Cloth diapers are very absorbent and durable, and can be used as burp rags and to clean up the numerous spills that occur. Receiving blankets can be rolled up to create nesting boundaries around your baby or to provide extra support in a car or infant seat.

A *small bassinet*. Many parents find a bassinet to be very useful in the first few months at home. Its smaller size makes it easier to provide the boundaries that give your baby a feeling of security. Bassinets have the added advantage of being portable. If you are more comfortable having your baby near you during the day and at night, you can carry his bassinet with you from room to room.

A *stroller or baby carriage*. There are many styles and types of strollers and carriages. The one you choose depends on your personal preferences as well as how much money you want to spend. Keep in mind a couple of things when shopping for a stroller for your preemie. First, small babies do not get the support they need from an inexpensive folding umbrella stroller. Until your baby gets bigger and stronger, you will need to use a style that offers more back support or that allows your baby to lie flat. This is especially important if your baby has trouble breathing in a car seat. If your baby will be using oxygen or other equipment, try to get a stroller or carriage that has a roomy, sturdy storage area. It is much easier to stow these things below or beside your baby than to try to carry them.

Get a Car Seat or Car Bed for Your Baby

All infants and children under age four or less than 40 pounds are required by law to ride in car seats or car beds that meet federal safety regulations. Most preemies can ride in the typical semi-reclining car seats. However, as discussed above, a few babies have trouble breathing in this position, and should travel lying flat in a specially designed car bed until they are a little larger and stronger.

If your baby will be able to ride in a car seat, try to find the smallest seat you can, particularly if your baby still weighs less than six pounds. Seats designed specifically for infants under 20 pounds usually work better for preemies than the larger style, which can be used for infants and toddlers up to 40 pounds.

But even with a small seat, getting your baby strapped in for the first time can be a challenge. As one mother said,

"We put him in the car seat and he kind of disappeared. We put blankets around him to prop him up, but his feet barely reached the crotch strap, so it wasn't like we could actually place that strap between his legs. And the shoulder straps pretty much dwarfed the rest of his body. It didn't seem wonderfully secure but it was the best we could do."

In order to maintain your baby in a proper position in the car seat, place blanket rolls beside his head. Another roll can be placed between his legs and the crotch strap to keep him from slumping down in the seat. See the box below for ideas on ways to support your baby in his car seat.

Always secure the car seat in a place where an adult can keep an eye on the baby—the front passenger seat if you are driving alone and your car does not have passenger-side air bags, or the back seat if another adult is with you and can ride in the back. Infants always ride facing the back of the car. **No infant or child under the age of twelve should be placed in the front passenger seat of a car equipped with a passenger-side air bag. The force of the air bag deploying has caused serious and even fatal injuries to infants and young children.**

Bring your baby's car seat or bed into the hospital before the day of discharge to practice placing him in it. Many hospitals are able to give or loan car seats to parents. Your social worker will have information on such programs.

Continue Pumping Breastmilk

For mothers who want to supply breastmilk for their babies and eventually breastfeed, it is important to continue pumping milk regularly in order to maintain your milk supply. It may seem as though your freezer is filling with small bags of breastmilk, but resist the urge to cut back on pumping

Finding the Best Car Seat or Car Bed for Your Baby

CAR SEATS

Use a car seat specifically designed for infants weighing less than 20 pounds.

To get the most secure fit for your baby, the crotch strap of the car seat should be no more than 5 $1/2$ inches from the seat back, and the shoulder straps should be in slots that are no more than 10 inches above the seat bottom.

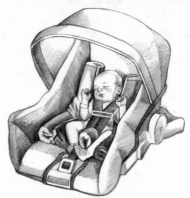

Car seats with shields, pads, or arm rests should not be used because a small baby can slip beneath the shield, or his face or chest could hit it in a crash.

Rolled blankets, cloth diapers, or a car seat insert can provide extra support for your baby in his car seat.

You will probably need to provide extra support and padding for your baby, using rolled-up cloth diapers or receiving blankets. These can be placed along the sides of the seat, around your baby's head, and between the crotch strap and your baby's bottom (but never under his bottom or back).

Be sure that your baby's head rests against the back of the car seat and doesn't fall forward when the car seat is strapped into the car. A firm roll of cloth or newspaper can be wedged under the car seat to make it recline more if necessary.

CAR BEDS

For babies who need to lie flat in the car, there are basically two types of car beds.

- One type uses straps to harness the baby in the bed, which is then secured with seat belts.
- The other type uses a bunting bag into which the baby is zipped. The bag itself is attached to the car bed.

In either case, the harness or bag should fit snugly, and the baby's head should be placed toward the center of the car. Use extra blankets or diapers to support the baby.

or to throw out the excess milk. That supply will come in handy during the first weeks your baby is home. If your milk supply seems to be dwindling, you may want to pump more frequently the week before your baby comes home in order to build your supply. Chapter 8 contains more detailed information on preparing for breastfeeding at home.

Choose a Pediatrician

If you have not already done so, find a pediatrician to take over your baby's care after he comes home. Your baby's doctor does not need to be a specialist in prematurity, but some familiarity with the special needs of preemies helps. Friends, family, and the hospital staff can provide information on pediatricians in your area. In some locations and hospitals, your pediatrician will be able to participate directly in your baby's care while the baby is still in the hospital. If that is not the case, your pediatrician can get an overview of your baby's condition and any ongoing medical or developmental problems from the neonatologist who has been supervising your baby's care. Your pediatrician will probably want to see your baby within a week or two of his discharge.

Set Up Any Necessary Follow-up Appointments

In the week before your baby is discharged, meet with his care team and find out if you need to make any follow-up appointments with specialists or hospital clinics. If possible, call to make these appointments before your baby comes home. It will be one less task to worry about during those first tiring weeks at home.

Contact Your Local Early Intervention (EI) Program

Early intervention programs provide services to infants and toddlers up to age three who are at risk for developmental delays or who have identified disabilities. In some states, preemies are eligible for services because they are at higher than normal risk for developmental delays. In other states, preemies are eligible for EI only if they have an identified disability or delay. EI programs can provide valuable services for your child, and can also put you in touch with other parents of preemies. Your hospital nursery staff or the social worker can give you information about the EI program that serves your area. Contact them before your baby comes home so that they can send you information about their program and registration forms. You won't be billed for any services that your child receives. Early intervention programs are supported by federal and state funds, and by your health insurance.

Special Situations

If you will be bringing home more than one baby, or your baby will be coming home from the hospital with continuing medical needs, your preparations for discharge will be more complex. As your baby's (or babies') health begins to improve in the Level II nursery, begin discussing his (or their) discharge during your weekly meetings with the care team. It is never too early to begin this planning process. Your baby's needs will still be changing, but you can get a general idea of what might be required or what your options are.

In some hospitals, a specific individual known as a discharge planner will work with you to identify your baby's needs, locate the necessary medical supply companies or home health care agencies, and guide you through the maze of insurance coverage paperwork. In others, you will work with a nurse or social worker. If you are a member of an HMO, you may have a company case manager or discharge planner assigned to your baby.

Depending upon your baby's needs, where you live, and your insurance coverage, you may have a number of medical supply companies from which to choose. Or you may be restricted to only one or two. Whichever situation you are in, you may want to ask the company that you will be working with some of the questions in the boxed section below. You will also find more information about planning for and living with babies with ongoing medical needs in Chapter 7.

One other very important aspect of planning for your baby's homecoming is to make sure you arrange for extra help. Caring for multiples or babies with ongoing medical needs can be very demanding and exhausting. Your friends and family may be able to provide some relief, but they may not be comfortable caring for babies with medical needs. You may qualify for a certain number of hours of nursing care per week—your baby's doctor will write orders for this before your baby is discharged. But you might want to hire additional help as well, at least for the first few weeks.

Questions to Ask Your Medical Equipment or Home Care Company

- What training and supports do you provide for parents? Will someone come to the house on a regular basis to check that the equipment is functioning properly? If my baby is on oxygen, how do you monitor his oxygen saturation levels?
- Are you specifically a pediatric home care company, or do you care for both adults and children?
- What training or experience does your staff have in providing care to preemies?
- Is someone available 24 hours a day, 7 days a week to answer questions? How do you handle emergencies or equipment failure?
- How often and on what schedule will deliveries be made? Can special deliveries or deliveries on short notice be arranged?
- If we need to travel, can you help us make arrangements for supplies or equipment in other cities?
- Are your services covered by insurance? Do you bill the insurance company directly or will we need to do the paperwork?

Ask your hospital social worker for information about nursing agencies or companies that specialize in caring for newborns at home. Although expensive, these services may be a worthwhile investment for a short time.

Arranging for Equipment

If your baby will be using oxygen, a monitor, or other medical equipment and supplies at home, have it delivered several days before your baby is scheduled to be discharged. If the equipment differs from that used in the hospital, bring it in and practice with it in the nursery.

Babies on Medications

Before you leave the hospital, make sure you have detailed instructions about any medications your baby needs to take at home, including:

- the name of the medicine and its purpose
- the dosage and how to measure it

- the schedule for giving medications
- how to administer the medicine
- what to do about missed or vomited doses
- possible side effects such as jitteriness, irritability, stomach upsets

If you find you have questions about these or any other matters after you get home, don't hesitate to call the nursery or your pediatrician.

Bringing Home Twins or Multiples

If you have more than one baby to bring home, it is unlikely that they will both or all be discharged at the same time. Having one baby in the hospital and the other at home presents some new complications in terms of visiting and child care. But this transition time also offers several benefits. It allows you a chance to ease more slowly into the realities of parenting multiple infants. In addition, it gives you the opportunity to practice your skills with your child at home while one or more of your babies are still being cared for in the hospital. As questions and concerns arise, your continuing relationship with the staff of the nursery can be very comforting and helpful. In the unlikely event that your babies are ready to come home at the same time, you may want to request that their discharges be staggered, even for a day or two, in order to give yourself this valuable transition time.

Going Home!

The day finally arrives when you can take your baby home! Before leaving the hospital, you'll meet with your baby's nurse or neonatologist to review and sign his discharge summary. This form summarizes your baby's medical history, lists any ongoing problems, and specifies plans for his follow-up care. During this meeting, ask any remaining questions you may have about your baby and how to care for him. Make sure you know how soon you should take your baby to the pediatrician and whether or not you need to make appointments with any specialists for follow-up care or testing. Because the last day in the nursery can feel hectic and disjointed, you may want to bring with you a list of questions or concerns for this final meeting.

Before You Leave: A Final Checklist

- Review your baby's discharge summary with his nurse or neonatologist, sign it, and get a copy.
- If your baby has had respiratory difficulties, get a copy of his most recent chest X-rays to take with you.
- Ask about your nursery's policy on phone calls after discharge, including times that are or are not good for calling.
- Be sure you know how soon to see your pediatrician and whether or not your baby needs to see any specialists in the coming weeks.
- Don't leave the nursery without a good supply of nipples, formula, small feeding bottles, pacifiers, preemie-sized diapers—anything that you and your baby are accustomed to using. Try to get enough of these critical supplies to last you for the first few days at home.
- Ask the neonatologist how much formula your baby should consume in a day, how often to feed him, and what the maximum length of time is that he should go between feedings. If you need to add supplements to his formula, make sure you have the recipe written down.
- If you have any breastmilk in the nursery freezer, remember to bring a cooler with you to transport it home.
- Bring your baby's car seat or car bed to the nursery and place your baby in it before you leave the nursery.

You will be given a copy of your baby's discharge summary. This summary is an important document, especially for a baby who has had a complicated time in the hospital, who continues to have medical problems, or who has been identified as being at particular risk for problems. One mother recommended keeping a copy of it in your diaper bag or some other handy place. On the two occasions when her son needed to be readmitted to the hospital, she was able to provide the hospital staff with his discharge summary so that they were immediately aware of his history and could treat him appropriately.

For some parents, the discharge process proceeds quickly and smoothly. Others find that hospital protocols—the need for one last test or test result, a discussion with the billing office, a meeting with the

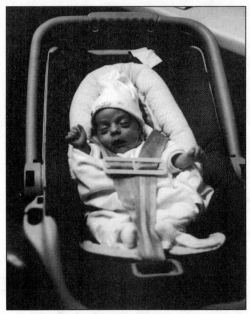

Ready for the ride home—at last!

neonatologist—cause delay after delay. But no matter how smooth or rocky your last moments in the nursery, or how nervous you feel about taking your baby home, remember that this is a day of celebration. You may want to dress your baby in a special homecoming outfit, take some pictures, and say good-bye to any staff members to whom you have become close. Some parents bring in cookies or flowers for the staff, or write them a thank-you note. Before you leave, one of the nurses will probably take your baby's picture to add to the collection in the nursery. And then, with your baby strapped into his car seat and looking, as one mother described it, "like a little baby bird in a big nest," it is finally time to go home.

CHAPTER 6

As Your Baby Settles In

$\mathcal{S}$

MANY PARENTS WISH THAT as they leave the hospital with their infant, they could close the door on the previous weeks or months and start a fresh life with their child at home. One mother summed up these feelings when she said, "I just wanted it to be over. I want to think of her as normal." And in many important ways, your baby is just that—a normal baby with all the normal needs of any newborn.

But she is also a preemie. She has had a different start in life, and her development and experiences have not been the same as those of a baby born at the end of a full-term pregnancy. This means that her behavior, her needs, and some of the ways you care for her will differ somewhat as well.

In general, most preemies are less mature when they come home than their full-term counterparts. This is particularly true now that hospital stays are cut as short as possible, and many preemies are discharged weeks ahead of their due dates, weighing less than five pounds. In addition, some babies leave the hospital with continuing medical needs, and require specialized care for a time. But even a baby who had few problems during her hospitalization will not have completely recovered from her early birth by the time she is discharged. She has, however, reached a point where—even if she continues to have medical needs—she is better off at home with you.

In this chapter, you will find information on how to help your baby adjust to home, and on typical ways that preemies behave in their early weeks and months at home—in other words, on what is normal for preemies. A section called Special Handling covers some of the ways in which you can provide extra support for your baby as she continues her recovery at home.

But preemies aren't the only ones who must recover from an early birth. You and your family face adjustments as well. The last section of this chapter covers some of the common issues faced by families of preemies.

Even though you must be feeling relieved and pleased to finally have your baby home, you are probably feeling some anxiety as well. As you begin your life at home with your baby, it may help to remember that she has already proven herself to be a strong and determined individual, and has come an enormous distance since her early birth. And during her hospitalization, you have undoubtedly discovered new strengths and abilities of your own. Appreciate all that you and she have accomplished so far, and have confidence in yourself and in her.

Helping Your Baby Adjust

There is no way to predict how your baby will react to the transition from hospital nursery to home. Some babies hardly notice the change, sailing through the first days at home much more easily than their anxious parents. Some babies act tired and sleepy for a few days, while others are fussy and irritable. A number of parents said that their babies stayed on the schedule they had been on in the hospital for a week or two, waking to eat every three to four hours, and then became less predictable as they settled in. Others reported that their babies spent most of their time sleeping until they got closer to their original due dates, at which point they seemed to wake up.

Easing the Transition

Depending upon how your baby reacts and what her needs are, the following suggestions may help smoothe the transition to home.

Continue Some of the Routines Your Baby Is Used To. One of the benefits of having your baby home is that you finally get to be in charge of her care. However, as you and she are adjusting, you may find it helpful to follow the schedule or routines that your baby grew accustomed to in the hospital. There is certainly no need to recreate the nursery at home, but providing some continuity in your baby's care gives her fewer changes to cope with at one time. For babies who have ongoing medical needs or who are very sensitive and easily overstimulated, this approach can be particularly beneficial.

For example, you could continue feeding your baby on the same schedule she has been on in the hospital. Although you will probably want to move toward feeding your baby on demand, it may be easier to rely on a schedule during the first few days at home. Or, if your baby is accustomed to spending most of her time sleeping in her bassinet, you may want to continue this routine at home. You may long to hold her for hours to make up for the separation you have endured—and some babies may be able to handle this—but others may find such a change to be stressful.

Leave a Night Light or Radio On During the First Few Days. After the noisy, bright nursery, some babies seem to have trouble settling down in the relative quiet and darkness of home. If your baby seems very fussy at home and is having trouble sleeping, she may be soothed if you leave on a dim light at night or have a radio playing softly. You can phase these things out over a few days.

Keep a Log or Chart of Your Baby's Daily Activities. Although this isn't a necessity, many parents find it useful to record information about feedings, medications, body temperature, or sleep patterns for the first few days or weeks. You can make a simple chart by drawing columns on a piece of paper, you can just jot notes as you go through the day, or you may need to keep more detailed notes.

A log makes it easier to see any patterns that exist in your baby's behavior, or to monitor anything that you may be concerned about. If your baby's care is complicated, if she is on several medications that must be given on different schedules, or if you are worried about something in particular, such as how much formula or breastmilk she is consuming, a log can be particularly helpful. On the next pages are two examples of logs developed by a family with triplets. These logs helped them keep track of three complicated medication and feeding schedules as well as other important information.

DATE _____

I N F O

Alex				Ellen				Gwen		
Last Poop				Last Poop				Last Poop		
Last Bath				Last Bath				Last Bath		
Last Weight		kg	10 lb. 4 oz.	Last Weight		kg	10 lb 4 oz	Last Weight		kg

F E E D I N G S

Alex						Ellen						Gwen				
Time	diap	oz	cum	cal/r	comment	Time	diap	oz	cum	cal/r	comment	Time	diap	po	pg	cum

M E D I C A L

Alex	Ellen	Gwen	2.5 Sterile Water	BRE

Ellen:
1:00 [ ] 0.50 Cisapride
8:30 [ ] 0.50 Cisapride
9:00 [ ] 0.30 Iron
      2.50 Bactrim
5:00 [ ] 0.50 Cisapride

Alex:
9:00 [ ] 0.30 Iron
      2.50 Bactrim

Gwen: 2.5 Sterile Water
5:00 [ ] 1.50 Steroid -- EVEN days only
8:00 [ ] 1.10 Duiril   0.30 Ranitidine
      1.73 Potassium   2.40 Corn Oil
                        0.20 Iron
11:00 [ ] 0.80 Cisapride
2:00 [ ] 1.50 Bactrim   0.30 Ranitidine
                         2.40 Corn Oil
                         0.20 Iron
5:00 [ ] 0.80 Cisapride
8:00 [ ] 1.10 Duiril   0.30 Ranitidine
      1.73 Potassium   2.40 Corn Oil
                        0.20 Iron
11:00 [ ] 0.80 Cisapride

A C T I V I T I E S

	Alex			Ellen			Gwen		
	Time	Loc	States	Time	Loc	States	Time	Loc	States
Start Laundry									
Tidy Nursery									
Alex's bath [ ] or Tip & Tail									
Ellen's bath [ ] or Tip & Tail									
Gwen's bath [ ] or Tip & Tail									
Clean Kitchen									
Start Dishwasher									
Clean Feeding Bag									
Move Laundry									
Disenfect Counters									
Boil Water									
Fold Laundry									
Put Away Laundry									
Empty dishwasher									
Ellen's & Alex's Bottles									
Prepare Gwen's Formula									
Draw up day's meds									

DATE _____

Alex's info					Ellen's info					Gwen's info				

Last Poop		Weight	lb	oz	Last Poop		Weight	lb	oz	Last Poop		Weight	lb	oz
		10/16	18.0	1.5			10/16	17.0	12.5			10/16	17.0	12.0

Alex's Feedings / **Ellen's Feedings** / **Gwen's Feedings** / **Gwen's PO**

Time	diap	vol	total	meds	Time	diap	vol	total	meds	diap		meds	Time	vol	total
				BD					BD		7A	CO			
											11A	CKP			
											4P	CO			
				D					D		10P	CKPF			

Gwen's Stats					Gwen's pump			Goal		Kid's temps		

Time	O2	SAT	HR	RR	Time	Pump	Total			Child	Time	Temp
					night			8A	960			
								10A	79			
								12P	159	Gwen's vomits		
								2P	238	Time	vol	total
								4P	317			
								6P	396			
								8P	476			
								10P	555			
								night	405			

Notes

Help Your Baby Learn the Difference Between Night and Day. Because nurseries operate 24 hours a day, most babies come home not knowing the difference between night and day. Although it will take a while before your baby is able to sleep for long unbroken stretches at night, you can begin teaching her the difference between night and day as soon as you get her home. Keep night-time feedings as brief and businesslike as possible. Keep lights low, and do not talk or play with your baby. If possible, try to settle her back to bed as soon as the feeding is over. Do most of your socializing with her during the day.

Of course, this approach will not work immediately. Some babies need to be fed so often during the early weeks at home that there is little difference between night and day. And some babies never seem to sleep for more than a brief catnap at any time. But, in general, if you try to make a clear difference between day and night, your baby will gradually respond and become more organized over time.

Arrange for Extra Help. Sleep deprivation plagues parents of preemies during the first weeks at home. If your baby is a typical preemie and needs to be fed every two to three hours and each feeding takes 30 to 45 minutes, you'll find it hard to get even a minimal amount of sleep. Parents can help each other by taking turns with feedings so that each can get at least one stretch of four to five hours a night. However, this can also result in both parents becoming exhausted after a few days. You may find that you need more help, particularly if you have other children to care for during the day.

- For the first few weeks, consider having a family member move in with you or come one or two nights a week to help out.
- Although hiring help is expensive, it may be worth the investment to help you get through the first few weeks. If you have twins or more, or a baby with multiple medical needs, extra help may be a necessity.
- Try to simplify your life as much as possible until your baby begins to sleep for longer stretches of time. Most housekeeping chores can be postponed or skipped altogether, and friends can help with meals, shopping, or child care. Grab moments of rest whenever you can.
- You may be able to doze for a few precious minutes by settling your baby securely on your chest as you lie down on your bed or couch.

Getting through your days on minimal amounts of sleep is extremely difficult, but this period in your baby's life is relatively short. In the coming weeks she should gradually begin to sleep for longer periods of time.

What to Expect from Your Baby

Although most newborns are unpredictable in their habits at first—sleeping and eating at variable times, crying for unknown reasons—preemies tend to be even less predictable than their full-term counterparts. To a large extent, this reflects their general immaturity at the time they are discharged.

It may take more time for your baby to get organized than it would a full-term newborn. In the meantime, you may need to do a lot of experimentation to find out how best to comfort her, feed her, and help her sleep. And you will probably have to wait longer for her to become sociable—to spend more time awake, to smile at you, and to enjoy watching what is going on around her. As one mother described it,

"I felt like I had a very short pregnancy followed by a very long infancy. Those first few weeks with any newborn are tough; you feel like you work and work and get very little in return. With a preemie that period seems to go on for a lot longer."

Using Your Baby's Adjusted (or Corrected) Age

As you settle in at home with your baby, it is very important that you adjust your expectations about her behavior and abilities because of her early birth. In order to do this, you should calculate your baby's adjusted, or corrected, age. This is the age she would be if she had been born at the end of a full-term, 40-week pregnancy rather than several weeks or months early. Your baby's corrected age provides a more accurate indicator of her stage of development than does her actual or chronological age (the number of weeks or months since she was born). Most experts recommend using your baby's adjusted age to judge her development for the first two to two and a half years. If your baby was born very early or was very sick, you may need to use her corrected age for a longer time than this.

To calculate your baby's corrected age, subtract from her actual age (the number of weeks since her birth) the number of weeks she was born early. For example, if your baby was born 14 weeks ago but was 11 weeks premature, she is now the equivalent of a 3-week-old. She needs to complete the development that should have occurred in the womb for those final 11 weeks before she can be considered to be the equivalent of a full-term newborn. So even though she has been in the world for 14 weeks, her behavior and development will much more closely resemble that of a 3-week-old baby, rather than a 14-week-old one. Another simple way to figure your baby's adjusted age is to use her original due date as your starting point. If you are one month past that date, your baby has an adjusted age of one month.

When your baby reaches the age of two or so, she is said to have caught up to other children with her same chronological age and it is no longer necessary to use her adjusted age. This is not exactly accurate since there is actually no reason that your child should be expected to "catch up" to these children; development begins at conception and your child will always be slightly younger than full-term children born on her birth-

---

A New Definition of Adjusted Age

People were always asking me how old Jenny was, particularly in the beginning when she was so tiny. At first I would tell them her real age and explain about how she was premature and everything. After a while I got tired of these long conversations with strangers and started using her adjusted age since that matched her size more closely and didn't lead to long explanations.

As she grew, that didn't seem exactly right either so I started making up an age that I thought seemed about right—it was usually somewhere between her adjusted and her real age. I would sometimes realize that I had said she was a certain age for several months and I'd have to make a leap forward and adjust her age again. I guess I developed a new meaning for the term "adjusted age."

---

day. The real reason that children are said to have caught up is that as they get older, the difference between their actual age and corrected age becomes much less significant, and at some point can no longer be measured. For example, there is not nearly as much difference between a 24-month-old and a 27-month-old as there is between a 3- and a 6-month-old. There is only one time past infancy that you might want to keep in mind the difference between your child's adjusted and actual ages, and that is when your child reaches school age; many professionals who work with preemies advise that children start school based upon their adjusted ages (i.e., use your child's original due date) rather than their actual age.

Many parents find that their child's adjusted age has another use beyond its generally recognized one. It can help you deal with what might be called "grocery-store questions," the inevitable questions about your baby that occur when you take her on outings (see box above).

Common Preemie Behavior Patterns

Using your child's adjusted age provides useful insight into her development and behavior in the early part of her life. However, preemies also have a set of behaviors that differ from those of full-term babies. Although each baby is unique, the following patterns are typical of many preemies in the early months at home.

Sleeping Patterns

Most preemies have less mature sleep patterns at discharge than full-term newborns. They spend less time in deep, quiet sleep and more time sleeping lightly. When they are sleeping lightly, they may move, grunt, jerk, and even fuss, and be more easily disturbed or awakened by noises. In general, they tend to have shorter sleep cycles and wake more often. In fact, many preemies wake and fuss every two hours until they are three to four months old (adjusted age).

Feeding Challenges

Babies are not discharged from the hospital until they are able to take a bottle or breastfeed (or a combination) well enough to gain weight steadily. But many parents report that feeding was the single most difficult and time-consuming aspect of caring for their baby at home. There are a number of reasons for this. First, your baby's stomach is still quite small and may only be able to hold an ounce or two of milk or formula. Second, your baby may not have a lot of energy yet, and her nursing muscles may not be very strong.

In general, most preemies need to be fed smaller amounts more frequently. And each feeding may take longer—your baby may feed very slowly, or may need to take breaks in the middle of a feeding. You may also need to experiment with nipples, formula, and feeding positions to help your baby feed well. In addition, a number of other problems can add further challenges.

- In some cases, a baby's need for sleep seems to override her desire to eat. Some babies tend to sleep for long periods, are difficult to rouse, and fall asleep before finishing.
- Other babies have not yet fully mastered the suck-swallow-breathe sequence. These babies get so intent on sucking that they periodically hold their breath for too long as they are sucking.
- Some babies become easily distracted with any extra stimulation, such as noise, lights, rocking, eye contact, or talking.
- Babies who have been on respirators or had other unpleasant oral

experiences may dislike having anything, even a nipple, placed in their mouths.

Not every baby will have problems with feeding. But feeding is such a big concern to parents, and feeding problems are common enough, that Chapter 8 is devoted to this topic.

Crying and Irritability

Although many premature babies are sleepy and hard to rouse in the early weeks at home, others are quite sensitive, fussy, and hard to comfort. Like all newborns, preemies may fuss and cry because they are hungry, wet, too hot or cold, or uncomfortable. But a preemie's immature nervous system can cause her to overreact to stimulation, become more easily overwhelmed, and have a harder time relaxing and calming down. Babies with ongoing respiratory problems or on certain medications such as stimulants for apnea prevention or bronchodilators can be particularly irritable.

A full-term newborn will spend an increasing amount of time fussing and crying in the early months, reaching a peak of two to four hours a day at about six weeks of age. A preemie typically reaches a peak a little later, about three to four months after her original due date.

Since crying requires strength and energy, an increase in your baby's fussiness or crying signals that she is growing stronger. On the other hand, excessive crying is difficult to cope with and can be very tiring for your baby. And if you have a baby who spits up frequently, particularly when she is upset, or a baby with ongoing respiratory problems, you may need to try to minimize her crying as much as possible. Tips on ways of calming your baby are covered in the next chapter.

Immature Behavior Patterns

Most preemies are less mature in their behavior than full-term babies, even at their due dates. It can be harder to read their cues, and to know when they are tired, hungry, or upset. And there may be little predictability in their days. One day your baby may sleep well, wake regularly every three to four hours to eat, and fall back asleep easily. The next day, she may wake often, be hungry but spit out the nipple almost as soon as she begins feeding, and be difficult to comfort.

A common manifestation of a preemie's immaturity is in an area called state regulation. Newborns have six distinct states of alertness which they move through during each twenty-four-hour period, ranging from deep sleep to alert activity (see box). Most full-term babies move from one state to the next fairly smoothly, while preemies have more difficulty with the transitions.

Preemies may make sudden unexpected leaps from one state to the next, or may get stuck in one and be unable to move to the next. For example, many preemies have particular difficulty moving easily to sleep when they get tired, as this mother describes:

"With Bobby, the dividing line between being awake and happy to being over-tired and screaming was really thin. It took me a long time to figure out what was going on with him. As he got tired, it seemed like he started moving faster and faster rather than slower. He'd start waving his arms and kicking his legs, and then all of a sudden he'd just have a melt-down. He'd be crying and stiff, and it could take an incredibly long time to get him calmed down. Finally I learned that as soon as he started to get wound up I needed to put him in bed, turn out the light, and leave him alone—quickly. No patting him on the back, no singing, no nothing. What might be soothing for other babies was just more stimulation to him at that point and was too much. If I did it right he would fall asleep before melt-down occurred."

As your baby matures, she will begin to make smoother transitions, and her behavior should become more predictable. Like the mother above, through a lot of experimentation you may also learn to read your child's confusing signals and avoid some of these melt-downs.

Special Handling

By the time your baby is ready to come home from the hospital, she is no longer the fragile infant she once was. But her immaturity means that you may want to care for her a bit differently and take a few extra precautions in her early weeks and months at home. Most importantly, preemies need to be protected from overstimulation and from exposure to illness. Some suggestions on ways to provide this extra protection to your child are described below.

Not every child will need to be handled in these ways. As is true with

The Six States of Alertness

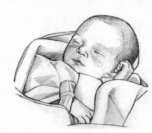

Deep sleep
Your baby is motionless, her breathing is regular, she shows no eye movements, and her arms and legs are relaxed and limp. It can be very hard to rouse a baby from a deep sleep state.

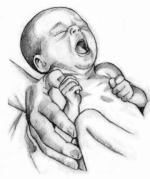

Light or active sleep
Your baby is still asleep but is beginning to move around. She may make sucking movements with her mouth, you see her eyes moving beneath her closed eyelids, and her breathing is more irregular. While in this state, your baby can be more easily awakened if it is time for a feeding, or, if left alone, she may move back into deep sleep.

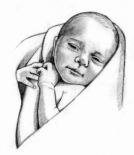

Drowsiness
Your baby's eyes may be open but she looks sleepy and doesn't focus on anything. She may move a little but is quiet. From this state, she may go to sleep or wake up more fully.

any infant, part of the challenge of parenting a preemie is learning what works best for your own child and for you. Your pediatrician can also give you specific guidance about these matters.

Protect Your Baby from Too Much Noise or Activity

Most preemies remain quite sensitive to stimulation such as noise, handling, lights, and movement. The noise and bustle of a normal household

The Six States of Alertness, continued

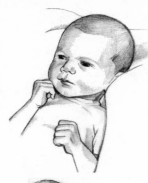

Quiet alertness

Your baby is fully awake and attentive, her eyes are open, and her arms and legs are fairly quiet. While alert and quiet, your baby will be most able to feed well and to interact with you.

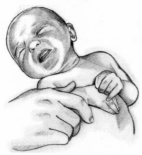

Active alertness

Your baby becomes more active, waving her arms and kicking her legs. She may become a bit frantic, in which case her movements may get jerky, and her eyes wide and staring. You may be able to calm her down with swaddling or by decreasing stimulation around her, or it may be time for a nap.

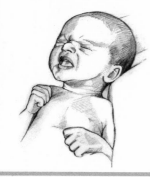

Crying

At this point your baby has become upset, overtired, or overstimulated. As you get to know your baby better, you may be able to avoid some crying periods. But most babies develop regular crying periods as they grow older.

may present your baby with much more stimulation than she was accustomed to in the hospital and may be difficult for her to handle at first.

Some babies are more sensitive to noise, and others to movement or to visual stimuli. Activity levels that would present no problems to full-term babies, such as being rocked, fed, and sung to, can be overwhelming to preemies. Others seem to find that the mobiles or visual patterns designed for babies (such as those black-and-white geometric designs or simple faces) are too much.

As your baby is settling in at home, watch her for signs that indicate she is becoming overstimulated or overwhelmed. Different babies react differently. Some babies show the classic signs of stress that you learned in the hospital—finger splaying, hiccuping, yawning, arching, startling. Others begin to fuss and cry inconsolably, and others shut down and fall asleep. Your baby may outgrow this sensitivity fairly rapidly. But others, particularly those born before about 32 weeks, continue to be easily overwhelmed for much longer.

- If your baby seems very fussy, try reducing the amount of stimulation she is exposed to. This may involve turning down the TV, stereo, or radio; moving her crib to a quieter location; lowering lights.
- Keep your baby's environment simple: do not surround her with too many bright objects or toys, music boxes, toys or mobiles that move. A brightly decorated nursery may present your baby with more stimulation than she is comfortable with at first.
- Keep feeding times as simple and quiet as possible, and limit the amount of stimulation you give your baby as she eats. You may need to feed her in a quiet, darkened place away from the noise of television, radio, or playing children.
- Limit how much your baby is handled. Don't allow her to be passed around from person to person, as this can be very tiring for her.

Protect Your Baby from Exposure to Illness

Many people, both friends and family, will want to come see your baby when you finally get her home. But you may want to limit the number of visitors you have in the early weeks—or at least limit their contact with your baby—to protect her from both overstimulation and exposure to illness.

Preemies are more susceptible to illness, especially respiratory infections, than are full-term newborns in the first six to twelve months (adjusted age) of their lives. This is especially true if they have had or continue to have respiratory problems. If your baby is discharged home during the winter months of November through March, take extra care since this is a time when there is more illness, including RSV germs (see box).

This does not mean that you must remain isolated inside your house. But it probably makes sense to take a few precautions, particularly during

What is RSV?

Respiratory syncytial (pronounced sin-sichial) virus, or RSV, is a common virus that almost all children will be exposed to before they are two years old. RSV infections usually cause a simple cold. But infants less than two months old, preemies born at 32 weeks or less, or those with respiratory or heart problems are particularly vulnerable to RSV. In these babies, RSV can cause a serious lower respiratory infection, i.e., congestion in the lungs, known as pneumonia, or bronchiolitis.

RSV outbreaks tend to occur during the winter, from November through March, although the timing varies slightly in different parts of the country.

• **What are the symptoms of RSV?** The first symptoms of RSV are those of a cold. Your child may have a runny nose, sneezing, fever, and cough, but not seem particularly ill. However, the illness can quickly spread into the chest; your baby may begin wheezing (making whistling sounds during breathing), breathing quickly, seem to be working hard at breathing, and even turn slightly bluish or pale around the mouth. It is not uncommon for a baby with RSV to go to bed at night with very mild symptoms of a cold, but by the next morning seem very sick. If your child shows any of the symptoms of a lower respiratory infection, call your pediatrician immediately or take her to the nearest hospital emergency room. Because RSV is a virus, antibiotics are not effective in treating it. Babies with RSV may need to be hospitalized, given extra oxygen, or even be placed on a respirator during the worst part of the illness. Other treatments, such as the use of anti-viral medicines, have had some limited effectiveness.

• **What can you do to protect your child?** RSV germs are spread primarily on the hands, so hand-washing is the simplest, most effective way of preventing its spread. In addition, keep your baby away from anyone who is sick, and out of crowded places, especially during the winter. There are also two medicines available that can help to prevent RSV infection, or lessen its severity. The most commonly used, Synagis, is an injection given once a month during RSV season. The other, Respigam, is given intravenously, i.e., directly into a vein, once a month. More detailed information on these two immunizations and who should be treated can be found in Chapter 7.

the first three to six months. Depending upon your child's health, you may need to be careful for a longer period of time.

- Healthy adult friends and family can certainly visit, but ask anyone with a contagious disease—a cold, fever, or cold sore—to postpone their visit until they are well.
- Ask anyone who is going to touch your baby to wash their hands first. Hand-washing with regular soap is a simple and effective way to protect your baby since many germs, particularly cold germs, are spread primarily by the hands. Typical cold germs can remain alive on your hands for about 25 minutes, and on surfaces such as counters for up to six hours. You may also want to take baby wipes to the store to clean the grab bar of the grocery cart that your baby may hold or suck on.
- It is best not to allow young children except siblings to get close to or hold your baby.
- Do not allow anyone to smoke in your home. This is healthy advice for all family members, but particularly for preemies, whose airways are small and easily irritated. If your baby is on oxygen, smoking can cause a fire.

Keep Your Baby Away from Crowded Places

Because your baby is more susceptible to illness, it is best not to take her into crowds or situations where she may be exposed to many people. For the first six weeks to three months, avoid bringing her to places such as malls, movie theaters, grocery stores, religious services, and schools.

Sometimes you can't avoid taking your baby into a less-than-ideal situation, and you may have to devise a creative solution. One family faced such a problem when they needed to attend a function at an older daughter's preschool a few days after their premature daughter came home. The mother recalled,

"There could hardly be a worse place to take a newly discharged preemie than a preschool but we didn't want to miss our daughter's program and we had no one to leave Emily with. Finally, what we did was put Emily in a baby carriage with mosquito netting over it. We parked the carriage in the

corner of the room, and my husband stood guard; I don't think he let anyone come within three feet of her that day."

Adjusting as a Family

After all the waiting, most parents expect to feel happy and relieved when they finally bring their baby home. But the time of homecoming is usually a difficult period as well, when you, your baby and the rest of your family must make many adjustments. You may be surprised at the range of your reactions during the first few weeks your baby is home. They may include joy, elation, sadness, guilt, anger, and depression. All of these feelings are normal and common. Just as your baby needs time to recover from her early birth, so do you. In fact, the periodic resurgence of these kinds of feelings is part of that recovery process. Although you will find that the strength of your emotions fades in time, certain times of the year or particular events will tend to reignite them. For many parents, these times include your baby's discharge, her original due date, her first birthday, or a rehospitalization.

Grief and Sadness

Many parents find their baby's homecoming to be a bittersweet time. Relief and joy are tinged with many other more difficult feelings.

> *"I thought I would be so happy once I got Joanna home. And I was, really. But then I started feeling lousy all the time, I cried a lot. I guess once all the excitement of her hospitalization was over and we got her home, I had time to get depressed about all the things that had happened. It was really a kind of delayed postpartum depression."*

The intensity and range of your feelings during your baby's early weeks at home may surprise you. You might find yourself reliving the events of your child's birth and hospitalization, wondering again if there was anything you did or didn't do that might have made a difference. Many parents, particularly mothers, continue to grieve over the loss of the pregnancy and birth experience they had imagined.

Recovering from the impact of your baby's early birth and NICU life can take a long time. "The first few months were pretty intense," said one mother, "but I thought I was pretty much back to normal by the time Sam was six months old. But looking back on it, I would say it really took a couple of years." You will probably find that as your baby grows, your anxiety will lessen, your confidence will grow, and your feelings will become more stable. However, if your baby continues to have medical or developmental problems, this process may take longer and be more problematic. Many parents find that talking with other parents who have had premature babies can help; your local early intervention program is often a good place to meet others in a similar situation.

If during or after your baby's hospitalization, you begin to feel overwhelmed by your emotions, you may want to get professional help. It's not a sign of weakness, and it may aid you in moving ahead more quickly. Your hospital social worker may be able to give you the names of therapists who are knowledgeable about the many issues that affect parents coping with premature birth.

Missing the Nursery

Another aspect of homecoming that surprises many parents is finding that they actually miss the nursery that they couldn't wait to leave behind them. The nursery staff have become part of your life over the last weeks or months, and have shared an intense experience with you that few other people in your life can understand. In addition, you probably established certain routines during your child's hospitalization that filled your days and lent some structure to your life.

When that changes with your child's discharge, it is common to experience a kind of post-nursery letdown during the early weeks at home. You may feel cut off, lonely, and isolated now that you no longer have the support that the nursery environment provided. Over time, you will establish new routines and support systems at home, but the first few weeks and months can be difficult. Some parents recalled that visits to the pediatrician or home visits from nurses were the main excitement and social outlets of their lives during this period.

Try to ease your feelings of isolation as much as you can. Have friends in to visit if you can't or don't want to take your baby out. If you are worried about exposing your baby to germs, sit with your friends in another room.

It will also help your spirits to schedule some time away from your baby if possible. Go for a walk, visit friends, go to the grocery store, or do anything you enjoy that gets you out into the world. "I used to stand by the door with my coat on waiting for my husband to come home," recalled one mother. "As soon as he walked in, I was out of there. No matter what the weather was or how cold it was, I went out for a walk every night. Without that, I would have gone nuts, I think."

Growing Attached to Your Baby

Many of the mechanisms that help parents grow attached to their newborns are disrupted when a baby is born early. Not only does your baby arrive before you are fully prepared either physically or psychologically, but your early contacts with her are limited by her medical needs, a lack of privacy, and physical separation. Spending time with your baby in the hospital can help you to overcome these initial barriers and become close to your baby. But for many parents of preemies, attachment comes slowly. As one mother said,

> "I spent as much time as I could with my son in the hospital, but I never really felt like he was fully mine. I kind of shared him with the nurses. When I got him home, I still felt weirdly detached from him, as if somehow he did not quite belong to me yet. It took a long time, probably several months, to really connect with him. It did finally happen but it took a while, and I wondered if there was something wrong with me."

What this mother experienced is quite common and occurs for a number of understandable reasons. First, the separation that occurs during the early days and weeks of your child's life puts you at an unnatural distance from her. In addition, you may subconsciously keep an emotional distance from her as a way of protecting yourself in case something bad happens. The challenges hardly end after you get home. Preemies can be difficult to care for in the first months at home. All of these things can slow down the process of becoming attached to your baby.

Most parents are able to surmount all of the challenges they face and develop warm, intense, and loving relationships with their premature babies. After you get home, give yourself time to get to know your child, gain confidence in your parenting skills, and recover from the emotional roller-coaster you have been on in the NICU. With time and patience, your feelings for your baby, and hers for you, will grow and strengthen.

Are You Being Overprotective or Realistic?

All parents of infants and young children get helpful and not-so-helpful advice from relatives, other parents, professionals, parenting books, and even strangers. And parents of preemies often feel that they receive more than their share of this advice. Because most preemies need extra care when they come home, or need to be protected from too much stimulation or from exposure to illness, you may find that others think you are being overprotective, or neurotically watchful and anxious.

In the face of advice or criticism of this sort, it is important to keep in mind that you know your own child and her needs better than anyone else. You see her in her good times and her bad, you care for her when she is healthy and sick, and you have a better chance of being realistic about her needs than just about anyone else. In the famous words of Dr. Benjamin Spock, "Trust yourself. You know more than you think you do."

Many preemie parents admit that during the early years of their child's life they may go easier on the child, perhaps to make up to them for everything they've been through; perhaps they aren't as strict about behavior, mealtimes, or bedtimes, or they let their kids sleep with them since they were alone in an incubator for so long. As long as this indulgence does not become excessive and lead to spoiled, rotten behavior on your child's part, it may be that it helps both parent and child feel better.

On the other hand, it is important to develop a balanced, realistic view of your child as she grows. While some parents may continue to view them as frail or vulnerable, another mother said that she was left with a very different view of her former 28-weeker:

"I thought he was such a super-baby after everything he'd gone through. I had this sense that nothing would ever phase him. One day when he was about two, another child yelled at him and he burst into tears. I was so surprised. It made me realize just how out of whack my perceptions of him were. He wasn't a super-baby after all, he was just a normal little kid who could get scared and hurt like any other kid."

For many reasons it can be difficult to see your child as "normal," and if your child has ongoing medical or development problems, the challenge is even greater. But it is important for you and your child that you try to balance whatever special needs she has with the fact that she is, at heart, a normal kid with a normal kid's needs for play, adventure, friends, structure, guidance, and love.

Helping Your Other Children Adjust

How your older children adjust to your infant's homecoming depends on their ages, but all children need some extra support during this period. For example, your children may expect that life will return to normal once the baby is home. Most are upset to discover how disruptive a new baby can be. They may also worry that you no longer love them as much, and that they are being supplanted by the young intruder who does nothing but sleep, eat and cry.

Your toddler may become more demanding and difficult, she may begin to wet her bed or pants again, suck her thumb, or want a bottle. Although it can be difficult to deal with these annoying behaviors, they should soon disappear with patience from you.

You may want to ask your older children to help you care for the baby so that they feel involved. Even a young child can get a diaper or spread out a blanket for the baby. Older children can hold the baby or even feed her. If feeding times pose a problem, put together a basket of special activities or books for your other child that you bring out only then.

Throughout the adjustment period, make sure to give your older children some special time and attention separate from the baby. An extra story or game at bedtime, a special outing, or just a few minutes talking after lights out can make a big difference. Recognize that your children's feelings for their new sibling will take time to grow. Don't expect them to instantly love the new baby, and don't be surprised by their negative behaviors or words. Soon they will not only adjust but begin to enjoy the addition to their family.

Taking Time for Yourself and Your Partner

Premature birth takes a toll on relationships. The demands on your time, stress, anxiety, financial and job pressures, and differences in coping styles can all cause distance to build up between partners. Try to make some time for each other during the hectic first few weeks and months your baby is home. Take a short break from home periodically or focus on talking together for a few minutes at the end of each day.

Each of you also needs to take some time for yourself. No one can care for a baby, especially a demanding one, without a break. Your ability to cope will improve after a short walk, or getting out to the movies or a meal. You may feel more comfortable leaving your baby with your spouse or another family member at first. Eventually, you may want to find a babysitter who can give you regular breaks. If your baby has special needs, you may qualify for a state respite care program (see below) which will provide you with a trained home care worker. Other places to look for sitters may include a local college, or programs in early childhood education, nursing, or physical or occupational therapy.

Finding Help in Your Community

After the intensive support and care your baby received in the hospital, you may feel almost abandoned once you get home, as this mother experienced:

> *"I was nervous about taking my daughter home but I was also so happy that she was finally well. What I didn't expect was feeling as though I had fallen off a cliff. One day we were part of this sophisticated system that took care of our baby and even us to a certain extent. The next day, we were home alone."*

Ironically, this feeling of being abandoned is particularly true if your baby comes home healthy. Babies who come home with continuing medical needs tend to be tied in more tightly to health care providers and the transition to home may feel less sudden and dramatic. Although your pediatrician will probably become your main source of information and support, a number of other resources in your community may also be able to provide you with help or specific services.

Visiting Nurse Associations (VNA)

Depending upon your baby's needs and your health insurance coverage, your baby may qualify for nursing services from your local VNA after she is home. If your baby needs these services, the VNA receives a formal referral from your baby's neonatologist. A healthy preemie may qualify for only one or two visits in the first couple of weeks at home for weight checks or help with feeding issues. If your baby has complicated medical needs, she may qualify for more extensive services, such as a specified number of hours of nursing care per week. Many VNAs also have a private pay group which can provide you with nurses or home health aides whom you can hire and pay directly.

Private Nursing Agencies

Other nursing agencies in your area may provide baby nurses to help you at home during the early weeks. Your hospital social worker should be able to provide you with their names. Be sure that any nurse you consider hiring has had experience with newborns, preferably preemies, if possible.

Early Intervention (EI) Programs

Before you were discharged from the hospital, you were probably given the number for your local early intervention program. They can monitor your baby's progress, provide you with information, offer services such as physical or occupational therapy, and connect you with other parents of preemies. Chapter 10 provides more information on EI programs and the services they offer.

Programs from State Human Services Departments

Although governmental budget constraints have led to many cutbacks in human services, your state may offer family support services for which you or your baby qualify. For example, in Massachusetts, the Department of Mental Retardation provides a number of services for children at risk for or with developmental delays. One of these services is respite care, in which the Department provides someone to care for your child so that you can take a break. Your hospital social worker or local EI program should be able to give you information on useful programs in your area.

Infant Follow-up Clinics

Many of the major urban teaching hospitals where Level III NICUs are located operate follow-up clinics for graduates of their nurseries. These clinics usually see babies periodically, typically every three to six months up to about three years of age, and provide a comprehensive assessment of your baby's health and development. The wide range of professionals who staff these follow-up clinics include neonatologists, nurses, psychologists, social workers, physical and occupational therapists, and speech and language therapists.

Infant follow-up clinics don't replace your regular pediatrician, but provide additional services and usually report their findings to your doctor. They are familiar with many of the issues facing growing preemies and can be a wonderful resource, particularly if you have special concerns about your child.

Parent Support Groups

Support groups for parents of preemies exist in many areas. Some are sponsored and supported by a hospital and some are independent, primarily volunteer-run, organizations. Because the problems and concerns of preemie parents can be so different from those of the parents of regular newborns, finding a group of preemie parents can be very helpful and comforting. Each organization operates differently. Some will link you with a specific parent who has been through experiences similar to yours for one-on-one telephone support. Other groups sponsor regular meetings or parent gatherings. Many publish newsletters and sponsor educational evenings. Again, ask your hospital social worker or EI program for the name of local support groups.

Internet Connections

The growth in resources for parents of preemies on the Internet over the past several years has been astounding. You can find chat rooms where you can converse directly with other parents of preemies; there are bulletin boards where you can post questions and receive answers from other parents; and there are numerous sources of information on every aspect of preemie care.

Because the resources on the Internet keep growing all the time, there is no way to give a comprehensive listing of those currently available. The best way to find the sources or services you are looking for is to do a search, using the keywords *preemie* or *premature baby*. This will give you a large listing of websites to choose among, and each of these websites will link you with others. In Appendix E you will also find a listing of websites of particular interest to parents of preemies. To get started, you might want to try these two comprehensive sites:

- **Mary Searcy's Resources for Parents of Preemies:**
  http://members.aol.com/maraim/preemie.htm. This site contains one of the most comprehensive listings of resources for parents of preemies, including books, clothing, websites, development, information on medical conditions, and more.

- The **Preemie-L** website:
  http://www.preemie-L.org. This is one of the first websites established for parents of preemies. Through it you can get access to an email support group of parents of preemies, a discussion forum (that is, you post a question and other parents answer you), an online newsletter called *The Early Edition*, and much more.

CHAPTER 7

Caring for Your Baby at Home

ℒℴ

THIS CHAPTER COVERS some of the most common aspects of caring for your baby at home that may be particularly problematic or worrisome to parents of preemies. In the first section you will find information on basic matters such as sleeping arrangements, keeping your baby warm, taking him on outings, immunization needs, and other aspects of his care. The second section covers some of the common concerns voiced by many parents of preemies, particularly around the issues of apnea and SIDS. The third section focuses on the special needs of babies with continuing health problems.

There is always a great deal of trial and error involved in learning how to care for any new baby, and methods that work for one baby will not necessarily work well for another. Or, what works well for your baby at one time may not work the next. Don't be discouraged if the first weeks or even months at home are rocky and confusing. Most parents of full-term newborns feel that way, too.

The Basics

The information here is meant to supplement what you know or have read about regular newborn care in order to help with some of the special concerns or challenges presented by your preemie.

Where Should Your Baby Sleep?

This question has no single right answer. Over the first few weeks you will probably need to experiment with different options; what works best will vary as your baby grows and his habits change.

Most parents of preemies start out sleeping in the same room with their baby, either by placing the crib or bassinet in their own room or by sleeping in their baby's room. Having your baby close to you during the night may ease some of the anxiety you naturally feel during the early weeks at home. Some parents prefer to bring their infants into bed with them to sleep, while others prefer having their baby in a separate bed. If your baby is on oxygen, an apnea monitor, or other specialized equipment, your options may be more limited. Your baby will probably need to be in his own bed and may need to be in a separate room.

Keep several things in mind as you experiment with sleeping arrangements. First, young preemies tend to be noisy sleepers. They spend a great deal of time in a state of light sleep during which they move around, startle, twitch, grunt, and even fuss. Because their nasal passages are still quite small, even small amounts of congestion or mucous can cause them to snore, snuffle, and sneeze. They also commonly breathe in an irregular pattern known as periodic breathing. You will hear your baby take several rapid breaths, pause for several seconds, and then take a deep breath. This pattern is completely normal for all newborns and particularly common for preemies. It is unrelated to any apnea spells that your child may have experienced earlier during his hospitalization.

But these things can make sleeping in the same room with your baby a challenge. After the first few weeks, you may want to move him into his own room. To listen in on him you can use a nursery monitor, an inexpensive intercom system that can be purchased at your local baby store. Even if your baby sleeps in your room, you may want to feed him in a different room so that your partner can get some uninterrupted sleep.

Back to Sleep . . . or Not?

Since the early 1990s, the American Academy of Pediatrics (AAP) has recommended that healthy newborn babies be placed on their backs to sleep. Their recommendations reflect a number of studies that strongly suggest that babies who sleep on their tummies are at higher risk of Sudden Infant Death Syndrome (SIDS). As more babies are being routinely placed on their backs to sleep, the death rate from SIDS has fallen.

But what about your premature baby? The AAP recommends that a healthy premature baby be treated like any other newborn at discharge and be placed on his back to sleep. A few exceptions temper this guideline. Babies with the following conditions may be better off sleeping on their tummies:

- premature infants with active respiratory disease,
- infants who vomit or spit up excessively (gastroesophageal reflux), and
- infants with facial deformities that may make it harder for them to breathe on their backs.

If you have any concerns about which position is right for your child, ask your pediatrician.

Most babies become accustomed to the position in which they are placed during the early weeks and months of their lives and sleep quite happily on their backs. However, others may dislike this position. If this is the case with your baby, you can try positioning him on his side. Place his back against the side of the crib or bassinet and position his lower arm out at right angles to his body to help keep him from rolling onto his stomach.

Some babies begin to roll over at a very early age and are impossible to keep on their backs or sides. Don't feel as if you need to go in to check on your baby constantly. In fact, the risk of SIDS is quite low no matter what position your baby sleeps in.

For further information about your baby's sleeping position, ask your pediatrician or call the Back to Sleep campaign at 1-800-505-CRIB. They can send you informative brochures and a video in English or Spanish. The Back to Sleep campaign is a public service education effort sponsored by the AAP, U.S. Public Health Service, SIDS Alliance, and Association of SIDS Program Professionals.

Helping Your Baby to Sleep

Although some preemies seem to spend most of their time sleeping, many others are poor sleepers. They tend to sleep for short amounts of time, wake frequently, and get disturbed easily. If your baby has trouble sleeping, you can try some of the following:

- Keep night-time feedings as short, simple and business-like as possible. Keep lights low, don't play or talk with your baby, and settle him back to sleep as soon as possible.

- Your baby may sleep better if he is swaddled, placed close to the side of his crib or bassinet, and given boundaries of rolled blankets or diapers against his feet for security and to help keep him in a flexed position. But leave his hands free so he can touch his face and suck on his fingers or fist.
- Kangarooing or carrying your baby in a sling close to your body may also help him sleep.
- Place his crib or bassinet in a quiet, dark location.
- If your baby sounds snuffly at night, raise the head of his crib or bassinet so he is lying slightly uphill. A humidifier may also be helpful, particularly in winter when indoor heated air tends to be quite dry. Check with your pediatrician for his recommendations, however, since humidifiers can become sources of germs if not used properly.

Calming Your Baby

Learning how best to comfort your baby can take a great deal of experimentation and some plain old luck. If your baby tends to be fussy or irritable, try some of these techniques:

- Swaddle him, keeping his hands free so he can touch his face and suck on his thumb or fist.
- Hold him in a flexed position, with his arms and legs tucked in.
- Limit the amount of stimulation around your baby: darken the room; stop talking to him or moving him; hold him, but don't pat him.
- Hold him upright on your shoulder, and walk with him or rock him.

Some babies are particularly challenging and require unusual approaches. One mother reported that the only way to calm her baby once he became upset was to swaddle him firmly, take him in a dark closet, and hold him close. Another baby was soothed by the sound of a vacuum cleaner. Some babies find riding in the car soothing.

No matter what you do, some crying is inevitable. Some babies seem to need to rid themselves of excess energy by crying before they sleep, others cry at regular times during the day, and others simply have days when nothing you do seems to help. As your baby grows and matures over the next several months, and begins to interact with you socially, you will notice the amount of crying and fussing decreasing.

Keeping Your Baby Warm

Your baby's body temperature was probably monitored often during his stay in the hospital, and you may wonder whether you should continue to watch it closely when you get him home. The answer is both yes and no. As long as your baby is dressed properly, he will have no trouble staying warm by the time he is ready to leave the hospital. But until he weighs about eight pounds, your baby won't have much fat to insulate him. He also will not be able to shiver or sweat very effectively, so he will have a harder time adjusting to very cold or warm temperatures, or wide swings in temperature. Although this isn't a big problem, you may want to take a little extra care in dressing him and in keeping his surroundings warm until he gains some weight.

Household Temperature. You don't need to keep your house as warm as the hospital nursery; a normal temperature of 68°F to 72°F should be fine for most babies. If your baby still weighs less than five pounds, you may want to keep your house a bit warmer, between about 72°F and 75°F. Until your baby weighs eight or ten pounds, try to maintain a constant temperature in your house. After that he can more easily tolerate changes in temperature, and you can let the night-time temperature dip to about 60°F as long as he is dressed properly.

Dressing Your Baby. The usual rule-of-thumb for dressing babies is to dress them in one more layer of clothing than you are wearing. For example, if you are wearing pants and a long-sleeved shirt, you will probably want to dress your baby in a footed sleeper-type outfit with an undershirt, and add a blanket. If your baby is under about six pounds, you may want to have him continue to wear one of the knit hats he has been wearing in the hospital, particularly at night. When the temperature is very warm, over about 85°F, your baby will need to be dressed only in a T-shirt and diaper, with perhaps a light covering to protect his legs from drafts. In the summer, be careful not to place your baby near an open window, a fan, or an air conditioner. He could become chilled even if the weather is very warm.

Judging Your Baby's Temperature. Overheated babies get red in the face, their skin feels quite warm and possibly sweaty, and they may fuss. A cold baby will become pale and fussy, and his hands and feet may look mottled or bluish. Because even a properly dressed baby usually has cool hands and feet, feel your baby's arms or legs or the back of his neck for a more reliable sense of his body temperature.

During the first few days your baby is home, you may want to take his temperature periodically just to reassure yourself that he is dressed properly. You will probably find that he has no problem maintaining the right temperature (98.6°F), and you will soon forget to think about it.

Bath Time

If you regularly bathed your baby in the hospital, you may feel confident about handling this task at home. But if you feel nervous about giving your tiny, slippery baby a bath by yourself, you have several options.

First, remember that babies do not have to be bathed every day. In fact, many preemies have thin and delicate skin and shouldn't be bathed more than once or twice a week at first. Between baths, simply clean your baby's diaper area, face, neck, and any creases where milk and dirt accumulate.

When your baby does need a bath, you may want to start out with a sponge bath instead of a tub bath. Sponge baths are easier since you don't have to wash and hold your baby at the same time. They may also be less stressful for your baby. Although some babies love tub baths, many others dislike being naked and become very upset during baths. To give a sponge bath, lay your baby on a padded surface (a folded towel on the kitchen counter works fine) and uncover and wash each part of his body separately. Then dry that part and re-cover it before moving on.

When you are ready to try a tub bath, choose a warm, draft-free room. The air temperature should probably be around 75°F to 80°F. You can bathe your baby whenever you want to, but it is probably best not to do it right after a feeding since all the extra handling may cause your baby to spit up. Use only a few inches of water at first, and test that the water is comfortably warm by dipping your wrist or elbow into it before slowly lowering your baby into the tub. Not all babies enjoy baths at first. If your baby seems tense or upset, try leaving his undershirt on and supporting him with a folded towel or piece of foam. Be sure to spread warm towels nearby to wrap him in after his bath.

Holding and washing a tiny infant can be challenging. The most secure way of holding your baby during a bath is to rest your baby's head on your wrist and encircle his upper arm (the arm farthest from you) with your thumb and fingers. That way your baby's head is firmly supported against your arm, and he cannot slip from your grasp. Wash him with your other hand. Since regular soap is drying, use only water on his face and a mild baby soap for the rest of his body. Soap his body with a baby-sized washcloth or your hand. Some parents have found it helpful to wear soft cotton gloves while bathing their babies; the gloves help you hold your baby securely and also make good washcloths. Cotton gloves can usually be found at the drugstore.

Never leave your baby unattended during a bath, even for a second. If you must turn away to reach for something, always keep one hand on him. Or, if you need to answer the phone or doorbell, wrap him up in a towel and take him with you.

Taking Your Baby Out

Taking your baby out for a walk in the fresh air and sunshine can be a great way to pick up your spirits, and often seems to help babies sleep better as well. As long as your baby weighs eight pounds or more, and the temperature outside is in the upper 60's or above, there shouldn't be any problem taking him for an outing. However, if your baby weighs less than eight pounds, or the weather is very cold or very hot, you should check with your pediatrician for his advice. Even if your baby has come home on oxygen or an apnea monitor, you can get out for walks using a small portable bottle of oxygen or a portable monitor. To hold any equipment your baby needs, your stroller should have a sturdy storage area below or behind the seat. In the car, wedge the bottle or monitor under the seat or secure it so that it won't become dislodged during a sudden stop or accident.

Although there are many benefits to getting out into the fresh air, watch your baby's reactions when you are outside. For some babies, the combination of movement, changing light patterns, air temperature, and noises may be stressful or overwhelming at first. My own son could only tolerate short walks in a baby carriage on smooth ground when he was young. If we walked too long or the road was bumpy, he would begin startling, and get very uncomfortable and tense. Sometimes I had to stop and hold him to help him relax.

As mentioned in Chapter 6, it is best to keep your baby away from crowded places for the first several months he is home.

Protecting Your Baby from the Sun. The best way to protect your baby is to stay out of the sun during its strongest hours from 10 a.m. to 3 p.m. If you will be out, keep your baby covered and have him wear a broad-brimmed hat or bonnet. Remember that your baby may be exposed to more sunlight than you realize on snowy or cloudy days, or at the beach where light reflects off the water and sand. Sunscreen is generally not recommended for babies under the age of six months, but check with your pediatrician for specific guidelines.

Kangarooing at Home

Kangaroo care continues to be beneficial for preemies after they come home. Dr. Susan Luddington-Hoe, a nurse-researcher who has studied kangaroo care extensively, recommends kangarooing your preemie at least one hour a day until he is three months past his original due date. Kangarooing seems to help babies sleep more soundly, fuss less, and eat better. It is also extremely useful if you are trying to breastfeed; with easy access to your breasts, your baby can nurse or even just nuzzle whenever he wants.

Here's how to kangaroo at home: after washing your hands and showering, place your diapered baby next to your skin with a loose-fitting shirt, smock, or robe over you both. If you use a sling or baby-carrier, you can wear your baby as you go about your normal activities. But for safety, don't wear your baby when you are cooking, or drinking hot liquids. And never wear him in a car. When you kangaroo, be alert for signs of stress such as fussiness, arching, or jerking. If your baby seems stressed as you move about, you may be more successful if you simply sit quietly while you are kangarooing.

Check with your doctor before kangarooing a baby on oxygen or a monitor. In these situations, you may want to kangaroo only while sitting down. Some parents even learn to sleep in a semi-upright position with their babies nestled securely on their chests.

You may be more comfortable with a modified form of kangarooing in which you carry your baby outside your clothes in a sling or baby-carrier.

The baby experts, William and Martha Sears, call this "babywearing." They advocate using a simple sling, which can be used to carry your baby in a number of positions.

Knowing When Your Baby Is Sick

When babies are sick, their behavior or appearance usually changes. They become lethargic or fussy, don't eat well, and look pale or flushed. Some of the most common signs of illness include:

- a fever of over 99°F axillary (armpit) or 100°F rectal
- coughing, sneezing, watery eyes, or dripping nose
- changes in behavior: your baby seems especially sleepy, lethargic, or fussy
- difficulty breathing: your baby may start breathing more rapidly, seem to be working harder at breathing, or have noisy or raspy breathing
- vomiting all or most of his feedings
- diarrhea: frequent, watery stools that may be greenish in color and foul-smelling
- fewer wet diapers and dark-colored urine
- changes in skin color: your baby may become pale or flushed.

However, preemies often act in unpredictable and confusing ways even when they are feeling fine. At times, this can make it difficult to tell if there is a problem. One mother told of such an experience:

"One day, out of the blue, when he was about three or four months old, Eric started screaming. He'd never done that before and nothing I did seemed to help. He'd been having trouble with constipation for a few days so I was worried that something serious was wrong. After he'd been scream-ing for about two or three hours, I started getting panicky and took him into the doctor's. It turned out there was nothing wrong, but I think when you have a preemie, it's hard not to worry."

If you are ever concerned about your child's health, don't hesitate to call your doctor. Particularly in the first few months, you may end up mak-ing more calls or visits than are strictly necessary. But you will soon become better at judging your child's health. You spend the most time with him, and will be the first one to notice when things are not right.

And as your baby grows, his behavior will become more predictable, making it easier to tell when he isn't feeling well.

Visiting the Pediatrician

If your baby has had a long hospitalization, weighs less than five pounds, or has continuing medical problems, you will probably see your pediatrician during your first week at home. Otherwise, bring your baby to the doctor within two weeks. This visit gives you a chance to ask questions and discuss any concerns you have. It also gives your doctor an opportunity to examine your baby and review with you his stay in the hospital. Be sure to take along your baby's discharge summary as well as care plans or other pertinent medical records.

Healthy preemies usually see the pediatrician on the same schedule recommended for full-term newborn babies. Although individual pediatricians may suggest a slightly different schedule, these regular well-baby checkups generally occur during the first year at one, two, four, six, nine, and twelve months (chronological age). You may want to see your pediatrician more often than that, particularly in the first several months at home, in order to ask questions or check on your baby's progress or weight gain. Post the pediatrician's phone number by your telephone and find out the best time to call with questions. If your baby has ongoing medical problems, you will probably see your doctor more frequently and have appointments with specialists as well.

When you take your infant to the doctor's (or for any outing), be sure to bring along a bag of basic baby supplies, including one or two changes of clothing, bottles, pacifiers, and extra diapers. As one mother recalled,

> "I was so nervous about getting Katie to the doctor's the first time, I forgot to bring the diaper bag. Of course, she chose that time to poop all over everything and all they had at the doctor's office were large-sized diapers. I had to take her home in a diaper that practically covered her whole body. It wasn't a big deal, but I felt like such a dope. I knew so much about all the special things that go into caring for a preemie, but I'd forgotten basic, simple baby stuff."

If your pediatrician's waiting room is full of sick children when you take your baby in for his checkups, ask if you can wait in an empty examining room or out in the hallway in order to avoid exposing him to germs.

Immunizations

Your baby should receive all the standard immunizations recommended for infants. Premature babies are immunized on the same schedule as full-term newborns based upon their chronological age. Your baby will receive his first DPT (diphtheria, pertussis and tetanus) shot and a dose of oral polio vaccine (OPV) when he is two months old as calculated from his actual date of birth. If he is still in the hospital at this point, he will receive his first DPT shot there but will not be given the OPV until discharge. In Appendix D, you will find the immunization schedule recommended by the AAP.

The immunization recommendations for preemies vary from those for full-term babies in a few situations.

- Babies with chronic lung disease should receive annual **flu shots** after they reach six months of age. Any adult involved in caring for a baby with CLD, as well as siblings and other family members in close contact with your baby, should also receive a flu shot each winter.
- The **hepatitis B vaccine,** usually given at birth to full-term babies, appears to be more effective in preemies if given at a later date. The AAP currently recommends postponing the initial inoculation until hospital discharge if the baby weighs 2,000 grams (4 pounds 7 ounces) or more, or until two months of age. This recommendation is only for infants of mothers who test negative for the hepatitis B antigen; babies born to mothers who test positive should receive an initial shot at birth.
- **Synagis** is an immunization that became available in the summer of 1998 to help prevent RSV infection, and lessen the severity of any RSV illness that does occur. At the present time, the AAP recommends that its use be considered for babies under two years of age with CLD who are currently on oxygen or have received oxygen in the last six months. Treatment with Synagis may also be worthwhile for premature babies without respiratory problems. Babies born at 28 weeks or less should receive Synagis during the winter until they are 12 months of age, while babies born between 29 and 32 weeks should be treated until they are six months old. Your baby should be given her initial Synagis injection a month before RSV season starts in order to give her time to build up a good level of resistance, and injections are

given once a month throughout the RSV season. Because Synagis is so new, it is quite expensive, costing approximately $900 per injection. Many pediatricians do not stock Synagis, and you may need to be referred to a hospital clinic or infant follow-up program to get your baby's injections.

• **Respigam**, or respiratory syncytial virus immune globulin intravenous (RSV-IGIV), is an earlier form of RSV-preventive that has now been largely supplanted by Synagis. Respigam is given intravenously (directly into a vein) throughout the RSV season, generally November through March, and costs about $4,000-$5,000 per season. Some babies are given an initial dose of Respigam in the hospital, and then given subsequent injections of Synagis once they are home.

• Preemies should receive their **measles-mumps-rubella (MMR)** and **chickenpox (varicella)** vaccinations at the regular time unless they are being treated with Respigam. Respigam interferes with these live vaccines and makes them less effective. The AAP recommends waiting for nine months after treatment with Respigam has ended before vaccinating your child with the MMR and varicella.

Common Questions and Concerns

In this section, you will find information on some of the questions that are of particular concern to many parents of preemies.

Can I call the NICU or special care nursery with questions after I've brought my baby home?

Most nurseries encourage parents to call with questions or concerns during the first few weeks at home. Since the nursery is open and busy 24 hours a day, there is usually someone to talk to, even in the middle of the night. Some hospitals even send one of their nurses out for a home visit during the first week or so. Unfortunately, a few hospitals discourage continuing contact between parents and nursery staff out of concerns for legal liability, so be sure to check your hospital's policy before you leave. Also, ask if there are regular times when it is better not to call, such as during shift changes or rounds.

Even though the nurses welcome your calls, remember that their primary responsibility is to care for the babies currently in the nursery so they may not be able to spend a great deal of time with you on the phone. In addition, their expertise lies in caring for hospitalized babies; they are less familiar with the many issues that arise as your baby grows and develops.

If you have become close to a particular nurse or nurses during your baby's hospitalization, you may feel like calling or visiting the nursery simply to stay in contact. A phone call, a note with pictures, or even a quick visit to the nursery are all appropriate ways of keeping in touch. The nurses or doctors you have become close to will appreciate news about your baby's progress. Some parents express their gratitude by putting together pictures of their infant to be hung in the nursery. These collages documenting a baby's progress from his early days in the nursery until discharge or later can really bolster the spirits of parents with new babies in the NICU.

My baby had many spells of apnea and bradycardia, and was on a monitor the whole time he was in the hospital. How can I be sure that he won't stop breathing once he's home?

If your baby has experienced episodes of apnea and bradycardia in the hospital, it is natural to worry about the possibility that this will happen again at home when there is no monitor to warn you. And the fact that most hospitals continue to monitor babies up until the time of discharge can give you the sense that your baby is still at some risk, even if your baby's nurse or doctor has reassured you that this isn't so. One mother whose baby had a long series of respiratory problems during his three months in the hospital reported that she was so anxious, she spent her son's first night at home sitting by his bassinet, watching him breathe. Another parent checked on her baby every two hours day and night for months to reassure herself that he had not stopped breathing.

A great deal of research has been conducted to investigate whether or not preemies continue to be at risk for apnea spells after they have outgrown the apnea of prematurity that so many experience in their early lives. After looking at all of the studies, the National Institutes of Health in 1992 concluded that there was no evidence to suggest that a baby who has experienced apnea of prematurity has an increased chance of having a later serious apnea attack. They also found that apnea of prematurity is not a separate risk factor for SIDS. Although premature babies in general have a higher rate of SIDS, this is unrelated to whether or not they have experienced apnea of prematurity.

In other words, once your baby has outgrown his apnea of prematurity which he indicates by having no episodes for a certain number of days, he is at no greater risk than any other baby for having a serious apnea episode at home. Knowing this may help to assuage some of your anxiety, but it takes many parents several weeks or months before they truly stop worrying about this problem.

Some babies continue to have apnea attacks as they near their original due dates. If your baby is otherwise ready to be discharged, he may be sent home on apnea-controlling medication, and sometimes on a home monitor. Most babies outgrow their tendency to have apnea and their need for the medication by the time they have been home for several months.

What About SIDS (Sudden Infant Death Syndrome)?

Most parents of new babies worry at least a little about Sudden Infant Death Syndrome (SIDS). Parents of preemies, particularly of those who have had respiratory problems or apnea spells in the hospital, probably worry more than most.

Here are the facts. SIDS, the sudden unexplained death of an infant under a year old, claimed the lives of approximately 2,700 of the approximately four million babies born in this country in 1997. The number of babies who die from SIDS has been declining steadily since 1992 when the American Academy of Pediatrics issued recommendations that babies sleep on their backs rather than their stomachs. In 1992, the SIDS rate was 1.5 per 1,000 live births; by 1997, the rate had dropped to less than half that, or .69 per 1,000 live births.

SIDS occurs more often during the fall, winter, and early spring months, and more boys than girls are affected. Most SIDS deaths occur between one and six months of age, with the highest incidence between two and four months. With preemies, the high-risk period appears to extend a little longer, possibly until about ten months of age.

Certain groups of infants, including premature babies and babies born weighing less than 2,500 grams (5 1/2 pounds) are at higher than normal risk, and the risk of SIDS increases as birthweight goes down. Preemies with bronchopulmonary dysplasia (chronic lung disease) are at highest risk, but some of the SIDS deaths reported among these children may actually have been caused by other illnesses.

The causes of SIDS have not yet been identified, but there are certain actions you can take that will lessen your child's risk. The most important of these is to place your baby to sleep on his back as explained earlier in this chapter. Other things you can do are:

- Make sure your baby sleeps on a firm mattress or other firm surface. Don't place your baby to sleep on a fluffy blanket, comforter, sheepskin, water bed, pillow or other soft material. Keep stuffed toys or pillows away from him while he sleeps.
- The temperature of your baby's room should feel comfortable to you. Your baby shouldn't be so heavily covered that he becomes hot or sweaty.
- Keep the environment around your baby as smoke-free as possible and never allow anyone to smoke near your baby.
- Breastfeed your baby if possible; babies who receive breastmilk have lower rates of SIDS.

The recommendations for keeping your baby on his back are for sleeping only. All babies also need to spend a certain amount of supervised time on their tummies while they are awake to aid in their physical development.

Your baby's chances of having a problem with SIDS are extremely small. For more information about SIDS and the Back-to-Sleep campaign, call 1-800-505-CRIB, or ask your pediatrician.

Special Situations

Babies on Oxygen

By the time a baby with continuing respiratory problems is discharged from the hospital, his need for supplemental oxygen is usually fairly slight. However, being on oxygen makes his life easier; he doesn't have to work as hard at breathing so he conserves calories and energy that can then be put into growth and development. In the past, doctors tried to wean babies off of oxygen as quickly as possible. Now, they tend to leave them on longer, although insurance companies sometimes push for earlier discontinuation. Babies on oxygen usually feed better, gain weight faster, and have an easier time recovering. Be sure to talk with your doctor or respiratory specialist before your baby is discharged about the plans for your baby, and their estimate of how long he will need to be on oxygen.

The respiratory therapist from the company that supplies you with oxygen will probably visit your baby on a regular schedule while he remains on oxygen. Review with the therapist how to set and read the flow regulator, how often to change the cannula, how to clean the cannula in case your baby spits up into it, how to secure the tubing to your baby's face, and how to get in touch with the company and/or a therapist in case you have questions or problems. Post their phone numbers near your telephone.

Travel: Your equipment company can provide you with a small portable oxygen bottle to take along on outings with your baby. This bottle can be carried in a sling or placed in the baby carriage or stroller.

Safety: Oxygen should never be used near an open flame, and do not allow anyone to smoke near your baby on oxygen. One couple found that the safety issue made it easier to ask people not to smoke in the house.

> *"We didn't want anyone smoking in our house anyway after all of the respiratory problems our babies had had, but having one of the twins on oxygen made it very easy to just hang up a sign saying* No Smoking. *No one could argue with us or give us any trouble, since it was a matter of safety."*

Babies on Monitors

Some babies who continue to have spells of apnea or bradycardia are sent home on apnea monitors. Others may come home on medications and be placed on a monitor after the medication is discontinued. Most families become accustomed to the use of a monitor fairly quickly, but false alarms can be stressful and tiring at first. One mother said,

> *"On the one hand we were glad to have it, but on the other it was a pain in the neck. It always went off in the middle of the night usually because Sammy had thrown up. You'd be standing there trying to push the button to*

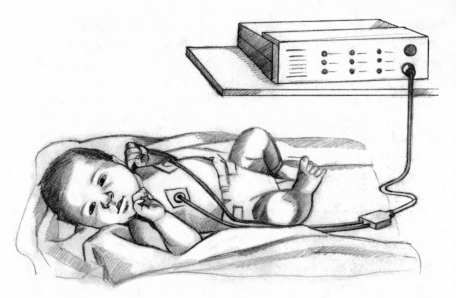

A typical home apnea monitor. Leads can be attached directly to the skin with sticky pads or held in place with a soft belt around your baby's chest.

shut the alarm off while trying to clean up the vomit and clear his cannula all at the same time."

Leave a small light on near your baby's crib at night so that if an alarm sounds you can easily check on him. If you find him sleeping peacefully with no change in his color, it's probably a false alarm. Common causes of false alarms include burping or vomiting, incorrectly placed or loose monitor leads, a baby's movement, and abdominal breathing, during which your baby uses his abdominal muscles more than his chest muscles to breathe.

But be sure you know what to do if you should find that your baby is unresponsive, pale, or dusky-colored. Post an emergency number near the phone and be familiar with infant CPR in the unlikely event that your baby has a serious apnea episode. You should also know whom to call for questions about the monitor. Someone should be available to you twenty-four hours a day, either at the equipment company or at the hospital.

Talk to your pediatrician or the specialist caring for your baby about when you can take your baby off the monitor. Obviously, you should disconnect your baby from the monitor before you bathe him. As long as you are directly watching or playing with him, it is usually safe to unhook him. Taking the electrodes off also gives your baby's skin a break if it is becoming irritated by the leads.

Travel: Even though your baby is on a monitor, you can easily take him in the car or for walks and outings. Most monitors are portable and your baby should remain monitored during trips. In the car, make sure your baby's car seat is located where someone can see and care for him. It's usually a good idea to have two adults in the car with a monitored baby, one to drive and the other to care for the baby if the alarm goes off. Make sure to wedge the monitor securely in the car so it can't be shaken lose in the event of a sudden stop. During walks and other outings, the monitor can be placed beside your baby in a stroller or baby carriage, or in the storage area.

Safety: Never leave a young sibling unsupervised with a monitored infant. All the wires and leads can be fascinating and dangerous. In particular, make sure that the monitor leads are securely connected to the monitor and that all wires are out of a child's reach.

Discontinuing Monitoring: It's natural to feel anxious about taking your baby off a monitor. When your doctor begins discussing plans for discontinuing the monitor, make sure you understand why it is now safe to remove it. You may want to wean yourself from dependence on the monitor by slowly increasing the amount of time your baby remains unhooked over several days or more. Leave him unmonitored for nap-times and then for sleeping at night. The transition can be difficult, and most parents find themselves checking on their baby frequently. But within a couple of weeks, you will probably feel more relaxed and enjoy not being awakened by false alarms in the middle of the night.

Babies on Medications

Many parents find it helpful to keep a log or diary of their baby's medications. If your baby is on multiple medicines or you have more than one infant to care for, keeping a log is almost essential (see sample log in Chapter 6). Include in your notes whether or not your baby spit up soon after being given the medicine or if you missed a dose. Some medicines can be given again to make up for a lost dose while others should not be.

Parents have come up with many different methods for keeping track of medicines. One mother of triplets gets organized at the beginning of each day by drawing up the different medicines her children take each day into small plastic syringes. She places these syringes into paper cups, each marked with the baby's name and the time the medicine should be given. Then she just has to grab the cup and she has everything her child needs at that particular time.

Another parent prepares all the bottles her child needs for that day in the morning. Into each bottle she places the medicines her child will need at that feeding, and marks each bottle with the feeding time. The formula or milk is added later. If your baby does not always finish a feeding, or if you are breastfeeding, you can place the medicine in a nipple with a small amount of milk or formula and feed it to your baby before his regular nursing or bottle. That way you are sure he has taken the full dosage he is meant to get.

CHAPTER 8

Feeding Your Baby at Home

ℬ

B Y THE TIME YOUR BABY
is ready to come home, she will have developed the ability to feed well enough by bottle, breast, or some combination that she is gaining weight consistently. But her feeding behavior and habits may still be quite immature and unpredictable. Her stomach is tiny so she may need frequent small feedings. She may feed slowly and tire easily, or be easily distracted and upset. It may be hard to tell when she is hungry; she may need special formulas, or extra help with her feedings.

In addition, you may be particularly anxious about feeding. Your baby may still be quite small or have ongoing medical problems that make it important that she consume enough calories every day. She may have had a hard time learning to take bottles or to breastfeed, and you may not feel totally confident of her abilities. On the other hand, feedings may have been going smoothly in the hospital, but your baby becomes fussy and difficult at home, and you are surprised at the change.

Not every preemie will have trouble, but, in general, these babies are more challenging to feed than full-term babies. In the words of one mother whose experience was echoed time and again by other parents, "The hardest thing [in adjusting to home] was feeding her. I was not prepared for how difficult it was." Fortunately, many of these problems are short-lived, and improve as your baby matures and gains strength, coordination, and energy. Others can be harder to solve or continue for a longer time. In the most difficult cases, you may need to seek help from a professional feeding specialist.

As with other aspects of preemie parenting, the more you understand about the common challenges presented by preemies, the more prepared you'll feel if problems do arise. The first section of this chapter focuses on issues that arise in feeding in the early weeks and months at home, including how often and how much to feed your baby, finding the right nipples and formula, subtle ways that preemies signal hunger, and common feeding problems. This section includes general information on feeding as well as issues specifically related to bottle-feeding. The second section is devoted to breastfeeding, including how to move toward more frequent or full-breastfeeding, how to tell if your baby is getting enough to eat, and methods of increasing your milk supply. The final section, Special Situations, provides information about tube feedings at home, how to add calories to feedings, colic, and finding professional help.

This chapter is meant to be used in conjunction with a regular child care or breastfeeding book; it does not aim to provide you with everything you need to know about feeding your baby, but focuses instead on the concerns specific to feeding a preemie. Always check with your pediatrician before trying something new, or when you are unsure about any aspect of your baby's feeding or behavior.

General Feeding Issues and Bottle-Feeding

During their first weeks at home, most preemies receive some or all of their feedings by bottle. This is true even for babies whose mothers are working toward partial or full breastfeeding. Because bottle-feeding is so common among preemies, this section is geared toward bottle-feeding, and includes detailed information on many of the concerns that preemie parents feel as they begin to feed their baby at home without the help and supervision of nursery staff. However, it also contains more general feeding information that is applicable to both bottle-feeding and breastfeeding.

Getting Started

Your first week at home may go more smoothly if you are able to plan ahead for some of the changes you will need to make in feeding your baby. The formulas, nipples, and bottles that are available in your local drugstores or grocery stores are probably different from those you and your baby have become accustomed to in the hospital. Some babies can switch from one to the other with no trouble, but you may want to prepare ahead in case your baby is one of those who doesn't react well to changes.

There are two approaches you can use. If you have time, you can buy several nipples and bottles from your local store and begin to feed your baby with them while she is still in the hospital. This way you can find a starter system for home that works well for your baby while you still have the security of the nursery and the advice of your baby's nurse to rely upon. However, if you are not able to accomplish this switch before your baby is discharged, bring home enough of the nipples your baby likes from the hospital so that you will not need to experiment much during the first week or two at home. Many parents prefer to continue using the small, graduated plastic feeding tubes at home, so you may want to bring home some of these also. "I was so used to measuring Katie's feedings in those tubes," said one mother, "even the small [4 oz.] bottles seemed too big and imprecise at first. I had no idea how much formula to put in them."

The same transition also occurs with formula. Before your baby leaves the hospital, try to get her established on the formula that she will be using at home. Most of the special formulas used in the hospital are not available commercially, so if your baby needs special formula or higher calorie formula it is even more important to try out her new formula before discharge. Again, if this is not possible, bring home enough of the hospital formula so that you can make the transition slowly, and have enough to fall back upon if your baby has any trouble with the changeover. One family stressed the importance of this:

> *"Our daughter was discharged on a weekend right before Christmas. She had been on 24-calorie formula in the hospital, and we were told to use regular powdered formula at home but to mix it to be more concentrated. We had the recipe and everything, but every time we tried to feed it to her she would throw it back up again. We didn't have enough of the hospital formula left, the stores were closed, and our daughter hadn't eaten anything in twenty-four hours. It was a bad way to begin at home."*

During the first weeks at home, you may need to experiment with different nipples, formulas, feeding schedules and techniques in order to find an approach that works well with your baby. Often there is no simple solution to getting your baby to eat well, nor is there one approach that will work well for your baby all of the time. Your baby's responses may change day to day, or within one day, and as she grows and changes, her feeding habits will change as well. You may stumble across something that works purely by accident, as this mother's story illustrates:

"Sarah fed beautifully in the hospital but when we got home she started to have trouble; she'd take a little bit of her bottle and then fall asleep. It was summer and very hot, so one day I took her down to the basement where it was cool to feed her. All of a sudden she started eating like a champ. I don't know whether it was the coolness or the relative darkness of the basement. I thought maybe the fluorescent lights might have reminded her of the hospital, but, whatever it was, it really worked. She and I spent a lot of time in the basement for the first few months at home."

Establishing a Feeding Schedule

In general, your baby will need to be fed six to eight times or more per day. Ask the neonatologist in the hospital or your pediatrician what the maximum length of time is that your baby should go between feedings. Usually, she should not go more than five hours without being awakened to feed, but if your baby is small or has ongoing medical needs, you may need to feed her more often.

Preemies are usually fed on a time-based schedule (such as every two or three hours), or on a modified demand schedule at first. To be fed on demand means that your baby is fed whenever she indicates that she is hungry, usually because she wakes up and begins to fuss. Using a straight demand schedule with preemies can be difficult at first, however, because they may not wake up or give clear signs that they are hungry. Using a modified demand schedule means that you watch your baby for signs of hunger so that you can time your feedings to her needs, but if she sleeps too long, you wake and feed her.

How Your Baby Tells You She's Hungry

The ways in which a preemie signals that she is hungry can be more subtle and difficult to identify than those of a full-term baby. Some preemies will wake and fuss or cry when it is time to eat, but there are a number of other signs that you can watch for, particularly if you have a sleepy baby or one

who seems not to wake regularly to feed. In order to detect these more subtle cues, you need to watch your baby closely. During the day, either keep
her bassinet near you while she sleeps or check on her every half hour or so
if she is in a different room. Don't worry about trying to do this at night;
simply feed her on a predetermined schedule.

Your baby may signal her hunger in the following ways:

- by beginning to move around in her sleep, possibly grunting, making
  faces, smiling, making sucking motions;
- by bringing her hands to her face or mouth, possibly sucking on her
  fist;
- by rooting, turning her head toward something, touching her cheek
  and trying to suck.

When you see any of these signs, and two or three hours have passed since
the last feeding, it probably indicates that your baby is getting hungry.
Gently try to bring her more fully awake before you begin feeding her. Pick
her up, unwrap her if she is swaddled, change her diaper, or brush her
cheek with your finger. Giving your baby a pacifier to suck on may help
her wake up and get ready to feed, but with some babies it can have the
opposite effect, causing them to fall back into a deeper sleep.

Knowing How Much to Feed Your Baby

Before you take your baby home, discuss with her neonatologist how much
formula or milk she should consume in one day. Since babies will not
always drink the same amount at each feeding, it is more helpful to know
the total volume your baby should take in a day rather than what she
should take at each feeding.

A baby who weighs between 4 and 5 pounds will need approximately
12 to 15 ounces of formula or breastmilk per day, or about 2 to 3 ounces
per feeding. As your baby grows, she will gradually increase her intake,
sometimes in rather sudden increments. If your baby finishes her bottle
quickly and almost seems to be looking for more, or begins to wake up earlier for her next feeding, increase the amount of formula you offer her. Do
not try to force her to take extra; simply put more in the bottle and see if
she wants it.

While your baby was in the hospital, you probably became accus-

tomed to measuring her feedings in milliliters (ml) or cubic centimeters (cc). At home, bottles are usually marked in ounces (oz). One ounce (oz) equals approximately 30 mls (or ccs). So if your baby has been taking between 45 and 60 mls per feeding in the hospital, this is equivalent to 1 1/2 to 2 ounces per feeding at home. Many parents continue to use the small feeding tubes at home; it is easier to measure small volumes with them and babies sometimes have an easier time feeding because they need to build up less suction to get the milk or formula flowing.

If your baby is getting enough to eat she will have at least six to eight wet diapers a day. If she has fewer than this—say you go to change her diaper before a feeding and it is still dry from the feeding before—or if her urine is strong smelling or dark yellow, she may not be getting enough to eat and is becoming dehydrated. If the dehydration becomes severe, she may seem listless and the soft spot (fontanel) on her head will become sunken. This is a serious situation and warrants an immediate call to your doctor.

Concerns About Weight Gain

Most babies will gain between about 1/2 and 1 ounce (15 to 30 grams) per day, or about 3 to 8 ounces per week. However, there is a great deal of variability among preemies. Some babies, particularly those born very early or small, or those with ongoing respiratory problems, gain very slowly. Some doctors will try to increase such a baby's weight gain by adding calories to her feedings, while others take a more passive approach. As long as the baby is the proper weight for her length, they will simply monitor her growth.

If you are concerned about your baby's consumption or her weight, speak to your pediatrician and see if you can drop in regularly to do a quick weight check. It may be possible to rent a baby scale from the same source that rents breast pumps. The nurse at your local early intervention program may be able to bring a scale over for a quick check.

Choosing the Right Nipples and Bottles

Most babies have outgrown their need for the soft red preemie nipples and are ready for normal, newborn-type nipples by the time they go home. In fact, the rapid flow of milk through the red nipples can cause some babies to choke or hold their breaths. If you are worried about your baby's ability to handle a tougher nipple, you can judge the strength of her suck by placing a clean finger, nail side down in your baby's mouth and letting her suck on it. A baby with a strong suck will almost pull your finger down her throat.

There are a number of different types and shapes of nipples available on the market today and you may need to experiment to find one that works well for your baby. Most nipples are marked as having a low, medium, or high flow rate, and your baby will probably do best with a low flow rate nipple at first. These may also be called newborn nipples. If your baby is still quite small or has low muscle tone, you may want to try the preemie nipple made by Evenflo. Just be sure that the flow rate is not too high—milk or formula should drip slowly from the nipple at about one drop per second when the bottle is turned upside down. Another company (Avent) makes a nipple that combines all three flow rates into one nipple. As the bottle is turned, the flow rate of the nipple changes. The side of the nipple has markings on it which indicate the flow rate.

There are preemies who like all types of nipples, although the nipples that come with disposable plastic nursers seem to be the most difficult to use. If you prefer these nursers but your baby doesn't do well with the nipple, there are adapter rings available in most drugstores that allow you to put other types of nipples on these bottles.

If your baby tends to swallow air or spit up a lot, you may want to try the disposable nursers or the angled bottles. Otherwise, choosing bottles to use is strictly a matter of personal preference or availability. It is probably easier to use the small 4-ounce bottles when your baby first comes home, or the small plastic graduated tubes used in the hospital.

Bottles and nipples can usually be kept sufficiently clean by washing in hot, soapy water or in a dishwasher. Some pediatricians recommend sterilizing them for the first few months, so check with your doctor for recommendations for your own child.

Finding the Right Formula

There are an amazing and confusing number of formulas on the market. Those that are readily available on drug- and grocery-store shelves can be divided into three main categories:

- milk-based formulas: Similac, Enfamil, and Good Start;
- soy-based formulas: Isomil, ProSobee, and Alsoy;
- special elemental formulas: Pregestimil, Nutramigen, and others.

Within the main categories there are further subdivisions, such as iron-fortified formulas and milk-based formulas that are lactose-free, in which milk sugar has been replaced by other sugars. The special formulas are designed to be easier to digest because their proteins have been broken down into smaller pieces. Good Start is also marketed as having smaller proteins and being easier to digest.

The basic formulas are usually available in three forms: ready-to-feed, liquid concentrate that needs to be diluted with water, and powder. The ready-to-feed is the most convenient but most expensive; powdered formula is useful if you only need to mix up bottles periodically or will be without access to a refrigerator. If you need to concentrate formula for added calories, use the liquid concentrate or powdered forms. Some babies seem to prefer the liquid forms of formula over the powdered forms.

Ross Products now offers a formula known as NeoSure, and Mead-Johnson has developed Enfamil 22. These formulas are specifically designed for premature babies for the first year of life. They contain 22 calories per ounce (regular formula has 20 calories per ounce) and higher levels of protein, calcium, and other nutrients that preemies need. If your neonatologist recommends that you use NeoSure or Enfamil 22, find out where you can get it before you leave the hospital. They are not always on drug- or grocery-store shelves at this time but should be available by special order through many of the large chains. Both of these formulas are available only in a powdered form.

Sometimes it can be difficult to find a formula that seems to agree with your baby. Very few babies are actually allergic to cow's milk, but your baby may seem uncomfortable on regular formula. It isn't clear whether this is just another sign of preemie sensitivity or whether the formula is difficult for them to handle. However, it probably makes sense to start with a regular milk-based formula, preferably iron-fortified (Similac, Enfamil, Good Start, NeoSure, or Enfamil 22) unless your neonatologist or pediatrician recommends otherwise. Then if your baby seems to be having trouble, you can try another formula, such as a lactose-free or soy-based formula. If a formula switch is going to help, you will usually see an improvement in your baby within about 48 hours. The special elemental formulas are marketed as being helpful for severe cases of colic; they are much more expensive, but if your baby has colic, you may want to try one for 48 hours to see if her symptoms improve.

Be sure to discuss any feeding problems your baby is having with your pediatrician before you make any changes in her formula.

Your Baby's Need for Nutritional Supplements

The recommended daily needs of premature infants for nutritional supplements (vitamins, minerals, fluoride) are the same as those of full-term infants, according to the guidelines of the American Academy of Pediatrics. Your pediatrician can advise you on the best way to meet those needs.

The one area in which preemies are particularly at risk is in their need for iron. Because they have less iron stored in their bodies at birth, they run out more quickly when they begin to manufacture red blood cells. In order to avoid further problems with anemia, preemies should receive iron supplements starting two months after birth. This can be in the form of iron-fortified formula, multivitamin drops with iron, or ferrous sulfate drops.

Common Feeding Problems and How to Handle Them

There are a number of common behaviors or problems that many babies show that can make feedings more difficult or frustrating at times. These are discussed below along with suggestions for ways of handling them. Your baby may have none of these problems, or may have one or two on a short-term basis. Some babies have a very difficult time feeding and you may want to consult your pediatrician or feeding specialist for advice and help.

The Sleepy Baby

For many preemies, the need for sleep seems to override the need to eat. Left alone, these babies do not wake regularly or often enough for feedings. As one mother recalled, "I tried to move my daughter toward a demand schedule, but she would sleep for six hours at a time and I would panic."

If your baby falls into this category, you will probably need to set up a regular schedule for feedings for a while, or use a modified demand schedule (described above). Learn to recognize some of the more subtle ways in which your baby signals that she is getting hungry. Ask your baby's neonatologist or pediatrician how long to allow your baby to sleep between feedings. Commonly parents are advised not to let a baby go for more than five hours. If your baby is still very small or has increased need for calories, you may need to wake her more often.

Some babies wake regularly for feedings but fall asleep again so quickly that it is difficult to complete a feeding. Several things may be happening in this situation. Your baby may simply not have the energy yet to finish a large feeding, and you may have more success if you feed her smaller amounts more frequently. If your baby is on oxygen, the extra effort involved in feeding may be causing her oxygen-saturation levels to drop slightly. Although this drop is not dangerous, it will cause her to become tired and sleepy (she is probably feeling a little woozy). After talking with your pediatrician or respiratory therapist, you can try boosting the flow rate of oxygen a bit during feedings to see if that helps. Some babies recently off oxygen may need some blow-by oxygen during feedings.

Finally, your baby may be falling asleep because there is too much going on around her while she feeds and she is reacting by falling asleep to protect herself. The act of feeding is full of stimulation—being held, having milk flowing into the mouth and throat, coordinating sucking, swallowing and breathing. For many babies, adding anything else, such as talking, movement, noise from TV, radio, or other children, or bright lights, interferes significantly with their ability to focus on feeding. Look at the environment when you feed your baby and see if there are ways that you can cut down on excess noise or other types of stimulation.

The Baby Who Holds Her Breath

Learning to feed orally requires that your baby be able to coordinate sucking, swallowing, and breathing. While she is mastering this sequence, your baby may become too intent on sucking and forget to breathe. Or the flow of milk into your baby's mouth may be so fast that she is having a hard time handling it. Breath-holding makes feedings somewhat nerve-wracking for you and tiring for your baby.

If you notice that your baby is sucking intently without taking a break and begins to slow down, or look pale or sleepy, she probably needs to breathe. Pull the nipple from her mouth and let her catch her breath. One lactation consultant recommends removing the nipple regularly after every three to four sucks to prevent this situation from developing.

If your baby's mouth is full of milk and she seems to be having difficulty handling it, turn her onto her stomach across your knees to help it drain from her mouth. This, along with breath-holding, may be a sign that the nipple you are using is too soft or has too high a flow rate. Find one that is firmer or has a lower flow rate and see if your baby has an easier time. Babies usually outgrow the tendency to hold their breath while feeding by the time they reach their due dates or a few weeks after.

Fussy, Difficult-to-Feed Babies

Some babies seem to fight having a nipple placed in their mouths, or take a few sucks and then begin to fuss. This makes feeding extremely difficult and frustrating. Babies with ongoing respiratory problems or those who have had a rough time in the hospital can be particularly challenging. If your baby falls into this category, try feeding her in a darkened, quiet place, avoid making eye contact or talking, and do not rock her as you are feeding her. She may do better if she is swaddled (leave her hands free so she can touch her face). It may also help if you change her diaper after the feeding rather than before to cut down on activity.

Babies who have had early unpleasant experiences with their mouths such as suctioning, the endotracheal tubes of respirators, or feeding tubes often develop a strong dislike of having anything around or in their mouths. This is called an oral aversion and can clearly make feeding difficult.

To help counteract these early unpleasant associations, try to give your baby as many pleasurable experiences with her mouth as possible. Touch her around her face and mouth with gentle, firm strokes. Encourage her to touch her own face, particularly around her mouth. You may get her to suck on her fist or on a pacifier. Not only will this help her experience some pleasurable sensations with her mouth, but it will also help build her sucking muscles. She may have a strong preference for one type of nipple; try not to change nipples too often or experiment with too many different kinds. If you continue to have real trouble getting her to eat, ask for a referral to a feeding specialist.

Babies with a Weak Suck and/or Low Muscle Tone

Some babies, such as those with low muscle tone who are very soft and floppy feeling, or who are young and small, have little muscle strength in their cheeks and around their mouths. They tire easily when they feed and may have trouble maintaining suction around a nipple. You can help them feed by providing gentle support with a finger under their jaw, or with your thumb and forefinger pressing gently on their cheeks. You may have to experiment with different types of nipples and bottles.

It is important for your baby to build up the muscle strength around her mouth and in her cheeks. Try to move her away from nipples that are too soft such as the red preemie nipples as soon as possible. Feeding her small amounts more frequently may allow you to use a firmer nipple and build her strength. It would probably be valuable to talk with a feeding specialist for further strategies.

Spitting Up or Gastroesophageal Reflux

Spitting up, also known as reflux, is another very common trait among premature babies. Although rarely serious, it can make life difficult, as this mother describes:

> *"My son spit up so much, I basically spent the first year of his life sitting in a chair in the kitchen, twenty-four hours a day. I never knew when he would spit up and I didn't want it in the living room or bedroom....I felt like I was constantly covered in throw up."*

Spitting up is most often caused by an immature or weak muscle at the bottom of the esophagus where it enters the stomach. This allows the contents of the stomach to get pushed back up into the throat and out the mouth. Sometimes the milk will only come part way up the throat so that the baby does not actually spit up. Because stomach acids can irritate the esophagus, your baby may act uncomfortable after feedings, or cry and squirm if this is happening.

In most cases, reflux is not a serious problem. As long as your baby continues to eat well, gain weight, and not seem too uncomfortable, medical treatment is usually unnecessary. If you are concerned that your baby is losing too much of her feeding, try pouring a tablespoon or two of milk on a counter to see what it looks like. Most reflux amounts are not significant and amount to a teaspoon or two of milk mixed with stomach juices and mucous. In most cases, spitting up decreases gradually as your baby grows, and is usually gone by about 6 to 12 months of age.

There are a number of things you can try that may help to decrease the amount of spitting up your baby is doing. First, try not to jostle her during or after a feeding, hold her in more of an upright position, burp her often, and make sure she isn't sucking in air with the milk in the bottle. Angled bottles or those with collapsing disposable bags may help decrease the amount of air she takes in. Holding your baby upright against your shoulder for about 30 minutes after a feeding may help the milk settle and reduce spitting. You can also place your baby on her stomach with the head of her bed raised so that she is lying at a 45° to 80° degree angle for 30 to 60 minutes after a feeding. If you worry about placing your baby on her stomach, position her on her right side instead; this helps the food pass more quickly through her stomach. Sitting her in an infant seat may actually put more pressure on your baby's tummy and cause more spits.

Some pediatricians suggest that you thicken your baby's feeding with one or two tablespoons of infant rice cereal per ounce of formula. You will have to cut a cross-hatch in the nipple in order to get the thickened formula to flow and it can be quite frustrating to get this to work right. If you are breastfeeding, you can give your baby some rice cereal before or during her feeding. Smaller, more frequent feedings may also help.

If your baby seems extremely uncomfortable after feedings, is not gaining weight, or begins to vomit more forcefully so that the vomit shoots over your shoulder and lands some distance away, talk to your doctor immediately. Something more serious may be going on, or your baby may need some treatment to help her be more comfortable or to help her digestion.

Starting Solids

Parents of preemies are generally counseled to begin introducing solid foods into their baby's diet on the same schedule used for full-term infants, but based upon their baby's corrected rather than their chronological age. In most cases, this means starting small feedings of infant rice cereal or mashed fruit when your baby is between 4 and 6 months old (corrected age). By this time, many babies can hold their heads up fairly well and are beginning to show an interest in what is going on around them, including mealtimes, food, and eating. In addition, the tongue-thrust reflex which causes babies to push solid foods out of their mouths automatically begins to disappear. All baby books provide guidelines on how to begin feeding your baby solid foods, and your pediatrician can give you additional guidelines as you get started.

But as with many other aspects of preemie care, you may find that there are some additional complications associated with starting solid foods. For example, the timing may not seem very clear. Because of the unevenness of preemie development, some babies seem ready to start solids based more on their chronological than their adjusted age. Others, particularly those with low muscle tone, oral aversions, or continuing lung problems, may need to wait longer than usual.

You may want to look for other indications of readiness for solids rather than to rely solely on age. For example, even if your child is on the young side, if she seems interested in food and has good head control, you can try giving her a spoonful or two of thin rice cereal, or mashed ripe banana thinned with formula or breastmilk (with your pediatrician's okay). Although most babies are surprised by the new tastes and textures presented by solid foods, they generally begin to get the hang of this new skill within a few days if they are developmentally ready. If, on the other hand, your baby has a lot of trouble handling even thin cereal or fruit puree, wait for a few more weeks and try again.

Another common difficulty reported by parents of preemies is trouble with lumpy foods, such as those found in stage 2 and 3 baby foods, or with foods containing different textures such as peanut butter on toast. This occurs particularly among sensitive babies who dislike having anything placed around or in their mouths. The mixture of textures seems to be particularly repugnant or difficult for them to handle. If your baby falls into this category, she may do better with individual foods than with mixtures. You can try small pieces of soft cooked vegetables, dry foods such as Cheerios or small toast squares, and smooth cereals and yogurt. You will probably need to do a lot of experimentation and exercise a great deal of patience in order to find foods that are acceptable to your child. You may also want to get some ideas from an occupational therapist, nutritionist, or feeding specialist. Even the most difficult and fussiest eaters slowly develop an ability to handle foods of different textures as they grow, although many continue to show strong likes and dislikes for years. Meanwhile, you can add calories to the few foods that your child does enjoy (or at least tolerate) to assuage some of your concern over her intake (see "Adding Calories to Formula and Solid Foods" in the Special Situations section at the end of this chapter).

Breastfeeding Your Baby

If you pumped milk and did some initial breastfeeding while your baby was in the hospital, you are probably hoping to move toward more frequent or even full-breastfeeding at home. You should know at the outset that for many mothers and preemies the transition to complete breastfeeding is an extremely challenging goal. It takes time, commitment, energy, work, and luck. This is not meant to discourage anyone from trying, but to let you know from the beginning that it is not easy.

There are mothers who have surmounted all kinds of odds in order to successfully breastfeed, including one mother who was able to fully breastfeed quadruplets born at 34 weeks (in the first month after the babies came home from the hospital she breastfed between 12 and 34 times a day). And these mothers generally feel that breastfeeding was worth all the time and effort involved. Your chances of being successful are greater if your baby was born no more than five weeks early, if you have the help of a lactation specialist who is experienced with preemies, and if you and your baby have had a lot of practice nursing in the hospital before you came home.

But for many babies and mothers, including Philip and me, an intermediate approach is more realistic. Although I tried for weeks to increase the number of feedings Philip took directly at the breast, he was never an energetic nurser. Finally, while not exactly giving up, I decided to nurse him only once or twice a day, but to continue to pump milk, and bottle-feed him breastmilk or a combination of milk and formula for the remaining feedings. As he grew, he slowly outstripped my milk supply and moved gradually toward all formula feedings. I think our experience is a common one among preemies and mothers. However, I knew little about how to increase the chances of success with a preemie. In this section of the chapter, you will find a number of methods that you can try to improve your ability to breastfeed your baby.

Before You Leave the Hospital

To prepare for breastfeeding your baby at home, breastfeed as much as possible while your baby is still in the hospital, keep your milk supply high by continuing to pump regularly, and get a copy of a good, basic breastfeeding book.

The more experience both you and your baby have with nursing directly at the breast before you come home, the greater your chances of being successful at breastfeeding at home. Ideally, your nursery will have a lactation specialist who can help you learn the basics of breastfeeding a preemie, including how to position your baby at your breast and how to gradually move toward more frequent breastfeeding. Unfortunately, the support for mothers who want to nurse their babies is often fairly limited and you may find yourself pretty much on your own. Research during the last decade by Dr. Paula Meier and her colleagues at the University of Illinois has shown that breastfeeding a preemie is actually less stressful than bottle-feeding, and the support for and knowledge about the special challenges of breastfeeding a preemie have improved dramatically, but is still lacking in many places.

In order to breastfeed your baby frequently in the hospital, you must spend a good portion of your day there. This may not be possible if you have gone back to work or have other children at home to care for. In this situation, try to breastfeed at least once a day, if possible. One mother suggested having a nurse take a Polaroid picture of your baby properly positioned and latched on: "Once I got home I could look at the picture to make sure I was doing it right."

Keeping your milk supply high is almost as important as practicing feeding your baby. Preemies often come home before their due dates and do not have the energy for long feedings. The higher your milk supply, the easier time your baby will have getting an adequate volume of milk. She will be able to get most of what she needs during the initial milk let-down and not have to work hard at nursing. In addition, you can pump the extra and use it in supplemental feedings after or between breastfeeding sessions. Many mothers find that their milk supply begins to dwindle after weeks or months of pumping. Two weeks or so before your baby is scheduled for discharge, begin to rebuild your supply, if possible.

As you get started at home, many of your questions and concerns will be similar to those of any mother learning to breastfeed a baby. Even when a baby is born full-term, breastfeeding is not something that mothers and babies know how to do instantly and instinctively; it takes time, practice, and patience to develop your skills and confidence. As you learn, referring to a breastfeeding book can be enormously helpful. See Appendix E for a list of books for nursing mothers.

Increasing Your Milk Supply

It can be very difficult to maintain your milk supply over weeks and months of pumping. Most mothers find that their supply gradually dwindles so that by the time their baby is ready to come home they are not producing enough milk. You can estimate how much milk you are producing by keeping track of how much you pump during one twenty-four-hour period. Since pumps are not as efficient as nursing babies, you are probably producing slightly more than it appears, but you will have a general idea of your supply. Compare this amount with the amount your baby is being fed in the hospital.

You can also calculate how much milk your baby needs by multiplying her weight in kilograms (1 kg. = 2.2 pounds) by 22.5. This will tell you how many milliliters of milk your baby needs per day. To convert this amount to ounces, divide the total by 30. If your supply is much lower than your baby needs, try to build it up before she comes home.

Increase the Number of Times You Are Pumping. Your milk supply will grow in response to more frequent pumpings rather than longer ones, so try to pump at least seven or eight times per day if possible. Some mothers pump every three hours during the day and reserve a five-hour stretch at night to sleep. Unfortunately, it probably isn't possible to give yourself a break of eight hours at night when you are trying to increase your milk supply.

Use a Double Pump Set-Up. Use a double pump set-up so you are pumping both breasts at the same time. This not only saves you time but also stimulates higher prolactin levels, which helps to increase your supply. Pump until you are producing only drops of milk, approximately 10 to 15 minutes.

Get Enough Rest, Eat Well, and Drink Plenty of Fluids. Try to keep nutritious foods around to snack on during the day, and drink eight to ten glasses of water or other fluids a day. If you are not sleeping much at night, try to put your feet up for a few minutes several times a day. Continue to take your prenatal vitamins while you are producing breastmilk.

Consider a Dietary Supplement. You can try a dietary supplement to stimulate milk production. In particular, many mothers have found fenugreek to be helpful when they are trying to build their milk supply. Fenugreek is a harmless substance used to flavor artificial maple syrup; it is available as a tea or in capsules at most health food stores. The usual dosage is two or three capsules a day. While you are taking it you may notice that your urine and sweat have a maple syrup odor. Some women find that brewer's yeast is helpful also. It is available as a powder that can be mixed into a drink or as a capsule, and can be found at most health food stores. A prescription drug, Reglan, helps stimulate milk production but has been known to cause stomach upsets in some nursing babies.

Basically, it takes time and effort to build a milk supply. As one mother cautioned,

> *"In most nursing books, it tells you that when your baby hits a growth spurt and needs more milk, it only takes a couple of days of nursing him more frequently before your body responds and starts to make more milk. In my experience it wasn't nearly that fast, maybe because pumping isn't as efficient. It always seemed to take me about two weeks of really working at it before I would see an increase."*

Your body may respond more quickly than this, but if it takes you longer than a couple of days, try not to become discouraged. If you keep pumping, in most cases, your breasts will eventually respond. It will be easier once your baby can do more of the work for you.

Storing Your Milk at Home

At home, your freshly pumped milk can be safely stored for the following amounts of time:

At room temperature:	6 to 10 hours
In a regular refrigerator:	24 hours
In a freezer compartment inside refrigerator:	2 weeks
In a freezer with a separate door:	4 months
In a freezer below 0°F:	6 months

When you want to use some of your frozen breastmilk, thaw it in the refrigerator or under running water. Once it is thawed, it will remain safe to use for one hour at room temperature, or 24 hours in the refrigerator. Never refreeze thawed milk.

The Early Weeks at Home

Very few preemies are able to breastfeed fully at the time they are discharged. Many come home several weeks before their due dates, weighing less than five pounds, and do not have the necessary stamina to take in all of the milk they need from breastfeeding. You will need to gradually increase the amount of time your baby spends at your breast over the first several weeks at home, and slowly decrease the amount of supplemental feedings she receives.

Never go "cold turkey" with a preemie, that is, suddenly stop all supplemental feedings and rely solely on breastfeeding. While this approach may work with a full-term newborn, it is too risky with a preemie. Most will not be able to take in enough milk from breastfeeding alone during the first few weeks at home and may lose weight and become dehydrated.

The following suggestions may help your efforts at successful breastfeeding.

Find a Lactation Consultant or Other Sources of Help and Information. As you begin breastfeeding at home, you will undoubtedly have many questions and concerns. It can be very helpful to find a board-certified lactation consultant who is familiar with the special challenges of breastfeeding premature infants. Your hospital may be able to give you names of lactation consultants in the community, or call your local La Leche League for recommendations. In addition, ask your local La Leche group leader if she knows of any other mothers who have successfully nursed a preemie who might speak with you. La Leche League meetings can also be good places to talk about concerns and get support for your efforts.

Unfortunately, it can be difficult to find someone who has had much experience with breastfeeding a premature infant, and it can be expensive to hire a lactation consultant. Be wary of advice given by those who are only familiar with nursing full-term babies. The problems faced by mothers nursing preemies are different from those faced by mothers of full-term infants, and approaches that work with full-term infants may not be effective or appropriate for preemies. Some hospitals and HMOs provide ongoing support for breastfeeding mothers, but this is not very common at this stage.

Check Your Baby's Weight Frequently. Take your baby to your pediatrician within a couple of days of discharge for a weight check, and continue weighing her at least weekly or more often until you are confident that your baby is nursing effectively and gaining weight consistently. Your pediatrician's scales may vary somewhat from those in the hospital. Your first weight check can establish a baseline weight for your baby on your doctor's scales, and can also be compared with your baby's discharge weight. If you are doing a great deal of breastfeeding, do not wait for more than a couple of days after you have come home from the hospital to weigh your baby.

Utilize Kangaroo Care as much as Possible. Kangaroo care is very helpful when you are trying to establish or increase breastfeeding. Not only does your baby benefit in many ways from this skin-to-skin contact, but it also provides unlimited opportunities for her to breastfeed when she feels like it. She may not always latch on and actually nurse, particularly in the beginning, but you are giving her the opportunity to nuzzle, smell, lick, and become familiar with your breasts and the sensations of breastfeeding. She'll gradually develop the ability to latch on and suckle more effectively.

"Triple-Feed" Your Baby. When you triple-feed, you nurse your baby first, then offer her a supplemental feeding of expressed milk or formula, and then pump your breasts. Using this regimen, your milk supply will gradually increase, your baby will become more adept at nursing, and the volume that she takes from a supplemental feeding will decrease until you no longer need to offer it. This is obviously a time-consuming regimen and you may not want to use it for every feeding at first. With the help of a lactation specialist in the hospital, or a lactation consultant at home, work out a schedule in which you gradually increase the number of times you put your baby to breast during the day.

Continue Pumping Milk. Continue to pump every three to four hours in order to keep up your milk supply during this transition phase. Your baby will have an easier time nursing if your milk supply is on the high side, and you will have extra milk for supplemental bottles. You will probably need to pump for at least the first few weeks that your baby is home. Some mothers are unable to make progress toward full breastfeeding but continue to pump and feed their babies breastmilk from bottles for months.

Check Your Baby's Intake with a Before- and After-feeding Weight Check. According to Dr. Meier's research, the only reliable way to measure a baby's intake during a nursing session is to weigh her before and after a feeding in her same diaper and clothing. This is known as test weighing. In order to get an accurate measurement, you need to use an electronic scale that measures weight in grams; a 1 gram change in weight indicates your baby has consumed 1 milliliter of milk. Medela, Inc. manufactures a scale of that accuracy, known as the BabyWeigh scale, for use in the home. Some suppliers of breast pumps have these scales available for rent. You may also be able to find a scale that is accurate enough at your early intervention program or in your pediatrician's office.

There is some controversy around the use of scales at home for test weighing. Some experts have worried that test weighing is too complicated and might increase a mother's anxiety. However, Dr. Meier and her colleagues found that the opposite was true. Because most mothers of preemies are very concerned about whether or not their babies are getting enough to eat, test weighing usually relieves much of their anxiety rather than heightening it. In addition, Dr. Meier found that the traditional signs that are used to judge how well a baby is nursing—including rhythmic sucking and breathing, sounds of swallowing, seeing the areola being drawn deeper into a baby's mouth, the length of time a baby nurses—indicate only that a baby is nursing, but do not accurately show how much milk a baby is getting. Test weighing is the only truly accurate method of measuring intake. You may only need to test weigh for a couple of days, or periodically, until you are more confident of your baby's nursing abilities and can see a steady weight gain.

Making Progress Toward Full Breastfeeding

The most important thing to remember as you work toward full-breast-feeding is that it is usually a very gradual process. Many mothers reported that they felt as if they made little progress during the first two or three weeks at home, and then, as they neared their baby's original due date, their babies seemed to suddenly catch on and begin nursing well. Others found that although their babies always seemed to enjoy their time at the breast, they never nursed with any real interest or energy and did not make much progress over time.

Keep Your Milk Supply High. A high milk supply means a greater volume at let-down and easier feeding for your baby.

Make Sure Your Baby Latches on Properly. Bring your baby to your nipple and brush it against her lips. She should open her mouth wide enough to take in most of the areola, not just the nipple. If your nipples are particularly large or flat so that your baby has a difficult time drawing the areola into her mouth, ask a lactation nurse in the hospital or lactation consultant at home for some pointers. It may help to pump a bit first to help draw your nipples out and soften the areola. Or try compressing the area around the areola to allow your baby to get a better grip. You might also ask about temporarily using a preemie-sized nipple shield to help your baby latch on more easily. If your nipples are inverted, place your fingers around the areola and push your breast back toward the chest wall to encourage your nipple to protrude more.

Work on Increasing the Amount of Milk Your Baby Consumes. Many mothers comment that in the early weeks at home their baby seemed to latch on well but had a weak suck and did not take much milk during a nursing session. If this seems to be your baby's problem, there are several things you can try.

- Nurse your baby more often, every two and a half hours during the day and three to four hours at night. This will help her build her strength and increase your milk supply.
- Massage your breast when your baby pauses in her nursing. This helps to bring more milk down into the spaces behind the areola so your baby can extract it more easily. This milk, known as hindmilk, is higher in fat content and calories than the first milk your baby takes during a feeding.
- Keep feedings quiet and calm so that your baby is not overwhelmed by extra stimulation while she is trying to feed.

Best Positions for Nursing Preemies

The traditional position in which babies are nursed, cradled in the crook of your arm, does not work very well with preemies. The muscles in their necks are still weak, their mouths may be small relative to your breast, and they need more support than this position provides. Two other positions usually work better for preemies.

Cross-Chest or Cross-Cradle Position. If you are going to nurse your baby at your left breast first, place your left hand under your breast to support it. Your baby is laid across a pillow in your lap, chest to chest, and with your right arm and hand, you support your baby and gently hold the back of her head. You are then able to guide your baby to your breast and support her as she nurses. When she is ready for your other breast, you can either reverse your positioning, or simply slide her over to feed from the other side. The cross-chest position usually works best if your breasts are large.

Football Hold. If your baby is going to nurse at your right breast, you lay her along your right side, holding her head with your right hand, and supporting your breast with your left hand. Like the cross-chest position, you are able to guide your baby to your breast and support her as she nurses. For nursing from your left breast, reverse your position. Hold your baby along your left side with your left hand under her head, and support your breast with your right hand.

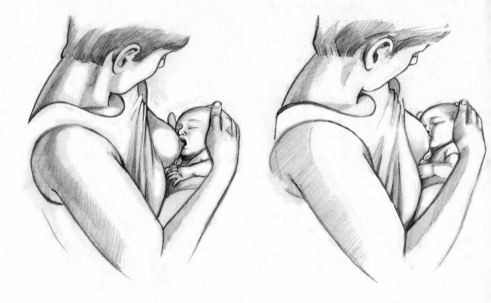

The cross-chest position

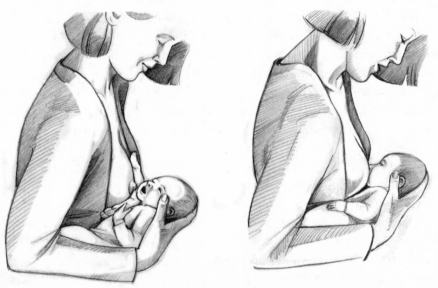

The football hold position

Other Nursing Aids

The following aids can make life a bit easier as you nurse your baby.

Nursing Pillow. Many mothers and lactation consultants recommend using a firm pillow to bring your baby up to the height of your breast and support her while she nurses. Special C-shaped or doughnut-shaped pillows are usually available from lactation consultants, La Leche League leaders, and baby stores. Make sure the pillow you buy is firm and will support your baby at a height that is useful. If you don't want to spend the $35 to $40 that a nursing pillow can cost, try using a firm cushion from a couch; bed pillows are generally too soft and thin to be of much help.

Supplemental Nursers. Many lactation consultants recommend using a supplemental nurser while your baby is learning to breastfeed. This device consists of a small bag that hangs around your neck and one or two small tubes that run to your nipples and are taped in place. As your baby suckles at your breast, she receives milk through the tube as well. This accomplishes several things at once: it helps to build your milk supply, it ensures that your baby is getting the volume of milk she needs, and it helps her build strength at your breast. As your baby's nursing skills increase and your milk supply grows, you put less milk in the supplemental nurser and your baby takes more and more directly from your breast. Supplemental nursers work beautifully for some people. However, others find them clumsy and frustrating to work with. They are something to consider though if you want to avoid using supplemental bottles.

Alternatives to Supplemental Bottles

If you wish to avoid using any bottles with your baby but she is not able to fully breastfeed as yet, there are a number of other feeding methods that you can use. These methods can also be used if someone else will be feeding your baby.

Supplemental Nursers. See above.

Cup Feeding. Use a small 28-cc. medicine cup. You can probably get a small cup while your baby is still in the hospital, or use one of the cups that

The tube of a supplemental nurser runs from the bag to your nipple so that as your baby suckles at your breast, she receives extra milk or formula.

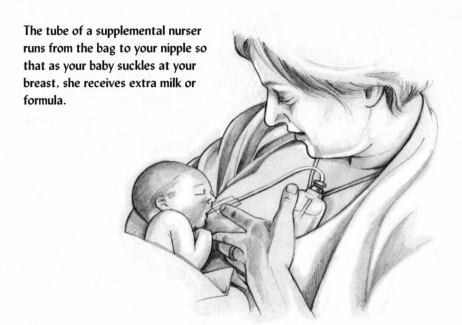

comes with liquid over-the-counter medicines. Fill the cup with milk and place it at your baby's lips, tipping the cup so that the milk touches her lips. Do not actually pour the milk into her mouth but let her suck from the cup.

Finger-Feeding. Attach the tubing from a supplemental nurser to the side of one of your fingers. Place your finger upside down, pad side up, in your baby's mouth up against the roof of her mouth with her tongue underneath. As she sucks on your finger, she will draw milk from the tube.

Eye Dropper. Eye droppers can also be used to feed your baby.

Sometimes these methods work well and help your baby avoid or overcome nipple confusion caused by switching between the breast and bottles. However, most people find it much easier and more convenient to use bottles for any supplemental amounts of milk that their baby needs. Although some babies do develop nipple confusion, you can lessen the chances of this happening by having your baby's first oral feeding experiences be at the breast. As long as you continue to breastfeed regularly, your baby should be able to switch back and forth with little trouble.

What If Breastfeeding Doesn't Work?

To hold your baby close, to see her grow and thrive on your own milk, to see her nurse contentedly at your breast—all of these aspects of nursing are extremely gratifying. Breastfeeding can help to build your confidence as a mother and counteract some of the anxiety and distress of your baby's first weeks or months. It also feels wonderful to be able to do something that mothers of full-term newborns do, or that you were planning to do originally.

But realistically, very few mothers are able to fully breastfeed their premature babies. At the present time, only about a third of mothers even begin expressing milk while their babies are in the hospital, and about half of these have stopped before their babies come home. Recently, a number of hospitals around the country have introduced new programs to provide intensive breastfeeding support to mothers of infants in the NICU. These have had greater success, with almost three-quarters of mothers maintaining their milk supply until the time of discharge. Hopefully, as this kind of support for breastfeeding preemies grows in the future, the number of mothers who can make the transition to full breastfeeding will increase.

But at the current time, with the minimal supports that are available in most places for mothers nursing preemies, greater numbers of very young preemies who are surviving, and early discharge of many of these babies, the success stories are the exception rather than the rule. If you had your heart set on breastfeeding your baby, or you have tried and tried and can't seem to make any progress, you will undoubtedly feel both frustrated and saddened at the loss of another dream, as this mother articulated:

"So much is taken away from you when your baby is born prematurely and there's nothing you can do about it. You jump on breastfeeding as the one thing that you can do, and that nobody can take away from you. But then it doesn't work and you feel doubly bad."

Although it is hard not to feel discouraged or let down in this situation, try to focus on the fact that you have given your baby your milk for as long as you were able, during a time when it was most important for her. Your goal is to help your baby eat as well as possible so that she grows and thrives. When you accomplish that you are a success whether your baby is fed breastmilk, formula, or a combination, and whether she nurses at your breast, cuddles in your arms with a bottle, or, in some cases, is fed by tube.

How to Mix Formula to Get Different Numbers of Calories

The standard mixture for formula results in 20 calories per ounce for regular formula, and 22 calories per ounce for NeoSure and Enfamil 22. Mix your baby's formula to a higher calorie concentration only if prescribed by your physician.

Desired Number of Calories	Using Similac with Iron Powdered Formula
20	2 scoops powder + 4 oz. water = 4 oz. formula
22	3 scoops powder + 5^1/$_2$ oz. water = 6 oz. formula
24	3 scoops powder + 5 oz. water = 6 oz. formula
27	3 scoops powder + 4^1/$_4$ oz. water = 5 oz. formula

	Using Similac with Iron Liquid Concentrate
20	2 oz. concentrate + 2 oz. water = 4 oz. formula
22	3 oz. concentrate + 2^1/$_2$ oz. water = 5^1/$_2$ oz. formula
24	3 oz. concentrate + 2 oz. water = 5 oz. formula
27	2 oz. concentrate + 1 oz. water = 3 oz. formula

	Using NeoSure
22	3 scoops powder + 5 oz. water = 5^1/$_2$ oz. formula
24	3 scoops powder + 4^1/$_2$ oz. water = 5 oz. formula
27	5 scoops powder + 6^1/$_2$ oz. water = 7^1/$_2$ oz. formula

Dilution formulas provided by Ross Laboratories, Columbus, OH. For questions or more information, contact Ross Laboratories, 1-800-515-7677.

Using Good Start Formula

Dilution formulas are released to health care professionals only (physicians, pharmacists, nutritionists). If you prefer to use Good Start, your pediatrician's office can obtain the information for you by calling Nestle/Carnation Infant Formulas at 1-800-782-7766.

How to Mix Formula, continued

**Desired Number
of Calories** **Using Enfamil with Iron Powdered Formula**

20   2 scoops powder + 4 oz. water = 4 oz. formula

22   3 scoops powder + 5^1/$_3$ oz. water = 6 oz. formula

24   4 scoops powder + 6^1/$_2$ oz. water = 6^1/$_2$ oz. formula

27   4 scoops powder + 5^1/$_2$ oz. water = 6^1/$_2$ oz. formula

Using Enfamil with Iron Liquid Concentrate

20   1 can concentrate (13 oz.) + 13 oz. water =
       26 oz. formula

22   1 can concentrate (13 oz.) + 11 oz. water =
       24 oz. formula

24   1 can concentrate (13 oz.) + 9 oz. water =
       22 oz. formula

27   1 can concentrate (13 oz.) + 6 oz. water =
       19 oz. formula

Using Enfamil 22

22   1 packed scoop powder + 2 oz. water = 2 oz. formula

24   2 packed scoops powder + 3^1/$_2$ oz. water =
       4 oz. formula

27   2 packed scoops powder + 3 oz. water =
       3^1/$_2$ oz. formula

Dilution formulas provided by Mead-Johnson Nutritionals, Evansville, Indiana. For questions or more information, contact Mead-Johnson's Consumer Resource Center, 1-800-BABY-123.

Special Situations

Adding Calories to Formula and Solid Foods

By the time they are discharged from the hospital, most babies gain weight on regular formula or breastmilk. However, some babies need formula containing more calories in order to grow and gain weight adequately. Others need to get their calories from a restricted amount of formula to avoid overloading their system with fluids. If your baby needs extra calories, be sure to talk this over with your neonatologist before your baby comes home. If you need to add nutrients such as MCT (medium chain triglyceride) oil, vegetable oil, or Polycose (a powdered form of easily digested sugars) to her formula, or mix it in greater concentrations, have the recipe written out and practice making it in the hospital. Make sure you know where you can get any additives or special formula that you will need before coming home.

Standard formula can be mixed in varying concentrations in order to boost the number of calories per ounce (see chart below). If you are breast-feeding or using expressed milk in bottles, ask your neonatologist or pediatrician how to supply the extra calories your baby needs. The hindmilk, the last milk your baby gets in a nursing, is rich in fat and calories. You may be able to boost your baby's calorie intake if you skim the rich hindmilk from an earlier pumping and feed it to your baby by bottle before you nurse her. The hindmilk will rise to the top if you let your pumped milk sit undisturbed in a bottle in the refrigerator. Powdered formula can also be added to expressed breastmilk. One scoop of powdered formula added to 10 ounces of breastmilk results in a 24-calorie- per-ounce mixture.

If your baby continues to need extra calories as she nears a year in age, you might add a high-calorie supplement like Pediasure, Instant Breakfast, or Ensure to her diet. You can also add butter or oil to foods, use cream instead of milk on cereal, and give your child high-calorie snacks such as peanut butter, bananas, custard, cheese, whole-milk yogurt, and muffins.

Feedings by Tube

Some babies come home from the hospital continuing to receive part or all of their feedings by tube. If this is a temporary situation, you may be able to use a gavage tube inserted through your baby's nose or mouth for each feeding. However, if your baby will need tube feeding for a prolonged period, she will probably need a gastrostomy tube, a tube that allows formula or breastmilk to be fed directly into the stomach. Other babies need to have a gastrostomy tube inserted later in infancy if they develop severe feeding problems that interfere with growth and development.

The common types of feeding tubes used with infants and young children include:

- **a gastrostomy tube (g-tube):** A g-tube is a plastic or rubber tube inserted by a surgeon directly through the skin into the stomach. A length of tubing through which the baby is fed extends outside the abdomen.
- **a button gastrostomy:** If a g-tube must remain in place for several months or more, it may be replaced by a button gastrostomy. With a button gastrostomy, only a short tube extends outside the skin of the abdomen. When not in use, the opening to the tube is covered by a small flap that is usually not noticeable under clothing.
- **a percutaneous endoscopic gastrostomy tube (PEG tube):** A PEG tube is a gastrostomy tube that can be inserted without surgery. Instead, a physician threads the tube down a baby's throat and into her stomach using an endoscope, a flexible tube with a light on the end. The end of the PEG tube can then be brought to the surface of the skin through a small incision.
- **a jejunal tube (j-tube):** Some infants with severe reflux or vomiting may do better with a j-tube, which is inserted into the second portion of the small intestine (the jejunum) below the stomach. The j-tube allows food to bypass the stomach altogether.

If your baby is fed by tube, make sure you understand how to insert a gavage tube or connect the gastrostomy tube, how to check the tube's placement, how to check for residuals in the stomach, how often and how much to feed, how to clean the tubing, what to do if the tube is accidentally pulled out, how to care for the skin around the tube, and where to get any special formula that you may need to use.

Most parents report that they become adept at feeding their babies by tube very quickly, and, although not an ideal situation, find that they are greatly relieved to know that their babies are getting the milk or formula that they need to grow. Babies on tube feedings can usually continue to take some of their feedings by mouth and will gradually move toward more oral feedings.

Extreme Fussiness or Colic

A baby with colic cries more often and for longer periods of time than most babies. The usual definition of colic includes crying that lasts for three hours or more at least three days a week for three weeks or more. Colic affects almost a third of all babies; it isn't clear whether more preemies have colic than full-term babies. If your baby develops colic, it will usually show up two to four weeks after her due date and disappear by about three to four months of age (corrected). Despite the fact that many colicky babies are hard to feed, they are generally healthy and continue to gain weight throughout their colicky period.

Although colic is not strictly a feeding problem, it is included in this section because babies with colic tend to be gassy, their tummies may seem tense and bloated, they often refuse to eat, or they begin to cry shortly after they begin feeding.

There have been many theories advanced about the causes of colic and the best ways of treating it. Although it often appears related to feeding, in reality few babies get colic as a result of sensitivities to milk or formula. Most doctors recommend that if you are breastfeeding, you do not stop nursing; you can try eliminating milk products from your diet for two weeks to see if your baby seems more comfortable. If you are using formula, you can try a different kind (lactose-free, soy-based, Good Start, or even one of the elemental formulas like Pregestimil or Nutramigen). Try feeding with an angled bottle or collapsible nurser. You may also want to ask your doctor about the possibility that your baby's discomfort is being caused by reflux into her esophagus.

Colic may be caused by a baby's hypersensitivity to her environment and by her overreactions to stimuli. You may be able to soothe your baby by using some of the techniques described earlier in this book. Some babies are soothed by white noise and movement, others by darkness and quiet, or by swaddling. Putting gentle pressure on your baby's abdomen by holding her face down along your arm or across your lap may be soothing. Gentle massage and warm baths help others. Sometimes, nothing you do seems to make any difference and your baby will simply cry.

If your baby develops colic, talk with your pediatrician so he can rule out any other possibilities or problems. It may help to keep a diary of your baby's behavior and habits to detect certain things that seem to set her off or soothe her, and to note what times of day she most often cries.

For most babies, the only sure cure for colic is time. This does not mean that you simply have to grin and bear it, however. With some help and experimentation, you should be able to find some techniques that help soothe your baby and shorten her crying jags, at least some of the time.

In the meantime, it is extremely important that you get regular breaks from your crying baby. If you can't get out, put your baby in her crib where you know she is safe, and do something that blocks the noise: take a shower, play the radio, or run the vacuum cleaner. When there is another adult in the house, step outside, go for a quick walk, and take some time for yourself.

Getting Professional Help for Feeding Problems

If feeding problems are particularly worrisome, you might want to seek professional advice from an infant feeding specialist. Feeding problems fall under the responsibility of two types of professionals: speech therapists and occupational therapists. Most early intervention programs have both types of therapists on staff. They can work with you to assess your baby's problems and provide some insight, ideas, and therapies to help. In addition, most large academic medical centers and children's hospitals have specific programs designed to handle feeding problems. These feeding clinics are staffed by a multidisciplinary team of feeding specialists, including occupational and speech therapists, nurses, nutritionists, psychologists, and others. You can either call the hospital, the nursery where your baby was cared for, the infant follow-up clinic, or your pediatrician to get more information about such a program in your area.

PART III:
AS YOUR CHILD GROWS

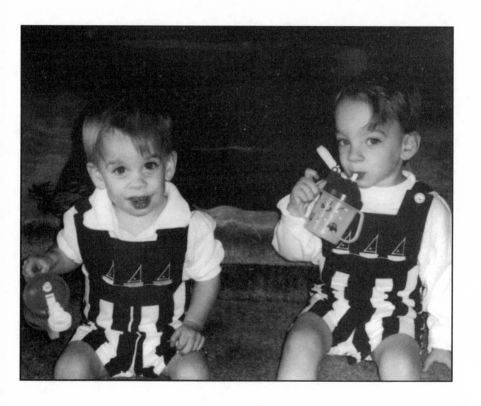

CHAPTER 9

From Infancy to
Age Three

ℱᴀ

 THE FIRST YEARS OF
any child's life are a time of dramatic growth, change, and development.
But because your baby has had such a rough start, it is natural to be concerned about what to expect in your baby's future. You may find yourself
full of questions: Is my baby going to be all right? Are there things I should
be watching for? How will I know if there is something wrong? Do I need
to do something special to help my baby, or will he outgrow his prematurity on his own?

In most cases, premature babies follow the same developmental course
that full-term babies do—but with some differences which are described
below. Many of these differences occur so commonly among preemies that
they can be thought of as being "normal" for them, and they generally
have little or no lasting impact on your child's development. Babies who
were born extremely early, had serious complications in the hospital, or
continue to have health problems may face greater challenges as they
grow and develop.

But preemies are more than just their beginnings. They are tough,
resilient, adaptable human beings. The care that you provide at home, the
environment in which they grow up, and their own inner resources make
a tremendous difference to their development. As nice as it would be to
know that everything is going to be fine, there are so many unknowns
involved that it usually takes some time to get a clearer sense of how your
child is doing.

In the first section of this chapter, you will find an overview of what
you can expect during the first three years of your child's life as he grows
from the tiny infant you brought home from the hospital to a relatively

independent child at three years of age. A brief summary of normal development during the first years is followed by a description of some of the common ways in which preemie development differs from that of typical full-term newborns. Included also are warning signs that may indicate that your child is having difficulties in some area of development. This is followed by a section which describes some of the health problems experienced by many preemies in their early years, and, finally, a discussion of some of the feelings and emotions that preemie parents commonly experience as their babies begin to grow.

As you read this chapter, keep in mind that normal development includes remarkable variations among children. Those who were born prematurely are often watched extremely closely as they grow, and many receive regular, detailed assessments of their development. Under such careful scrutiny many full-term babies and children would display some periodic differences in development. As you watch your child growing, trust your own instincts and your knowledge of him to round out the picture you may be given by doctors, therapists, or other child professionals.

Getting to know other parents of preemies can also be very useful and reassuring, but be sure to spend time with full-term children and their parents as well. This will help you keep a balanced perspective on your child as he grows. You may find that some of the concerns you have about your child are quite common among parents of other kids his age. Our children are special but they are also regular children, and, like other children, they will challenge us in many ways as they grow.

What to Expect During the First Years

Your expectations about your baby's development may come from a number of different places—your own parents or other relatives, books, friends, or from raising or watching other children. It is rare that any of those sources include experiences with a premature baby, and you will need to adjust your expectations a bit to take into account some of the general differences that preemies show in their development.

Preemies show more variation in development than do their full-term counterparts. Infants born prematurely are not a homogeneous group.

They are born at different gestational ages, have different types of complications and care in the hospital, and are discharged at different ages and in different states of health. Not surprisingly, they tend to show more variations in their development than full-term newborns.

Your baby's corrected age gives you a more accurate indicator of his developmental stage than his chronological age. As explained in Chapter 6, it is important to use your baby's adjusted or corrected age for the first two and a half to three years of his life. His corrected age is the age he would be had he been born on his original due date. Since development begins at conception, your baby's corrected age will give you a more accurate idea of what to expect from your baby than will his chronological age, his age from his actual birth date.

Preemie development tends to be uneven or scattered. Most parents find that using their baby's corrected age provides only a partial explanation of their baby's development and behavior. It is typical to find that your baby's development in one area correlates more closely with his chronological age, while in another area he more closely matches his adjusted age. In general, preemies' senses—their vision, hearing, alertness—tend to be ahead of their physical abilities.

Development may be slow at first. Even when you use your baby's corrected age, you may find that his development lags behind what you expect. Your baby is still recovering from his early birth, and may not have as much energy available for growth and development as would a full-term baby. If he is still struggling with medical complications, or if he was extremely young at birth, he may progress slowly for a longer time. These general delays, particularly in physical development, are very normal among preemies.

Your child will have his own unique personality. All babies follow a fairly predictable pattern and schedule as they develop. But within that expected sequence there are always variations. For example, some babies are very active and eagerly master physical skills such as sitting, crawling, and walking. Others are more sedentary and may use their hands, or talk at a younger age than those who are more physically active. Your baby has his own unique personality and approach that will affect the way in which he progresses, and his early birth is only one of many factors that will affect his development.

An Overview of Typical Development

In most cases, nothing magical or special is needed to help your preemie develop properly. The most important thing you can do is to provide him with loving, responsive care. By holding him, talking to him, letting him watch you, by feeding him, changing him, comforting him, and by providing him with opportunities to explore and play as he gets older, you help him to grow in the best way possible. It isn't necessary, and is usually frustrating and counterproductive, to push babies to achieve certain milestones before they are ready.

Over the first years of your baby's life your can expect him to develop the skills described below. I have not included ages for these milestones because of the wide variations that exist among preemies. Professionals who work with preemies continually stress that the age at which your baby acquires certain skills is not as important as the progress that he is making. Keep in mind that development tends to go in spurts. Periods of time when your child seems to be gaining many new skills will be followed by a plateau period in which nothing much happens. To see how your child is doing, look at his development over time; compare what he can do this month with what he was doing last month.

The most reassuring sign that your baby is developing well is his interest in you and his surroundings, and later his responsiveness to things going on around him. At first, your baby may tire easily and stay awake for only ten or fifteen minutes. You will need to pace your activities with him and watch for signs that he needs a break. As he develops and matures, he will be able to stay awake longer and tolerate more activity without becoming stressed.

Gross (or Large) Motor Skills

These include the major physical skills such as turning over, sitting, crawling, and walking. In general, babies develop from the head downward and from the middle of the body outward. First, your baby will gain strength in his neck and be able to hold his head up more steadily when he is held upright. On his stomach, he will learn to raise his head and then push the trunk of his body up with his arms. Once he can do this, he will start to roll from his stomach to his back, and later from his back to his stomach. As his back and the trunk of his body become stronger, he'll learn first to sit with support and then independently. Toward the end of the first year or early in the second, he will begin pulling himself up to a standing position, then begin moving along holding on to furniture or large objects. After he learns to stand for a moment or two by himself, he will begin to walk.

You can help your baby develop or practice his large motor skills in a number of ways:

- Hold him upright and let him look over your shoulder toward something interesting such as a mirror. Support his head and neck at first, then let him try it for a moment or two on his own as his neck gets stronger.
- Give your baby plenty of supervised time on his tummy. Place him on a blanket with interesting toys in front of him to encourage him to lift his head, push up, and later reach out. He may only tolerate being on his tummy for a few minutes at first. You can gradually work up to more time, or do a couple of short sessions in a day.
- If your baby hates being on his tummy, lie down on your back with your head slightly raised on a pillow or two. Put your baby on your tummy—he may enjoy looking up at your face more than looking at toys on the floor.
- When he is learning to sit, hold him on your lap supported under his arms, then at his waist, and finally at his hips as he gets stronger. Once he has mastered this, you can help him practice his balance and control by gently raising one of your legs so that he is slightly tipped. He should react by shifting his balance and trying to remain upright.
- When he is learning to crawl, let him practice climbing stairs (with you closely behind).
- **Do not put your baby in a jolly-jumper or infant walker.** Although most babies enjoy these, they encourage babies to straighten their legs and backs. Many preemies tend to be stiff through their legs and back and need to be encouraged to bend and flex rather than straighten (see discussion on high tone later in this chapter). For the same rea-

sons, do not encourage your baby to stand up on your lap before he has learned to crawl.

Fine (or Small) Motor Skills

Fine motor skills are those that involve using the hands and coordinating the eyes and hands. At first, your baby will keep his hands in tight fists. He may be able to bring them to his face or mouth to soothe himself. Gradually, he will begin to open his fists and be able to hold objects like rattles or a plastic ring of keys. Your baby will seem to discover his hands at some point and enjoy watching them, and then experimenting with them. He will bring them together in front of him, try to pick things up in his fists, transfer toys from one hand to the other, bang things together, and throw them. He will enjoy exploring objects with his mouth, as well. Finally he will learn to pick up small things with his thumb and fingers, and be able to scribble with a large crayon or pencil. As he is progressing through these skills, he may enjoy the following:

- Encourage him to bring his hands to his mouth. You may want to provide him with a pacifier to encourage him to use his mouth as well as his hands.
- Hang a mobile over his crib, or give him a bright object or two to look at in his crib.
- As he begins to bat at things, suspend a crib gym over him that makes noise when he hits it.
- When he can sit in a high chair or on the floor, give him rattles, rings, or other easy-to-hold toys to play with, bang together, or make noise with. Hold them out in front of him so he has to reach out. Encourage him to use both hands.
- Babies in the second half of the first year often enjoy putting things into other things. Give him a variety of containers and objects to put inside them (large enough so that they can't be choked on when he brings them up to his mouth).
- Give him toys or objects with different textures and that make different noises. Pieces of crinkly paper, or soft fuzzy materials may be interesting to him.
- Let him play in water or with pudding spread on his highchair tray. When he is learning to eat solids, Cheerios are a fun safe food for him to try to pick up and get to his mouth.

Language, Thinking, and Social Skills

Learning to understand spoken language and to talk are two different skills, the first known as receptive language, and the second as expressive language. Babies tend to understand what is said to them at an earlier age than they can express themselves with sounds and words. Thinking and social skills include learning to smile and respond to people, learning about the world around you, learning to play with friends, to drink from a cup, to feed and dress oneself, and become toilet trained.

At first, your baby will only watch you, and will be most interested in you when you are fairly close to him. As his distance vision improves, he will keep track of you as you move about the room. He will watch you intently as you talk with him and respond with smiles and coos, usually in the first six months. By the end of his first year, he may be saying a few simple words like mama and dada, and will understand much of what is being said to him. Your baby will begin to explore ideas like cause-and-effect, and the relationship between things as he grows. When he cries, you pick him up. When he drops something, it falls to the floor. When he bangs two things together, they make noise. He will enjoy putting objects into containers and dumping them out again. He will figure out how to fit shapes into a shape sorter, begin to look for a toy that he has dropped or that is hidden under something else, and do simple puzzles.

To encourage your baby or just to have fun with him, you may want to try some of the following:

- Let your baby spend time in a infant seat watching you during the day. Start with ten or fifteen minutes at first, then increase it as he can stay awake longer. (Be sure he is strapped into the seat and that it is stable and cannot fall from a table or counter.)
- Talk with your baby as you go about your daily business. Explain what you are doing when you care for him.
- Read simple books to him. Point out pictures and identify them with names.
- Teach your baby the parts of his body. Hold him up to a mirror and point out his nose, his mouth, etc.
- Smile at your baby, imitate the noises he makes at you, and have a conversation with him.
- Play peek-a-boo, pat-a-cake, and other simple games.

- Give him simple puzzles, shape sorters, containers, nesting toys, and blocks to play with. Simple household items, such as measuring cups and spoons, pot lids, plastic containers, and wooden utensils all make wonderful playthings for babies.

Common Issues in Development Among Preemies

Earlier in this chapter we discussed the general ways in which you should adjust your expectations for your baby's development. This section focuses on specific aspects of preemie development that often differ from that seen among full-term babies. In most cases, these differences represent an alternate path to the same endpoint in development. But if you ever have questions or concerns about how your baby is doing, don't hesitate to contact your pediatrician. Your local early intervention program or infant follow-up clinic may also be a good source of information about preemie development.

Will My Baby Catch Up in Size?

The stresses caused by being born prematurely temporarily slow down the growth of most babies. At their original due dates, almost all preemies weigh less than they would have had they been able to complete their gestation in the womb. Approximately 10 to 15 percent of preemies will remain small into their childhoods. But the majority will catch up, and their final size will be determined more by their genetics—that is, by how tall or short their parents are—than by the fact that they were born prematurely.

Babies who weighed over 1,500 grams (3 pounds 5 ounces) at birth, were the appropriate size for their gestational age at birth, and have no serious health problems usually have few problems with growth. Babies such as this often begin a growth spurt around their original due dates, and grow quickly in the first few weeks and months at home. Some soon catch up to the size they would have been had they been born full-term. Others grow more slowly, but gradually catch up over the first two or three years. Some babies with chronic lung disease have a growth spurt as their respiratory system recovers.

For babies who were born extremely early, were small for gestational age, were very sick in the hospital, or have ongoing health problems, growth is often more problematic. These babies are usually smaller at discharge, grow more slowly, and may remain small throughout their childhoods. They are often described as being "on their own growth curves". Most grow steadily but remain consistently at the low end (the 5th percentile or less) of the normal growth charts.

Recent research suggests that catch-up growth continues at least until a child is eight years old, with an additional spurt possible in adolescence.

Tracking Your Child's Growth. To determine how well your child is growing, your pediatrician will measure your baby's length, his weight, and his head circumference at every well-child check-up. For the first two and a half years, these measurements should be charted on the standard growth charts using your baby's corrected age, not his actual age. As preemies begin to catch up in their growth, their heads often grow the most quickly, followed by their weight and then length. This temporarily gives them slightly different body proportions than typical full-term infants.

Weight for Length Comparisons. One other growth measurement—a weight for length graph—should be used with premature babies, especially those who fall at the low end or below the standard growth charts. This graph indicates if your baby is the right weight for his length even if he is small. If he is in proportion, as indicated by falling near the 50th percentile on the graph, he is getting enough to eat and growing as well as he can. However, if he consistently falls below the fifth percentile, or if the proportion begins to decline, his growth is slowing down and you probably need to increase his caloric intake. If you are worried about your child's slow growth or small size, ask your pediatrician to track his progress using the proportion graph, and get a copy of the growth chart to use yourself.

Problems with Growth. A few children need extra help—supplementary calories or other nutritional supports—in order to improve the rate at which they are growing. Some preemies simply seem uninterested in eating, while others have health problems that use up a lot of energy, difficulties consuming enough milk or formula, trouble handling solid foods, or severe reflux. These complex feeding problems may be beyond the expertise of your pediatrician. If your child is having serious feeding problems, not gaining weight or gaining very slowly, or you are worried about any aspect of his eating, ask for a referral to a feeding disorders clinic, a pediatric feeding specialist, or a pediatric nutritionist. In other cases, your doctor may consider using a growth hormone to stimulate your child's growth.

Temporary Differences in Muscle Tone

One of the most common differences seen among preemies is abnormal muscle tone—being too stiff or too floppy. As many as three-quarters of preemies who weighed less than 1,500 grams (3 pounds 5 ounces) at birth are affected. In a few cases, a baby with abnormal tone is showing the first symptoms of a more serious problem like cerebral palsy, but most of the time this is a temporary condition that disappears gradually over the first year to 18 months of life.

High Tone. Stiffness, caused by an increase in the tone of the extensor muscles, is the most common of these differences. The extensors are the muscles that straighten your arms, legs, back, and neck. A baby with increased tone in these muscles will tend to keep his legs straight, arch his back and head away from you, and hold his shoulders back. Babies like this feel very strong when you hold them, and it can be difficult to get them to bend and snuggle into your body. The stiffness may be more noticeable in the shoulders and arms in the first six months of life, and in the legs in the second half of a baby's first year.

In the normal course of development, the extensor muscles start gaining strength when a baby is about four months old. This helps a full-term baby move away from the curled up or flexed position that is typical among newborns. Most preemies don't have as much strength in their flexor (or curling) muscles as full-term babies have, and as the extensors get stronger they begin to overwhelm the weak flexors. The baby becomes stiff—hard to curl—until the opposing muscle groups come back into balance later in the first year or early in the second.

Low Tone. Less commonly, preemies show decreased muscle tone, sometimes called low tone. These babies feel very floppy and soft when you hold them. Their heads tend to flop forward, and they have little strength

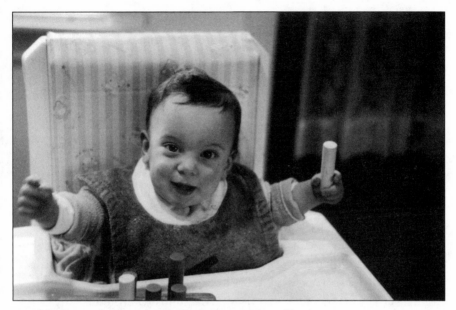

**High tone babies often keep their arms up and back; a toy encourages
your baby to bring his hands forward.**

in their backs. Babies who are still recovering from illness and do not yet
have a great deal of energy may have low muscle tone. If this low tone
continues, it may also be a symptom of developmental problems. Many
preemies have low tone in the muscles around their mouths, particularly
if they have had an endotracheal tube for an extended time. Because they
weren't able to suck while the tube was in place, the muscles in and
around their mouths do not have a chance to develop and get stronger.
This weakness may continue into the second year.

Mixed Tones. Finally, some babies will show a mixture of muscle tones,
the most common being high tone in the legs and low tone in the trunk of
the body. These babies may have a lot of strength in their legs but have a
hard time sitting by themselves and tend to slump forward.

The Impact of Tone Differences

Temporary differences in muscle tone pose a problem only if they interfere
with your baby's development. High muscle tone in the shoulders can

make it difficult for your baby to bring his arms and hands together in front of him. When the legs and back are stiff, your baby may have trouble learning how to crawl, since it makes it more difficult for him to bend his knees and pull them up underneath him. It can also cause other problems, as one mother reported:

> *"My son had a hard time sitting by himself. He had such a tendency to arch his back, he was constantly falling over backwards. He actually learned to belly-crawl before he learned to sit, even though babies are supposed to do it in the opposite order."*

On the positive side, high muscle tone enables some babies to control their heads and turn over at a younger age than is typical.

Low muscle tone can also slow down your baby's physical development, making it difficult for him to sit, stand, and walk. A physical therapist can work with your baby to help him strengthen weak muscles, or counteract the stiffness of high tone. This helps to minimize any delays that may occur as well as avoid some of the frustration felt by babies when they have trouble making progress.

If your baby has high muscle tone:

- Avoid using a jumper or infant walker. These devices make your baby stiffen his legs and back, which you want to avoid as much as possible.
- Try to keep your baby in a flexed position as much as possible. When you hold him, try to keep his back gently rounded, his shoulders slightly forward, his arms and legs bent, and his hands in front of him.
- Place blanket rolls behind your baby's shoulders in his infant seat to bring his shoulders and arms forward.
- Give your baby supervised tummy time every day. This helps strengthen his arm and shoulder muscles, and counteracts his tendency to hold his shoulders and arms back. If he has a lot of trouble raising his head, place a blanket roll under his chest with his arms in front of it.
- Place your baby on his side in a flexed position with a blanket roll under his head and one at his back to keep his shoulders forward. In this position gravity brings his hands together where he can see and play with them.

If your baby has low tone:

• Gently pull him by the arms into a sitting position from lying on his back. This helps to develop strength in his neck and trunk.

• While he is sitting on your lap facing you, gently raise one leg under him so that he has to shift his weight to stay upright. Provide whatever support he needs by holding him under his arms, at his waist, or at his hips. Physical therapists will often do these sitting exercises on a large ball as well.

• Help him to sit by spreading his legs, knees bent, with the soles of his feet together in front of him.

• Give him supervised tummy time as well. Place toys or a mirror in front of him to encourage him to lift his head, push up on his arms, and reach for things.

• When he is sitting, place toys in front of him to encourage him to reach. Help him move from a sitting position to a crawling position as he gets older.

Jitteriness, Startles, and Infant Reflexes

Preemies tend to remain jittery in their movements longer than do full-term newborns. And while full-term newborns outgrow infant reflexes within a couple of months, preemies may continue startling and arching well into the second half of their first year. My own son didn't outgrow his startles until he was about nine months old, whereas my two full-term children had stopped by the time they were about six weeks old.

Sensitivity and Sensory Integration Problems

Preemies generally continue to be quite sensitive to stimulation—noises, lights, movements, textures—well into the second year or beyond. Babies who have been sick, particularly those with respiratory problems, tend to be even more sensitive than healthy infants. You may find that your child has more trouble with one type of stimulus than another. He may particularly hate loud noises, while another child cannot stand the feeling of grass under his feet, lumps in his food, or tags in his clothing.

If your child continues to be extremely sensitive, or his sensitivity interferes with his development or behavior, you may want to talk with an occupational therapist. A discipline within occupational therapy, sensory integration therapy, specifically focuses on how children experience and react to stimuli. Sensory integration therapy includes a number of approaches that are used to help overly reactive children cope better with everyday sights, sounds, smells, touches, tastes, and movement. See Appendix E for sources of information about sensory integration problems.

Delayed Speech and Language Development

Many preemies begin talking at a later age than do typical full-term newborns. By the age of two, between 20 and 40 percent of preemies show some delays in language development. The delays occur more often in speaking than in understanding what is said.

Some babies begin to speak slowly because multiple colds, ear infections, and fluid in the ears have interfered with their hearing. Others have low muscle tone in the mouth and jaw, which can make it more difficult to form words. Rarely, delayed speech development indicates a more serious problem in development or a hearing loss. Most preemies have age-appropriate language skills by the time they reach school age.

If you are worried that your child is delayed in learning to talk, or if he seems not to respond to you or to sounds, talk with your pediatrician. He or your early intervention program can assess your child's hearing and language skills. Depending upon what they find, they may recommend your baby be given a hearing test, be seen by an ear, nose, and throat doctor (for chronic fluid in the ears), or work with a speech or occupational therapist. Or your child may have nothing wrong and will catch up to his age-mates within a reasonable amount of time.

Distractibility, High Activity Level, and Short Attention Span

Many parents are struck with how active their preemies are, particularly during the first couple of years. One parent's comments are typical: "She never stops moving during the day. She takes a few short cat-naps but otherwise she's all over the place. It's exhausting."

In fact, this type of behavior—a short attention span coupled with a high activity level—seems to be quite common among preemies. It may be caused by their sensitivity and immature nervous systems, and often goes away as they mature. Many parents of preemies worry that their children have attention deficit disorder (ADD) or are hyperactive (ADHD). Try not to worry about this yet. Although ADD and ADHD are more common among children who were born prematurely, a diagnosis cannot usually be made until a child is closer to school age.

In the meantime, you can try to help your child learn how to focus on one thing at a time and build up the amount of time he spends at any one activity. Try keeping your child's environment quiet and calm. You might want to limit the number of toys that are available to your child at any one time so he does not become overwhelmed with choices. Early intervention programs usually have circle time activities that help young children learn to sit and pay attention, even if it is just for a few minutes at a time.

If certain situations seem to aggravate your child's tendency to get disorganized and frenetic, you may want to avoid them until he grows older. For example, one mother said that she usually brought her son into his early intervention class after free-play was over because he couldn't handle all of the activity and children. Instead, he would join the group during circle time when it was quieter and there were fewer distractions.

The Quiet Observer

Although the active preemie seems to be a very common type, it is striking how many parents described their children as having a disposition that falls at the opposite end of this spectrum. These preemies are quiet children who seem to prefer observing others to entering the fray themselves. As infants they may spend a lot of time sleeping, or may fall asleep whenever there is too much activity around them.

As is true with many of the active preemies, a baby's quieter approach to life may simply be his natural personality, and not related to his prematurity. In other cases, it may be an indication that your baby is still very sensitive to noises, activity, to being touched or bumped. For example, if he dislikes being on a playground with many children, try to go at a time when there are fewer children around. Have him play with one friend rather than in a big play group. And as happens with many of the active preemies, your baby may simply outgrow this quiet reserved approach as he gets older. If sensitivity seems to be a continuing or increasing problem, you may want to talk with an occupational therapist trained in sensory integration theory.

When to Worry

Although preemie development tends to be slower and a bit different from that of full-term babies, certain delays and variations act as warning signs of more serious problems. You may be the first to notice problems with your child's development. You may have a vague feeling that something is wrong, or you may see definite problems. For example, your child's progress may seem to slow down or stop at a particular point, he may seem increasingly frustrated or cranky, he may not respond to sounds, or he may seem uninterested in his surroundings or in you.

In general, most serious developmental problems become evident during the first 12 to 18 months of your child's life. Although a lack of responsiveness on the part of your child is always a reason to worry, warning signs in the first year are usually physical and show up as delays in reaching certain milestones like sitting, crawling, or using the hands.

Using your child's corrected age, let your pediatrician know if your child is not doing the following by the ages indicated:

- By three months, your baby should be smiling at you, following you with his eyes, lifting his head and turning it from side to side when on his stomach.
- By six months, he should be reaching for, grabbing, and holding toys. He should be able to grab his feet when on his back, and when on his stomach hold his head and trunk off the floor with his arms extended.
- By nine months, he should be able to bring his hands together and transfer an object from one hand to the other, roll over from back to front and front to back, creep or combat crawl, and sit independently. He should be cooing and babbling.
- By twelve months, he should be able to pull himself up into a standing position, cruise along furniture, stand alone for at least five seconds, and take steps while holding onto your hands or a push toy.
- In the first year, your baby should not show a strong preference for using one hand over the other, and there shouldn't be a great differ-

ence in muscle tone between the two sides of his body with one side noticeably weaker than the other.

By the second and third years, developmental problems may show up as delays in language skills. Warning signs include:

- not responding to simple instructions at 18 months
- not putting two words together at two years
- having speech that is difficult for strangers to understand at two and a half years
- not speaking in simple sentences (more than two to three words) by three years

Keep in mind that there is a wide range of normal among both preemies and full-term babies, and that development does not always progress smoothly. But if your child does have developmental problems, the earlier they are identified the better. Therapy may be available to help your child overcome slight delays, or to help him develop as well as possible.

What Are the Chances My Child Will Have Something Seriously Wrong?

The most common serious disabilities that occur among premature babies are cerebral palsy, blindness, deafness, and mental retardation. In general, the disability rates are slightly higher for the smallest and youngest babies, and range from approximately:

- 20 percent for babies born weighing less than 1,000 grams (2 pounds 3 ounces)
- 14 to 17 percent for babies weighing between 1,000 grams and 1,500 grams (3 pounds 5 ounces)
- 6 to 8 percent for babies weighing between 1,500 grams and 2,499 grams (5 pounds 8 ounces).

Among full-term babies who weigh more than 5 pounds 8 ounces at birth, the rates of these serious disabilities are approximately 5 percent.

Cerebral palsy, a disorder of movement and posture that is described in Chapter 11, occurs among approximately 6 to 9 percent of preemies.

Blindness is more common among the smallest of babies, and develops in about 6 percent of those born weighing less than 750 grams (1 pound 11 ounces) and 2 percent of those weighing between 750 grams and 1,500 grams (3 pounds 5 ounces). Deafness occurs among approximately 2 percent of preemies, regardless of their birthweights. And approximately 20 percent of the smallest preemies (those weighing less than 750 grams) will have an IQ level that falls into the range of mental retardation (less than 70). Among larger preemies, weighing between 750 grams and 1,500 grams, the rate of mental retardation is about 8 percent; among full-term babies the rate is approximately 2 percent.

Remember that these statistics reflect the experience of preemies as a group and cannot be used to predict how any individual baby will do. Recent research has helped to identify some of the factors that seem to be associated with more serious problems among preemies. These include severe head bleeds (grades III and IV), periventricular leukomalacia (PVL), and chronic lung disease (CLD). The higher disability rates seen among the youngest babies are not caused by their young gestational age directly, but by the fact that these babies tend to have more medical complications and a longer, harder time in the hospital.

There are still many unknowns about why some preemies sail through their early births with few problems while others are affected more seriously. And looked at in reverse, the numbers seem much more positive, indicating that between 80 and 94 percent of preemies will recover without serious disabilities. As one neonatologist pointed out, the statistics tell only part of the story. "In the research, a child with cerebral palsy who cannot walk is identified as having a bad outcome. However, in real life, this child may be happy, healthy, and developing normally in all ways except for some of her physical abilities. Calling this a bad outcome is an oversimplification; it misses all the strengths and good things that are a part of this child and this family's life."

Common Health Concerns

Although most preemies will not have any serious health problems after they come home from the hospital, a number of aspects of prematurity put these children, as a group, at higher risk for illness and rehospitalization than full-term babies. The most common of these health concerns are discussed below.

Respiratory Infections

During the first two years, premature babies are particularly vulnerable to respiratory infections such as colds and flu. This vulnerability occurs because their antibody levels are low, particularly in the first six to nine months of life, and because their breathing passages are still quite small. Even small amounts of congestion or irritation can be problematic and, in some cases, cause serious illness. This means that your baby may seem to catch every cold to which he is exposed, his colds may make him sicker, and they may last longer. Even as toddlers and young children, many preemies seem particularly susceptible to colds.

Unfortunately, premature infants are also more susceptible to serious lower respiratory infections, such as pneumonia, bronchitis, and bronchiolitis, particularly during the first six to twelve months of life. These infections may develop after a cold or may occur suddenly without any preceding illness.

If your baby shows signs of a lower respiratory illness—fever, a decrease in appetite and activity level, rapid breathing, grunting or wheezing noises—contact your doctor immediately or take your baby to a hospital emergency room. Babies can quickly become seriously ill with lower respiratory illnesses and may need to be admitted to the hospital for treatment. Some babies will need supplemental oxygen or even a respirator during the worst part of the illness.

Premature infants who are discharged between September and January face the greatest risk of developing serious respiratory illnesses in their first winter at home and tend to be hospitalized more often (see explanation of RSV in Chapter 6). Babies who come home in the spring and summer are less likely to be exposed to RSV and other respiratory viruses during their first months at home. By the time winter comes, they can more easily fight off or cope with respiratory infections.

Because of your baby's increased susceptibility to respiratory illnesses, it is wise to take some precautions to limit his exposure to germs, particularly during his first winter. If at all possible, it is probably best to keep your baby out of large group day care settings during his first year. Family day care or care at home may help protect him from exposure to respiratory illness. And finally, if your baby needs to be admitted to the hospital for an elective surgical procedure, try to avoid scheduling it during the winter months when hospitals are full of children sick with RSV.

Vision Problems

The most serious vision problems among premature babies are those caused by severe retinopathy of prematurity (ROP). If your baby is discharged with active ROP, or before the retina in his eyes has matured completely, he should be followed closely by a pediatric ophthalmologist. In most cases, ROP regresses on its own without treatment. However, if ROP worsens, your child may need to be treated with one or more techniques designed to stop the ROP and save as much of his vision as possible (see Chapter 4).

But even preemies who never experienced any retinopathy of prematurity tend to develop more vision problems than full-term babies. These include:

- myopia, or near-sightedness, which occurs among 6 percent of preemies and only 2 percent of full-term babies;
- strabismus, in which the eyes do not work together in a coordinated way, which develops in 10 percent of preemies and 2 percent of full-term babies; and
- amblyopia, or lazy eye, which 4 percent of preemies develop compared to only .10 percent of full-term babies.

Luckily, all three conditions are usually very treatable, particularly when they are diagnosed early. Myopia can be corrected with glasses; the treatment for amblyopia involves strengthening the weak eye by temporarily covering the stronger eye with an eye patch; and strabismus is corrected with surgery on the eye muscles.

Because preemies are at higher risk for these problems, they should be seen by a pediatric ophthalmologist, or eye doctor, between six and twelve months of age (corrected age), and again at three years and five years. If everything is normal at your child's five-year-old checkup, he is no longer considered to be at any higher risk than any other child for vision problems.

Most babies with ROP that regresses by itself or with treatment have normal vision. However, some complications of ROP can develop years later. If there is scar tissue on the retina from the ROP, it can cause distortions and decreased vision. In some cases, as the eye grows, the scarring can cause the retina to tear or even detach. These types of retinal detachments tend to occur during adolescence or early adulthood. Luckily, these later detachments are much easier to repair than those that occur in infancy. About a third of infants with severe stage 5 (ROP) develop glaucoma, as well. Glaucoma is an eye disease in which increasing pressure within the eye itself can gradually destroy vision. This condition can usually be controlled with medication and sometimes surgery.

Hernias

More preemies than full-term babies develop hernias, a condition in which a portion of the small intestine pushes through weak muscles in the abdominal wall. The most common type among babies is an inguinal hernia which occurs more often among boys than girls. About one in six boys and one in 50 girls who weighed less than 1,200 grams (2 pounds 10 ounces) at birth develop inguinal hernias. Boys are particularly susceptible to developing hernias because of a weak spot that remains in the muscles of the abdomen after the testes have migrated from the abdomen down into the scrotum at about 32 weeks of gestation. The intestine will sometimes push through this weak spot, causing the scrotum to look quite enlarged or swollen. The swelling may increase when a baby is crying or active, and decrease when he is lying down or sleeping. Among girls, an inguinal hernia appears as a lump in the labia near the vaginal opening.

Hernias often appear around the time of your baby's original due date, so your baby may be home when a hernia develops. They are not generally serious but must usually be repaired surgically. If your baby developed a hernia while he was in the hospital, it may be repaired before he is discharged. But often surgery is postponed until a baby weighs between eight and ten pounds. Hernia repair surgery is usually done on an outpatient basis so your baby will not generally need to spend the night in the hospital.

The other common hernia, the umbilical hernia, occurs when the intestine pushes through weak places in the muscles around the bellybutton, causing a soft swelling. Umbilical hernias usually disappear by themselves sometime during the first seven years of a child's life as his abdominal muscles grow stronger, or they can be surgically repaired.

Scars, Preemie Head, and Other Reminders of the NICU

Most babies are left with some, usually minor, traces of their experiences in the NICU. Two are so common that almost all babies will have them. The first are tiny harmless lumps that develop in their heels, reminders of the many blood samples taken by heel sticks. The second is a characteristic shape to the head known as the "preemie head": the head is slightly flattened on the sides and the face is long and narrow. Preemie head develops because of the long hours your baby spent lying on firm mattresses instead of floating in the womb. The preemie head shape is sometimes more pronounced in babies who had trouble taking in enough calories and nutrients, especially calcium, for a prolonged time. This group includes babies with respiratory trouble, NEC, and those on diuretics. The preemie head shape does not affect a child developmentally; as babies begin to move their heads around more, sit up, and their hair begins to grow in, their heads round out and the shape becomes less noticeable.

Other babies who have had a long, complicated stay in the hospital may be left with more noticeable reminders, including scars from central IV lines, chest tubes, or surgeries. Scars often grow slightly larger as your child grows and may become more obvious in the first year or two. Then as your child's skin matures around age two or three, they will begin to fade and become less conspicuous. Gentle massage may help these scars from developing adhesions (attachments to deeper tissues) or from dimpling. If a scar is in a particularly bad spot or is very unsightly, talk to a dermatologist or Board-certified cosmetic surgeon about options for repairing or reducing it.

One family whose child had a number of scars mentioned a secondary problem caused by them:

> *"Any time we've seen a new doctor, we've gotten funny looks because of Emily's scars; they clearly think she's an abused child. We've learned to keep her discharge papers with us so we can pull them out to explain why she looks the way she does."*

Some babies who were seriously ill in the NICU and spent a long time lying on their backs have feet and legs that turn out a little more than usual. This condition is temporary and tends to disappear as the child learns to walk. And finally, some children are left with mild burns on their skin in places where tape or monitor leads were removed. These burns fade quickly but may show up later as lighter patches on dark-skinned children, or on light-skinned children as they tan.

Dental Problems

For reasons that are not well understood, many preemies have defects in the enamel, the hard outer covering, of their baby teeth. The defects appear as pits or grooves on the outside of the tooth, or areas where the enamel is missing altogether. These areas tend to collect plaque and develop cavities more easily. As many as one in three of all premature babies and about four out of five babies weighing less than 1,500 grams (3 pounds 5 ounces) at birth have these defects. Fortunately, the permanent adult teeth do not usually have any of these problems.

Some babies who have been intubated for long periods of time develop changes in their mouths such as highly arched palates and misshapen front teeth. Again, the adult teeth are usually fine, and babies adjust to the shape of their palates.

Prematurity does not usually affect the rate or timing of teething so you can use your child's adjusted age to give you some idea of when to expect his teeth to come in. Because preemies are at higher risk for decay in their baby teeth, it is recommended that they have their first dental examination after they have a few teeth or at least by the time they are two to two and a half years old, and regular checkups every six months after that. Fluoride treatments may be particularly helpful for preemies.

Ear, Nose, and Throat Problems

Preemies tend to get more colds and ear infections, which may be accompanied by an accumulation of fluid in the middle ear. This fluid muffles sounds so that your child's hearing is dramatically reduced. Unfortunately, ear infections and fluid in the ear tend to be most common in the second and third years of life, and can affect the rate at which your child learns to talk or cause him to mispronounce words and sounds. Having fluid in the ears is also uncomfortable. Your child may be more irritable, his balance may be affected, and he may be more prone to repeated ear infections.

Although many children between the ages of one and three develop ear infections with accompanying fluid in their ears, preemies seem to be at higher risk for these problems and to experience them more frequently.

Because of the potential impact on your child's speech development, you may want to have his ears and hearing checked regularly if he experiences these problems. Your doctor may put your child on a low dose of antibiotics to prevent ear infections, or may refer you to an otolaryngologist (ear, nose, and throat doctor). Your child may be helped with ear tubes, tiny tubes that are surgically inserted through the eardrum, that prevent the build-up of fluid. The operation is simple and takes only a few minutes, and is usually done on an outpatient basis. However, it does require that your child be put to sleep briefly with a general anesthetic.

Sometimes, fluid accumulates in the ear without a noticeable ear infection. One mother told of an appointment that she had with a neurologist in which she mentioned that her daughter seemed very slow to react and that she often had difficulty getting her attention. The neurologist seemed to feel that her daughter's slowness was probably due to developmental delays. However, a few weeks later at a routine checkup, the pediatrician discovered that her daughter had a lot of fluid in her ears. After ear tubes were inserted and the fluid drained, her daughter responded quickly whenever spoken to.

Preemies also seem to have more trouble with their tonsils and adenoids, glands that lie in the back of the throat and nose. These glands may become enlarged enough to obstruct breathing, cause chronic ear infections or snuffles, or become repeatedly infected. If your child snores or seems to breathe irregularly and noisily at night, you may want to talk with your pediatrician about the possibility that his tonsils and adenoids are enlarged. They may need to be surgically removed to provide relief.

The reasons that preemies have more trouble with their ears, noses, and throats is not clear. It may be due to the small size of their nasal passages and Eustachian tubes (tubes that connect the back of the throat with the middle ear), which can make drainage and congestion a problem. Some physicians feel that the problems are a result of minor damage or irritation caused by such things as ET or nasogastric tubes or oxygen cannulas. Reflux may also contribute to the problem. Most children outgrow these problems by the time they reach school age.

Asthma (Reactive Airway Disease)

Many preemies who have a history of respiratory problems experience episodes of asthma or asthma-like symptoms, known as reactive airway disease, when they get sick or when they are exposed to allergens or other irritants in the air. These symptoms, including difficulty breathing, wheezing, and coughing, occur when the air passages in the lungs become irritated and swollen, making breathing difficult. As these babies recover from their respiratory problems, they become less prone to these episodes, but many continue to have asthma even at school age.

If Your Child Needs to Be Rehospitalized

After all the time your baby has spent in the hospital, it is discouraging to face the possibility that he might need to be readmitted at some point. Unfortunately, preemies are twice as likely as full-term babies to be re-hospitalized during their childhoods. Most of these re-admissions occur during the first two years of life, but even into school age, preemies are hospitalized more often than full-term children. Almost half of the babies with respiratory problems will need to be readmitted to the hospital before their first birthday.

Among babies under two years old, most hospital admissions are for respiratory illnesses and problems with weight gain or dehydration. In later childhood, about half of the admissions are for surgical procedures, particularly for hernia repairs, ear tubes, tonsillectomies, and adenoidectomies.

Should your child need to be readmitted to the hospital, you can do a number of things to help his stay go more smoothly.

- Know in advance what to do if your child becomes seriously ill. Talk to your pediatrician and find out how to get in touch quickly. Know which hospital to go to in case of an emergency.
- Bring your child's discharge summary and any X-rays you have. This is particularly important if your child had or continues to have respiratory problems. Damaged areas of the lungs can be misdiagnosed as pneumonia; a radiologist who has the old X-rays for comparison can make a more accurate diagnosis of your child's current condition.
- If your infant needs to be readmitted to the hospital, he will not go

back into the NICU. A baby must be less than 28 days old at admission to be cared for in a NICU. He will be admitted either to a pediatric floor or, if he is very ill, to a pediatric intensive care unit (PICU). Like the NICU, these areas usually offer unlimited visiting hours for parents, as well as fold-out chairs or cots if you want to spend the night.

- If your child develops a lower respiratory illness, he may need to be treated with supplemental oxygen or even placed on a respirator during the worst part of his illness. This can be a tremendous psychological setback if your child has only recently been taken off this equipment.

- Illness and rehospitalizations usually cause a temporary slowdown in growth and development among babies. Among toddlers and older children, you may see a regression in behavior or a temporary loss of certain skills, such as toilet training. With time and patience, your child will catch up again.

Having a child in the hospital disrupts the entire family. Try to explain what is happening to other children at home. Don't be surprised if they act up or become angry with you or their sick sibling. Try to give them some extra attention when you can.

Your Changing Feelings

As your child grows and changes, your feelings about his birth and everything that you and he have been through also evolve. It takes most parents a long time—two years is probably an average length of time—to feel as though life is getting back to normal. And many parents feel that they continue waiting "for the other shoe to drop"—for something new or unexpected to show up—for years afterward. Some of the other common issues experienced by many parents are explored here.

Your Child's Birthday and Other Significant Dates

Your child's birthday, particularly his first one, can be a difficult, bittersweet time. As it approaches, you may find yourself reliving the events sur-

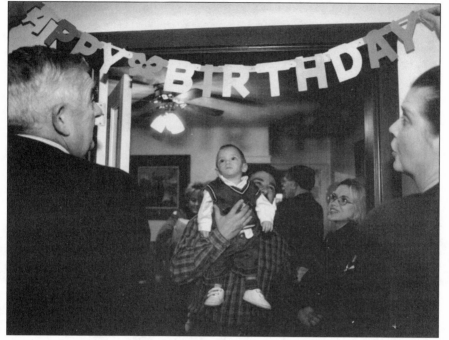

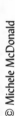

First birthdays are a time to celebrate, but can stir strong feelings and memories as well.

rounding his birth, and feeling a resurgence of all the strong feelings you had at the time. As one mother said, "I thought I was going crazy. I couldn't believe I was going through all this stuff again."

Your child's birthday marks the anniversary of so much in addition to your child's birth. You can't help but be reminded of things you've lost, including your dreams and expectations of a full-term pregnancy, an uneventful birth, and a healthy child. For some it is linked to the loss of one or more children who did not survive being born prematurely. And if your child has ongoing medical or developmental problems, the first birthday can be even more problematic. You may find yourself and your child still in the middle of an evolving situation, with more questions than answers, and with an unclear future.

On the positive side, though, your child's birthday is also a time for celebration, although some parents say that they are not quite sure whether to celebrate on their child's real birth date, or on his original due date. Despite your child's unexpected start in life, he survived and has made great progress in the year.

You will probably find that there will be other significant dates that stir up strong feelings and reactions as your child grows, although their strength usually begins to fade as time passes. However, sometimes your reactions may surprise you, as happened to this mother:

> *"I went to a routine teacher conference when my son was in second grade and the teacher asked me to tell him about my son. I opened my mouth to tell him something and, out of the blue, I said, "He's my miracle baby" and burst into tears. I had no idea beforehand that I was going to react like that. The poor teacher must have thought I was nuts."*

Waiting for Milestones

During the early months and years of your child's life, it is easy to fall into the trap of waiting for your child to achieve certain milestones as a sign that he is okay or has fully recovered from his prematurity. This might be called the "When he starts walking, I'll know he's all right" syndrome. Because preemie development tends to be somewhat different and is often slower than that of typical full-term newborns, waiting for milestones can set you up for anxiety, as this mother explained:

> *"Milestones have never been a particularly joyous time for me. I have always watched and waited with trepidation for whatever it was and once it was achieved I never felt excited. Rather, it was relief followed by anxiety as I waited for the next milestone."*

Another parent voiced a similar experience:

> *"Waiting for milestones has been especially hard on us. David has seemed to eventually come around and achieve each milestone so far, but just about when we are ready to give up and get very worried. The comparisons to other children and the constant questions from friends, relatives, and strangers alike is what makes it hardest for me. I'm willing to let him go at his own speed, because I have faith that he will be able to achieve each goal, but with constant questions as benign as 'How's he doing?' from people who don't really want a true answer, it can be very draining."*

The milestone issue is a big one for a couple of reasons. First, infant and toddler development is measured in terms of the achievement of very specific milestones. Every assessment and physical exam includes questions about what skills your child has acquired, and an analysis of where that places him on a developmental checklist. Since we all want concrete evidence that our children are progressing normally, it is almost impossible not to become focused upon these milestones.

However, many parents also talked about how important it is to develop a broader perspective, and to try to balance concern about milestones with an appreciation of all the things that your child can do.

"I would go into such a tailspin every time Joanna didn't reach a milestone, or she would reach one but our problems weren't over yet. Finally I learned to stop looking at my daughter in terms of milestones. I tried to appreciate all the things she could do and tried to worry less about the things she couldn't do. But it's very hard and I still find myself periodically falling into the same trap again."

This sentiment was echoed by another mother:

"The doctors could not tell us what effects the [brain] bleed would have in Katy. So because of this I am afraid I didn't take the time to smell the roses. In other words, I was so concerned about the next step that I didn't enjoy the little things enough."

Letting Go

For some parents, particularly those whose children have had a very rough time or those who have waited a long time for a baby, it can be extremely difficult to allow others to take over some of the baby's care, or to allow him to participate in a play group or early intervention group. It is natural to worry about whether someone else can care for your child as well as you can, especially if he has special needs or his behavior is erratic and difficult to interpret. Or if your child has had or continues to have respiratory problems, exposing your baby to a group of children who undoubtedly have germs seems like madness.

Finding a balance can be tricky. It is important for your own mental health to be able to take a break from your child, and as your child grows he needs the stimulation and socialization of being with other children. One mother talked about how difficult this transition can be:

"It's so difficult to know when you can let go. You tend to hover over them and it's hard to see that you're doing too much of it, that you really do have to let go a little....They have to learn social skills, they need to be around other kids. So at some point, you have to force yourself to start letting go."

Another mother felt similarly:

"If I want her to be normal, I have to let her go. This is very difficult for me. I have always been very overprotective of all my children, and am even more so with my preemie."

No one can tell you what is best for you and your child. Many parents of full-term children find it difficult to allow others to care for their children, or have trouble with the transitions to preschool or other group experiences. Because of your child's tougher start in life, you may find it even more difficult to cope with the normal process of letting go as your child grows.

But one mother had an interesting and different feeling about this issue:

"As opposed to other people with preemies, I think I am oddly less protective of my son. Not that I am not protective when it comes to something serious or when he could get hurt. But I feel that all the serious situations we have been through with him have made me lighten up about little things, about getting a scraped knee when he plays or misses a nap. Those kinds of things don't really matter to me."

Returning to Work

Like many other parents, preemie parents often face difficult decisions about when and whether to return to work after the birth of their child. Many parents have no choice about returning to work, but finding the right child care and balancing working and parenting can be difficult. When your child has been born prematurely, or has additional needs because of his early birth, the stresses of returning to work can increase.

Perhaps not surprisingly, many parents of preemies opt to stay home to care for their children, even when the financial impact is significant. However, many others have successfully combined working and being a preemie parent. These parents stressed the importance —and sometimes difficulty—of finding the right child care situation. If you are planning to return to work, you may want to consider using a sitter in your home or home day care, where there are fewer children for the first year while your child is more susceptible to illness.

Two mothers who have successfully returned to work shared their stories.

"When Adam was born, I was completing my residency at the hospital where he was born. Leaves of absence are very stringent in such programs, although I knew I would have been granted whatever I needed. When Adam was one month old, I went back to work for two months; I worked, however, in the hospital where he was. I used to visit at lunch and then again in the p.m. with my husband. I don't think I could have gone back to work so soon if I was not physically in the same building, knowing I could be there in an instant if there was a problem. A kind nurse once even paged me in the middle of the day to say they were changing Adam's isolette and he could be held for a while if I could get away to come to the NICU. When Adam came home at three months, I took another month off and then returned to work.

"I have continued to work full time since (except for maternity leave with my second full-term baby). Of course I often feel guilty and have the usual problems all working mothers have, but I believe this is what I would have done if Adam had not been premature. I know it is not for everyone, and maybe only for a few, but I hope that women who must or who desire to work know that it can be done."

~~~

"I realize I am probably in the minority here, but I went back to work when my preemie daughter was very young (four months). It is always hard to leave one's children with others, but I'm not sure I had that much of a harder time than other working moms. Part of it came from my desire to try to treat my daughter as normal and ours as a normal family, despite what we had been through. I have spent lots of time and energy checking into the best care situations for my daughter, and have been lucky enough to leave her with a babysitter and not at a day care center."

Deciding to Have Another Baby

Many parents find that they go through a period when they have a strong urge to have another baby in order to have a chance to "do it right," to experience all the aspects of a normal pregnancy, delivery, and infancy that they were cheated of this time around. Other parents report the opposite: the mere thought of putting themselves and another baby at risk for premature birth and all that it entails sends a shudder down their spines. Many parents vacillate between these two sets of feelings for quite a while.

Given the difficulty of this pregnancy it probably makes sense to wait for a year or so before trying to make this decision. Give yourself and your partner a chance to recover and to get a realistic sense of how your baby is doing.

But when the time comes that you begin to think seriously about having another child, a good starting place would be to get some information and advice from your obstetrician. You would want to explore with him some of the following issues:

- Why did this pregnancy end prematurely?
- What are the chances that such a thing would happen again?
- Would your next pregnancy be considered "highrisk"?
- Should you be cared for by an obstetrician who specializes in high-risk pregnancies?

There are a number of other questions to consider, some of which you probably thought about when you decided on this past pregnancy, and others of which are specific to preemie parents:

- Are you able to financially, physically, and emotionally care for another member of the family?
- Are both you and your partner ready for another baby?
- Do you have resources (either financial or family) to help you if your pregnancy becomes complicated and you must spend time in bed or in the hospital?
- If your prematurely born child requires extra care and attention, will you be able to handle the extra demands of a new baby?
- Are you ready to face the emotional strain that will undoubtedly be a part of this next pregnancy?
- Do you think you could cope with another premature birth?

CHAPTER 10

Getting the Most Out of Early Intervention and School-Based Programs

ℬℒ

A<small>FTER THE INTENSITY</small> of the NICU, many parents feel alone and unsupported when they get home with their baby. Their questions and concerns remain, but in many communities resources familiar with the special issues of preemie development may be hard to find. Three valuable sources for many parents are the infant follow-up clinics operated by urban teaching hospitals with NICUs, early intervention programs, and special needs programs offered by the local public school system. Infant follow-up clinics, discussed earlier in Chapter 5, are staffed with professionals familiar with preemies. They can examine your baby, evaluate her progress, and answer many of your questions. These follow-up clinics do not replace your pediatrician but provide additional preemie-focused services for you and your baby. In addition, early intervention programs provide services in many communities for eligible infants and toddlers up to age three. After age three, children with special needs are served by their local public school systems.

This chapter will orient you to the early intervention system and introduce you to school-based programs for children who need special education services after age three. Although not all preemies will need these services, the more you understand, the better you will be able to take advantage of them for your child, yourself, and your family.

Early Intervention Programs

Early intervention (EI) programs offer a broad range of services to infants and toddlers under three years of age who are at risk for or have problems with development. The purpose of EI is to:

- provide education, support, and therapeutic services to children with identified disabilities;
- prevent developmental delays or problems among vulnerable children, if possible;
- help each child develop to her full potential; and
- provide education and support to families.

The growth in the early intervention system in this country began after the passage in 1986 of federal law PL 99-457, which became known as the Individuals with Disabilities Education Act (IDEA) in 1990. Part H of that law, the Program for Infants and Toddlers with Disabilities, specifically targets children from birth to age three and offers federal money to states who establish EI programs that serve eligible children. This law has been amended several times, most recently in 1997; under the new amendments (known as PL 105-117), the regulations dealing with Infants and Toddlers became known as Part C rather than Part H. In order to qualify for federal funding, states must meet minimum eligibility and service standards as defined in federal regulations. But participating states are free to decide exactly who is eligible for services and how to provide those services. Thus, EI programs vary greatly from state to state.

Who Is Eligible?

According to the federal regulations, EI programs must serve two groups of children under the age of three: children who are developmentally delayed and children with an identified mental or physical condition that often results in developmental delay. Examples include problems with hearing or vision, neurological problems, congenital disorders, and prenatal exposure to drugs or alcohol. States may also choose to provide services to children who are considered to be at high risk for delays. Risk factors for delay include a low birthweight, brain bleed, and chronic lung disease, as well as certain environmental conditions such as poverty, parental substance abuse, or neglect.

At the current time, only nine states—Arkansas, California, Hawaii, Indiana, Massachusetts, New Hampshire, New Mexico, North Carolina, and West Virginia—provide services to "at risk" infants and toddlers in addition to those with an identified disability or delay. In those states, preemies may be eligible for EI services simply as a result of their early births, even if they have no developmental problems. In the remaining states, preemies qualify only if they have specific disabilities or if their development begins to lag behind by a certain, specified amount.

A Family-Centered, Multidisciplinary System

The EI system defines itself as being family-centered. Services are provided not just to eligible children but to their families, as well. As a parent, you will be involved in identifying and prioritizing the needs of your child, and in planning how those needs can best be met. EI programs often try to provide education and training as well as support groups for parents.

EI programs generally use a multidisciplinary approach, meaning that professionals with different types of training and expertise work together to identify your child's needs, and to design, with your help, services to meet those needs. These services may be provided by special educators, speech and language therapists and audiologists, occupational and physical therapists, psychologists, social workers, nurses, nutritionists, family therapists, orientation and mobility specialists, pediatricians, and other physicians.

Where Are Services Provided?

EI programs vary from state to state, and from program to program within each state. But one common approach is to provide services for qualified infants under one year of age in the home, or the infant's day care setting. Depending upon a child's needs, she may receive a specific service such as physical therapy, or her development may simply be monitored. Under a monitoring program, a nurse or other EI staff professional periodically comes to your home to assess your child's progress, and answer any questions you might have. If a specific problem is identified, the EI program

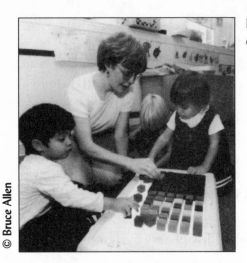

© Bruce Allen

EI therapists work on skills with children in small group play sessions.

must arrange for the necessary services—such as physical or occupational therapy—to be provided on a regular basis to your baby. If, on the other hand, a baby reaches the age of a year or so without developing any delays or specific problems, she may then be discharged from the program.

For children who are at least one year old, many EI programs offer center-based toddler groups. These programs resemble a play group or preschool program, but the staff includes special education teachers, physical and occupational therapists, speech therapists, and others trained to work with special needs children. In conjunction with these toddler programs, many programs operate parent discussion or support groups

In states that provide less comprehensive services, your EI program may assign you a case manager. This professional will identify your child's needs and coordinate services for your child from multiple resources in the community.

The latest rewrite of the federal regulations emphasized the importance of providing services to children in their "natural environments" if at all possible. A child's natural environment is where that child would be if she had no disabilities—at home, at a community preschool, a Head Start program, a day care center. In the future, EI programs will more commonly offer services to children in their community rather than bringing them into the EI center.

Who Pays?

Early intervention programs receive funding from the federal government, the state government, and health insurance (including private companies, Blue Cross, and Medicaid). You will never be billed directly for services, although, with your permission, your health insurance company or HMO will be billed. Even if you have no insurance, your eligible child must receive the services she needs at no cost to you.

Getting Started

Within each state, EI services are provided by a network of community-based providers. Your hospital nursery should be able to provide you with the name and phone number of the EI program that serves your area before your baby is discharged. It is a good idea to contact them before your baby comes home, but you can call them at anytime up until her third birthday. They will usually send you a description of their services and some initial paperwork, and arrange for a meeting with one of their staff members.

EI services are offered, but never forced, upon you and your baby. If you decide you are interested in accepting these services, you can expect to go through these steps.

Giving your permission. You must give your written permission before the EI program can do any assessments of your child or provide any services. During your initial meeting with a staff member, you should receive information about the program and services that your child may receive as well as your rights as a parent.

Determining eligibility for services. Once you have given your permission, your child will be evaluated to see if she qualifies for services. As mentioned earlier, states differ in their eligibility criteria. You can ask to see a copy of the eligibility standards used in your state.

Assessing your child's development. A multidisciplinary team from EI will assess your child's development as a first step toward planning the services that she will receive. This assessment may take place in your home or at the EI center. The team will ask you for information about your child and may use one of many possible assessment tests. Again, you can ask the team members to explain how your child's development will be evaluated.

Developing a Plan for Your Child:
The Individualized Family Service Plan (IFSP)

The services your child will receive from the EI program are specified in a document called the Individualized Family Service Plan, or IFSP (see sample form). You, your child's team at EI, and anyone else you wish to involve develop the IFSP together in order to set some common goals for your child in the coming months. The plan can include information about any or all of the following:

- Information about your child, including her medical history or other relevant information, the results of any tests or assessments made by the EI team, her identified needs and her strengths;
- Goals for your child and your family;
- How you'll reach those goals together with the EI team including methods and strategies;
- Which services will be provided—how often, by whom, when, and where;
- Who your service coordinator is.

Providing Information for the Plan

If you are new to the EI system, you may be unsure about what your baby needs and what the EI program can do for you. As one mother said,

> *"I remember the nurse from EI filling out a bunch of forms the first time we met. At one point she asked me what my son's strengths were. I wasn't quite sure what this question meant since he had been home only about a month and didn't do much except sleep and eat. The only strength I could think of was that he was cute. Then she asked me what my concerns were. My concerns were that I didn't know what to be worried about. I felt as if I was being asked to answer these questions in a vacuum. I didn't know enough yet to know what, if anything, I should be worried about."*

Excerpts from an Individualized Family Service Plan (IFSP) Form for a 31-Week Preemie at Two Months Corrected Age

From FAMILY PAGE

Child's Name: John Doe

Date of Birth: 9/25/99

Every family is different and has its own priorities, concerns, and resources. This is your family's opportunity to tell other members of the team about your child and family, and your involvement with other community providers. The information on this page is confidential and will not be shared without your permission. This page should be completed at least annually.

How would you describe your child and your family? What do you see as strengths as well as the concerns and priorities of both your child and your family?

John is eating well. He enjoys direct interaction, he smiles a lot. He is also developing social skills. Consistent growth has also been achieved (weight gain). He looks like he's thriving. Nighttime sleeping is good, as he will go for 5-hour stretches. He has become less fussy and more content.

We are concerned about all the movement; there seems to be exaggerated movement or excessive movement of his whole body. We would also like to explore the tremors recently observed of the foot. Furthermore, learn more about his organizational state (breathing patterns, sleep) and ways to facilitate his development any way we can. We'd like to learn exercises or activities that will enhance his development and that he would benefit from.

From DEVELOPMENT PROFILE

The Child's Development Profile summarizes the assessment/evaluation results and information gathered about your child's health and development. It may or may not include eligibility determination and function levels depending on the desires of your family and other team members. This section is designed to be shared with insurance companies, physicians, schools, and others as designated by the parent(s)/guardian(s).

Excerpts, continued

Summary and Recommendations:

John Doe presented as an adorable little boy who was referred to Early Intervention given his premature birth history. He is a 4 month old boy who was born at 31 weeks gestation. He was seen today during the late morning hours in the presence of his mother. He remained alert and content throughout the entire administration of the Early Intervention Developmental Profile (Michigan).

He has continued to improve at home though mom has concerns with feeding and sensory needs. Results of today's assessment indicated that most developmental skills are consistent with his corrected age rather than his chronological age. There were qualitative considerations that influenced his performance. Most notably, John's breathing appeared exaggerated and labored and he displayed a constant degree of movement. To what extent these indicate some degree of disorganization requires further investigation. It is imperative that these more subtle, but influential variables do not impede his ability to develop more refined skills and attention to details and learning. John is recommended for Early Intervention services based on a clinical judgement. He and his family would benefit from support to incorporate general therapeutic strategies into his daily activities and promote overall developmental gains.

From OUTCOMES AND STRATEGIES

This page outlines the specific Outcomes and Strategies that have been developed with the family as part of the Early Intervention Team based on the concerns identified throughout the evaluation process and family priorities. The Service Coordinator should discuss with the family what they hope to achieve through their Early Intervention experience.

Start date: 1/19/00
Desired Family Outcomes and Strategies:

1. **John will demonstrate more controlled patterns of movement.**
    a. Monitor and facilitate bilateral symmetry (head, hands, abdomen, etc.)
    b. John will be able to reach and grasp an object.
    c. John will assist with bottle holding and bringing his hands to midline, progressing to crossing midline and transferring objects from one hand to he next.

Excerpts, continued

d. John will be able to roll.

e. John will bring his hands / feet to his mouth.

f. John will tolerate prone (being on his stomach). This will encourage increased head and neck control, trunk rotation, arm strength, head turning and further prepares him for creeping and crawling.

g. Monitor recently noted tremors. Note whether there exist any consistent variables surrounding these episodes (fatigue, time of day, one foot or both, etc.)

2. John will demonstrate integration of questionable sensory integration concerns.

a. Explore sleeping and breathing patterns and whether they can be improved or modified through adult intervention.

b. Explore feeding skills and tolerance to surroundings during feeding. Encourage social interaction (eye contact) during these times.

c. John will tolerate his surroundings and demonstrated learning of more refined, mature skills (ability to maintain eye focus or gaze, etc.).

Some of the areas that you may want to consider as you develop your child's IFSP are listed here to help structure your thinking. You do not need to include information about all of these; use only those that seem useful or relevant.

Concerns about your child. You may simply want information about what to expect and what to watch out for as your child grows, or you may have specific concerns about your child's development in the following areas:

- movement and motor skills (gross and fine)
- speech and language development
- cognitive (thinking) skills development
- feeding, nutrition, and weight gain
- social skills
- learning to get along with other children
- difficult behaviors or emotions
- equipment or supplies

- pain, discomfort, or irritability
- vision or hearing problems
- health or dental care

Family characteristics. You may want to think about some of the aspects of your family, friends, or community that could affect your ability to care for your child. Some of these may be important sources of strength or support. In other cases, you may feel that a lack of resources creates a burden for your family. These characteristics include:

- support from family members, partner, or spouse
- communication with family
- support from friends
- support from community, social, or church groups
- relationship with your other children
- your parenting skills

Other concerns. The IFSP can also focus on your needs as a preemie parent, including:

- meeting other families whose children have similar needs
- finding or working with doctors or other specialists
- coordinating or making appointments, dealing with agencies
- coordinating your child's medical care
- finding out more about how different services work or how they could work for you
- planning for the future
- finding information about resources available in the community
- getting help with insurance, transportation, and child care
- finding a parent support group
- learning more about your child's particular disability or diagnosis
- identifying resources to help with the extra costs of your child's special needs

Setting Goals

The IFSP will specify goals for your child that you and the EI team will be working toward in the next three to six months. Goals can range from very general to very specific, and may include such things as working on a specific physical problem, learning a new skill, or getting support or training. You may want to set just one or two goals in your first IFSP; you can add other, more specific ones as your child grows and develops.

For example, you can set:

- specific goals for your child, such as: "I want Philip to learn to walk."
- goals for yourself: "I would like to meet other parents of preemies."
- goals for your family: "I would like to help my other children who are having a hard time coping with how time-consuming their preemie brother is."
- combination goals: "I would like to learn how to provide physical therapy for my child."

Once the IFSP has been written, and you have signed it to give your permission, your child will begin to receive services.

Changing Services

If you wish to change the services your child receives, or to have her team re-evaluate her needs, you have the right to make such a request at any time. If the EI program wants to change any aspects of your child's services, they must notify you in advance and explain the reasons for the changes. You must give written permission before any changes take place.

Resolving Disagreements

The initial packet of information you receive from your EI program should include a description of your rights as a parent in the EI system, and the procedures to follow in case you have a serious disagreement about any aspect of your child's eligibility assessment, developmental evaluation, or service plan. Many of these disagreements can be resolved through informal discussions with the EI staff or director. However, if this approach fails, you have recourse to formal procedures to resolve the differences. These may involve a hearing, mediation, or formal complaint to the state department that oversees EI programs.

Does Early Intervention Work?

The most comprehensive study of the impact of early intervention serv-ices on premature infants is known as the Infant Health and Development Program, which ran for three years in the early 1980s. Eight sites were selected to provide early intervention services to low birthweight (under 2,500 grams or 5 1/2 pounds) babies and toddlers. The children who par-ticipated were divided into two groups, both of which received regular pediatric follow-up services. In addition to these checkups, one group also received intensive early intervention services that consisted of regular home visits (0 to 36 months), a full-time center-based program (12 to 36 months), and a parent group program (12 to 36 months). These two groups were compared on three different measures: IQ, behavior, and health.

After three years, the group that received the EI services had signifi-cantly higher IQ scores than the group that received only medical follow-up services. The greatest impact occurred among the heavier low birthweight children—those who weighed over 2,000 grams (4 1/2 pounds)—and those whose mothers were less educated. Behavior seemed to be slightly improved among those children receiving the EI services, and health was the same in both groups.

These children were recontacted at the ages of five and eight—two and five years after the program ended—to see if the positive effects of the EI program had continued. The researchers found that the differences between the groups had largely disappeared by this time. They found no differences in behavior or health, and only slight differences in IQ, but only among the heavier group of LBW infants.

From this study, the authors concluded that EI services are effective and can improve the cognitive development of premature babies, but for those at highest risk—the smallest and those at lower socioeconomic lev-els—services probably need to continue throughout childhood in order to maintain the improvements in cognitive abilities and behavior.

The programs studied in this research project offered very intensive and comprehensive services. In reality, the quality and quantity of services available through EI programs vary from state to state, and even within a geographical area. Some parents find EI to be a wonderful resource, one that provides a broad range of coordinated services for their child as well as support for themselves. In other cases, it may be difficult to access services and you may need to act as an assertive advocate.

Potential Stumbling Blocks

As a parent you are at the center of the EI system of services for your child, a position that ensures your involvement in all phases of your child's program. This is one of the strengths of the EI approach, but, ironically, it can also leave you vulnerable to some potentially difficult experiences. The following issues were mentioned by a number of parents, and are included here not as criticisms of EI, but to emphasize the role that you as a parent play in providing perspective and balance to any program of services for your child.

Overemphasis on or Overdiagnosis of Problems. Children in EI tend to be watched carefully, and their development closely assessed on a regular basis. While this allows for early detection of specific problems, it can sometimes lead to an overdiagnosis of problems. Children show a vast range of development that still falls within normal bounds. Some of this normal variation may be misdiagnosed as developmental problems.

As a parent, you should be ready to use your own experience and knowledge of your child to balance what you hear from a therapist. EI personnel do their best to do complete and accurate assessments, but they see your child for a limited amount of time and in very specific circumstances. While their expertise often helps to clarify something that has been confusing or worrying you about your child, you may sometimes feel that they have taken a particular behavior out of context or placed too much emphasis on something that isn't a problem. One mother recalled:

"A speech therapist tested my son's language skills at about 18 months. Unfortunately, she tested him in an alcove in a busy hallway, using objects he was unfamiliar with. Not only was he distracted by people walking up and down, but he didn't recognize many of the things she was using. I wasn't surprised that he didn't do very well on the test. She recommended that he receive speech therapy, but I declined since I knew he was doing just fine. It was just a bad test situation that made it look otherwise."

Parent as Therapist. The philosophy of EI emphasizes the importance of actively involving parents in their child's care, so that they understand their child's needs and learn how best to help them. For example, if your child needs physical therapy, your child's physical therapist will probably teach you exercises to do with your child or therapeutic ways of playing. This is a positive approach unless you begin to feel overwhelmed by the multiple roles you end up playing: parent, teacher, and therapist. Try to balance these roles; don't let your child's therapeutic needs overshadow your natural role as a parent. You needn't turn every play time into a therapy session. Doing so will only frustrate you and your child.

Overemphasis on Progress or Achievement of Developmental Milestones. An emphasis on identifying problems and responding therapeutically can sometimes overshadow your ability simply to enjoy your child. You may find yourself focusing too much on your child's problems, and losing sight of her strengths and abilities. You may anxiously watch for certain milestones to reassure yourself that your child is going to be all right. If those milestones aren't reached on time, it's easy to become discouraged.

Too Much or Conflicting Information. Although most programs try to offer coordinated, multidisciplinary services, you may hear conflicting opinions from different therapists on your team. Each may have a particular, but differing, perspective on your child. Or you may hear more information than you want. Hearing that your child has a long list of problems in many areas can be quite discouraging and disheartening. If you find yourself in this situation, remind your child's team that you need to hear positive things about your child. You may want to use the IFSP to focus on the most important problems and let some of the minor ones go for the time being.

The Transition to School-Based Programs

When your child turns three, responsibility for providing special services for her shifts from the EI program you have been using to your local public school system. Not all children who have been in EI continue on into special education in the public school systems. Some children graduate into regular preschool programs, day care settings, or home day care, or attend no formal program at all. Children who continue may need different kinds of programs or services since their needs may have changed.

For many families this transition can be very anxiety-provoking. You've probably built up personal relationships with the professionals in your EI program, and you're familiar with how the system works. Now you need to learn a whole new system, including new individuals, programs, procedures, and locations. In addition, in a school-based program, your child will start mixing with a larger population of children from your community.

It is important to plan ahead for this transition. Because the school system takes over responsibility for your child when she turns three, you should begin the transition process when your child is two and a half at the latest. Doing so will give you and the school system time to accomplish all the tasks involved, explore the various options, and plan the best program possible for your child. If your child's birthday is in the summer, or if you think you may need to make special or complex requests of the school, it is a good idea to begin even earlier than that—sometimes up to a year in advance.

The more knowledgeable you are about your options and how the process works, the better are your chances for having the transition proceed smoothly and getting the services your child needs. One of the responsibilities of your EI program is to develop a plan to cover this transition. They usually know the public school systems in the areas they cover and should work closely with you as you approach your child's third birthday.

One of the crucial parts of working with your school system is knowing your child's rights and your rights as a parent. This information should be supplied to you at the beginning of the transition process. But every school system is unique, and special education services differ among schools within the same system. The process of learning how to work with the individuals within your school system to ensure the best services for you child can be a challenging task. Other parents are often the best source of information; find out how to contact your local Parent Advisory Council (PAC), a voluntary organization of parents of special needs children who can provide you with information, advice, and support.

The Differences Between EI and School-Based Programs

Eligibility requirements for school-based special education services are generally tighter than those for EI programs. While many states provide early intervention services for children at risk for developmental delays, special education services are always reserved for children with diagnosed special needs. As with EI programs, eligibility requirements vary from state to state. Request a copy of the regulations from your state department of education.

The focus of school-based programs shifts from the family-centered approach used in EI to a child-centered, educational focus. Your child will no longer be looked upon as a preemie, but will be assessed in terms of her identified problems and learning needs. Some of the other differences between the two systems are listed in the box below.

Differences Between EI and Public School-Based Services

	Early Intervention	Public School-Based
Responsible agency	various state agencies	state Department of Education
Ages served	0 to 36 months	3 to 22 years
Funding source	health insurance; state; federal	local taxes; state; federal
Location of services	varied: home-based, community-based	usually in the school
Focus	family needs	child's needs and education
Planning document	Individualized Family Service Plan (IFSP)	Individualized Education Plan (IEP)
Eligibility	identified disability, developmental delay, at-risk infant or family	diagnosis or identification of special needs
Cycle	year round	school year, with possible summer services

Adapted from "Turning Three." Used with permission from Federation for Children with Special Needs, Boston.

Types of Preschool Programs

Depending upon your child's needs and the resources available in your community, you may have a number of options from which to choose during the preschool years. Early in the transition process try to visit some of the programs in your community. Some of the most common types include:

An integrated preschool program. Your local public school system may offer an integrated preschool program for three- and four-year olds in which children with and without disabilities participate in the same classroom. Children without special needs may pay fees for these programs as they would for any preschool program, while children with identified disabilities participate free of charge as part of the special education services your town provides. In order to provide some of the special services needed by children with disabilities, an integrated classroom is staffed with more teachers and aides than a regular preschool. The head teachers usually have degrees in special education, and occupational, physical, and speech therapists may also participate in the classroom. This option offers advantages if your child has a number of problems for which she needs services. It also allows her to be in a regular preschool program and make friends with many different kinds of children.

Regular program with the addition of a specified service(s). If your child needs only one type of service, such as a weekly speech or physical therapy session, you may be able to get the school system to provide that specific service to your child while she attends the preschool, day care center, or Head Start program of your choice.

Separate special education classroom. Most systems are moving away from providing separate services to children with special needs in favor of the more integrated approach described above. However, some children may spend part of their day in a separate classroom with a teacher who can more specifically meet their particular needs.Out-of-district placement or collaborative program: If your school system cannot meet your child's needs, you may be referred to a program in another town or to a private school. In this case, the costs of the program will be covered by your local school system. Some smaller school systems join together to form collaborative programs that serve special needs children from several participating towns.

How the Special Education System Works

If you are seeking special education services for your child, you can expect to go through the following steps. The timing and exact nature of this process will vary by location, but this is the general sequence.

Referral. With your permission, your EI program will inform your local school system in writing that your child may be eligible for special education services. If your child has not been in early intervention, you can make this referral yourself by calling your local school department. If someone else such as a pediatrician or relative wants to refer your child, they must first get your permission to do so.

Notice. Within a specified number of days, the school system must send you a letter notifying you that they have received the referral. You then give written permission to the school to evaluate your child. At this time, you may want to request a preassessment meeting. In many systems, this meeting will not automatically occur unless you specifically request it.

Preassessment Meeting. This is an informal meeting with one or more of the people who will be involved in your child's evaluation. You can discuss the reasons for the evaluation, what types of professionals should be involved, and what you are hoping for your child. This meeting gives you a chance to meet some of the people involved in your child's evaluation, and lets you present your view of your child. At the meeting you can also let the school system know what types of evaluation tests have already been performed on your child by her EI team and provide them with the test results.

Evaluation. In the next step, your child will be evaluated to determine whether or not she is eligible for services. The evaluation also identifies her strengths and her specific needs for services. In some cases, the school will use evaluations done by your child's EI team. In other cases, they will want to do their own. Or they may be willing to collaborate on the assessment by participating jointly in your child's last EI evaluation.

The evaluation must be completed within a certain number of days after your written permission has been received, and you must be given a copy of it at least two days before your child's educational team meets. This gives you a chance to review it before you meet with the school officials who will help plan your child's program.

Team Meeting. At this meeting the results of your child's evaluation will be presented and discussed, and her Individualized Education Plan (IEP) developed. You are an integral member of your child's team, which will also consist of the people who did your child's evaluation and other school officials. This may include a teacher, a principal, and a representative of the special education department. You may also bring someone such as a friend, family member, or a representative from EI to this meeting with you.

Many parents find team meetings to be quite intimidating, particularly if you are not familiar with the individuals involved or this is your first time through the process. Your child's problems and special needs will be the topic of conversation, which can make it upsetting as well. Go into this meeting as well prepared as possible.

- Remember that you know your child better than anyone in the room and can provide important information that the others may not know. If you feel uncomfortable talking in front of the group, you may want to write up something about your child to share.
- Bring with you any relevant medical records, evaluations, and teacher reports.
- Don't be afraid to ask questions, or to ask for clarification about things you don't understand. You may want to bring with you a written list of questions or points that you want to make.
- Bring a friend or even a professional advocate with you to provide support and help you remember what is said. Some parents take notes or bring a tape recorder along, although recording can make other members of the team nervous. You can explain that you need it to help you retain important information.
- Most of the members of your child's team are on your child's side, and are interested in providing the best services possible for her. But some of them may be dealing with tight finances or a shortage of other

Components of an IEP

Although forms and requirements vary among states and school systems, the following basic components are included in most Individualized Education Plans (IEPs).

1. **Family Information.** Names, addresses, etc.

2. **Name of the individual within the school system who will act as a liaison between the family and the school.** The liaison may be the principal, a teacher, a therapist, or someone else within the school.

3. **Dates that this IEP covers.**

4. **Statement of student's performance level.** This includes a description of the student's areas of strength and current challenges, and is based upon formal and informal assessments, tests, and/or observations.

5. **Student's instructional profile.** The profile describes any adaptations or modifications that are needed to help the child learn, and can include adjustments to the classroom environment, equipment, or special instructional strategies. Any other pertinent information such as medication requirements, services the child is receiving outside the school program, etc. would be found here.

6. **Goals and objectives.** These can be as simple or extensive as necessary, and usually include both long-term goals and short-term objectives. An example of a long-term goal might be to improve expressive and receptive language skills. Short-term objectives would define specific benchmarks that would be used to measure progress toward that goal, such as using three or four word phrases by a certain date. Goals and objectives can be set in multiple areas, including cognitive, self-help, motor, and speech and language skills.

7. **Detailed description of service delivery plans.** The services that a student will receive under this IEP are described, including the type of services, how often, for how long, and where (inside or outside the classroom). The plan also specifies how information about the student will be shared between the classroom teacher, any therapists or special education teachers involved, and the team overseeing the IEP in order to ensure coordination and consistency among all the individuals involved. It may also include documentation of whether the child will need services that extend beyond the regular school year into the summer.

8. **Agreement page.** Finally, the IEP will contain a place where the parents and a representative of the school system sign off on the plan signifying their acceptance. The IEP cannot be implemented and services cannot begin until both parties have signed. Parents have a choice of accepting all components of the plan, accepting certain parts and rejecting others (in which case the child can begin receiving those parts of the plan the parents agree to), or rejecting the entire IEP.

resources that may affect their decisions. To counterbalance some of these pressures you'll need to provide a strong voice in support of your child's needs.

• Approach the team meeting with a positive attitude, and be assertive but not aggressive. In most cases, you will be able to come to an agreement about what type of services your child will receive. You may be working with the school system for a long time, and it is better to start on a positive note.

The Individualized Education Plan (IEP)

The outcome of your child's evaluation process is a document known as the IEP, the equivalent in the public school world of the IFSP in early intervention programs. The IEP spells out in detail what services your child will be receiving for the next school year, including how many times a week, for how long, by what kind of personnel, and where—at school, at home, or elsewhere. It also includes plans for transportation, if necessary, and special needs such as adaptive equipment. You must receive copies of your child's IEP within a certain number of days after the team meeting, and you have a certain number of days to respond.

When you get the IEP, you have a certain number of options. Hopefully, you will agree with it so that you can accept it as written, and services can begin for your child when she turns three. But you also have the option to accept parts of the plan and reject other parts, reject the entire plan, or to postpone a decision and ask for an independent evaluation from an individual outside the school system. If you reject part of the plan, or want to postpone a decision, you can still ask that the plan be implemented while you negotiate changes. In some school districts, your child cannot begin school until you have signed the IEP. If you disagree with parts of it, you can renegotiate it after your child has begun her program.

Smoothing the Transition

Some children adjust to changes more quickly than others, and you may find that your child has less trouble than you in making the transition from her EI program to a new preschool program. In order to smooth the transition, be sure to visit the program your child will be joining ahead of time. If possible, take your child to visit as well. Some programs may have a transition time in which your child spends a shortened time at school for the first several days. Some other suggestions offered by parents and teachers include:

- Schedule a teacher conference soon after your child begins.
- Use a communication book with your child's teachers. This can be a small notebook that travels back and forth to school in your child's backpack, in which you and the teacher regularly write notes or comments to each other.
- Drive your child to school periodically instead of using transportation. This will not always be possible, but it allows you to touch base with your child's teacher, to see the classroom, and to meet the other children and parents.
- Take advantage of opportunities to be involved in the classroom.
- Continue other support or play groups that you've been a part of, including seeing friends made through early intervention.

Potential Stumbling Blocks

A number of logistical and emotional stumbling blocks can interfere with the transition from early intervention to school-based programs, or can affect the services that your child gets.

Trouble Facing Your Child's Needs. For many parents, the meetings and assessments of their child that occur during the transition process bring them up against problems they find difficult to face. It is almost impossible to sit in a room full of people who are discussing your child's problems and not be upset by it. One coping technique is to try to include in these discussions a description of your child's strengths and talents as well as her needs and problems. Another is to bring a friend along who can listen with fewer emotional reactions and help you to think realistically about your child's needs.

If you realize later that you were unrealistic about the extent of your child's problems, or that you failed to provide certain information to the school that would have changed the nature or number of services that your child receives, remember that you'll be able to adjust her program over time. In the meantime, your child is benefiting from the services she is receiving, and her teachers are getting to know her better. For the next team meeting, all of you may have a much clearer view of her needs and be able to design a better program.

Difficulties with the Timing of the Transition. When your child turns three, the public school system becomes responsible for providing and paying for special education services for her. Unfortunately, few children have birthdays in September when this transition could occur most smoothly. If your child is moving into an integrated preschool program operated by your school system, the transition usually can be accomplished smoothly at any time during the year. But if your child will be moving into a private preschool program, making this transition in the middle of a year can be problematic.

Sometimes, interim programs can be worked out to cover these kind of transition periods. If your child turns three in the late spring and you do not want to switch her to a new program at the end of the school year, you may have several options. Depending upon the policies in your area, you may be able to switch her earlier and have the EI program pay for the program until she turns three. Or you may keep her in her EI program past her third birthday and have the school system pay for it. The earlier you start working on the transition process, the more time you will have to work on problems like this to ensure the smoothest change-over.

Disagreements with the School System. As your child grows and develops, her needs will change. For some children, this means that the school system will no longer feel that she needs special education services, or will propose that her program be cut back or changed. In some cases, your child truly has grown out of needing these extra services, and you can be pleased at this sign of progress. In other cases, you may disagree with the school's proposed cutbacks.

Unfortunately, most parents with children in special education find that they eventually clash with their school system over the content and structure of their child's program. Despite everyone's best efforts and intentions, the system tends to be an adversarial one, often because of the financial constraints that exist. Services tend to go to the parents who push the hardest and who know their rights. Becoming a pushy special education parent is something that most parents want to avoid, but you may find, as one parent did, that at some point "you have to put your kid first and put on your boxing gloves." Most of the time, these conflicts can be resolved to your satisfaction without resorting to unpleasant fights or legal battles.

CHAPTER 11

Caring for a Child with Special Medical or Developmental Needs

ℛ

IT CAN TAKE YEARS FOR a child to recover from some of the complications that occur as a result of prematurity, and his needs during that time can be complex and demanding. In some cases, the effects on growth and development remain unclear for a long time; in others, the impact of these complications continues throughout a child's life. Caring for these children can be quite complicated and stressful for parents and other caregivers.

This chapter focuses on some of the common chronic conditions that affect a sizable number of preemies—chronic lung disease, necrotizing enterocolitis, hydrocephalus, and cerebral palsy. You will find basic information on how the condition is treated, what types of complications can occur, and what to expect as your child grows.

If your child has an ongoing health problem, he will probably be followed closely by a pediatrician as well as other medical specialists and relevant therapists. These professionals are your best source of information and guidance on the specifics of your child's situation and needs. As in the earlier chapters on medical complications, use the information here to supplement what your child's providers tell you and to help you frame questions about your child's care.

Chronic Lung Disease (CLD)

The care for respiratory problems has improved over the years so that children who are discharged with CLD tend not to be quite as sick as in years past. However, babies with CLD still tend to be more difficult to care for in their early years; they usually come home on one or more medications and possibly supplemental oxygen, they often have feeding difficulties, less energy overall, and are particularly irritable. They often get sicker from any illnesses, particularly respiratory illnesses, and have a greater chance of needing to go back into the hospital during the first year or two of life.

The good news is that children with CLD gradually outgrow their respiratory difficulties, some within the first year, and almost all by the time they are three. As your child grows, his lungs grow and heal. The areas of his lungs which were affected by CLD become a smaller and smaller percentage of his overall lung capacity. The damaged areas will still show up on X-rays, but usually do not affect his ability to run and exercise as well as any other child. During the first two years, children with CLD have a tendency to develop bronchospasms or reactive airway disease similar to asthma with respiratory illnesses. This tendency usually lessens or disappears as they grow older.

Treatment

Most babies recovering from CLD come home on one or more medications, and/or on supplemental oxygen. The drugs used fall into three groups.

Bronchodilators. Bronchodilators help the lungs function better and make breathing easier by helping to open the airways. Sometimes a baby will need more than one bronchodilator, or will begin using one after his oxygen is discontinued. Some of these drugs are taken orally, and others are inhaled using a nebulizer, a machine that produces a mist to which medication can be added. Some common bronchodilators are theophylline (which also helps to control apnea and bradycardia), and a class of drugs known as beta agonists which includes Ventolin, among others.

Anti-inflammatories. Although these drugs do not open the airways like the bronchodilators, they help to control inflammation and swelling in the airways that can make breathing difficult. They are used in more severe cases of CLD or during acute illnesses if breathing becomes difficult. There are two types of drugs used for this purpose: steroids (such as prednisone) and cromolyn sodium (Intal). With some children, these drugs are sometimes used on a short-term basis, while for others they are prescribed for long-term therapy. If they are used on a long-term basis, your child will have to be weaned off them slowly.

Diuretics. Diuretics such as Lasix, Diuril, and Aldactone help the body get rid of extra fluid. Fluid build-up in the lungs and body can make breathing more difficult and cause the heart and lungs to work harder. While your baby is taking a diuretic, he may need to take potassium chloride supplements to counteract the loss of potassium that is a common side-effect of diuretics. As your baby improves, his diuretic will probably be the first drug that is discontinued.

Supplemental Oxygen

Some babies with CLD come home on supplemental oxygen, usually at a fairly low flow rate. A respiratory therapist from the company that delivers your oxygen should periodically measure the levels of oxygen in your baby's blood, which should remain at 95 percent or above. It is important that your baby be tested at different times during the day since many babies need slightly higher levels of oxygen when they are active, feeding, or asleep.

Over time as your baby recovers, his need for extra oxygen will decrease. However, there may be times when he will need slightly higher flow rates, or even to go back onto supplemental oxygen after he has been off for awhile. As babies grow and become more active, their need for oxygen sometimes increases for a time. Or if they become ill, they may need more oxygen also. Try not to become discouraged if this happens to your child. Providing your child with the extra oxygen he needs makes everything easier for him: he is able to put more energy into feeding, growth and development rather than into breathing; his respiratory system and heart will have to work less hard; if he is sick, it helps him to recover more quickly; and if he needs more oxygen as he becomes more active, you can take this as a positive sign that he is growing and developing.

If your baby continues to need oxygen as he becomes more active and mobile, you may find it difficult to keep the tubing from becoming tangled or interfering with his movements. Some parents recommend running the tubing down your baby's back under his clothing, under the diaper, and

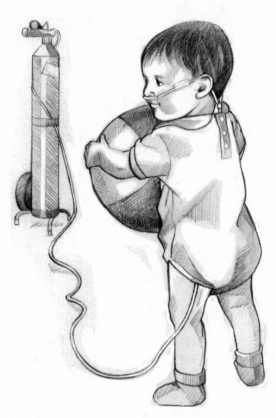

Running the oxygen tubing under the back of your toddler's clothing keeps it out of his way, and a jerk on the tube pulls him to a sitting position rather than over backwards.

out the bottom of his clothes. This keeps the tubing out of sight and easy reach, and if it becomes snagged, your child will tend to fall into a sitting position rather than be pulled over backwards. You can also begin to use longer pieces of tubing so that your child's movements are not restricted, although you may need to increase the flow rate of the oxygen in order to accommodate the longer length.

Weaning from Oxygen

Your doctor may begin to wean your baby off oxygen when his oxygen saturation levels are consistently above 95 percent and he is gaining weight steadily (15 to 30 grams per day, or $1/2$ to 1 ounce per day). Weaning usually progresses in a series of small steps that occur over a period of several weeks or longer. Your pediatrician or pulmonary specialist will oversee your child's weaning process.

In general, the first step is to decrease slightly the amount of oxygen your child is receiving during a period when he is awake but quiet. While he is feeding or sleeping he usually continues on the higher flow rate. If he is able to maintain his oxygen saturation levels at the lower rate of oxygen (his sats should be checked about 20 to 30 minutes after the oxygen is decreased and again a day or two later), the rate can be lowered for all times during the day and night (again your child's sats should be checked). This approach of lowering the flow rate slightly in a step-wise fashion continues until your child is no longer receiving any oxygen. Sometimes, your child will need his medications adjusted or will need to start a new medication, such as a bronchodilator, as his oxygen is decreased.

Although some insurance companies push to have babies come off oxygen as early as possible, it is important that your baby not be weaned too early. If he is unable to maintain his oxygen saturation levels or his weight gain slows down or stops as his oxygen is decreased, your pediatrician or pulmonary specialist should re-evaluate the weaning plan. It is possible that there are other medical problems that are slowing down your baby's progress, he may need extra calories added to his formula, or an adjustment to his medication.

Providing Enough Calories

Babies recovering from CLD need an increased number of calories. Unfortunately, getting those calories into them can be quite difficult since they tend to be hard to feed and may not be able to consume enough formula each day to get the extra calories they need. In general, babies with CLD need between 120 and 150 calories per kilogram (2.2 pounds) of weight in order to maintain a weight gain of $1/2$ to 1 ounce a day. For a $6\,1/2$ pound baby, this amounts to between 18 and 22 ounces of regular 20-calorie-per-ounce formula a day.

Many preemies with CLD are unable to consume this much formula in the early months or may not be able to handle all the fluid involved. Under your doctor's guidance, you may need to add additional calories to your baby's diet by concentrating or adding supplements to his formula. After your child reaches a year, you might add a high calorie supplement like Pediasure, Instant Breakfast, or Ensure to your child's diet, and high calorie foods (see Chapter 8 for ideas).

If your child continues to have trouble with feeding or gaining weight, you may want to consult a nutritionist or a feeding specialist for additional ideas.

Protecting Your Child from Illness and from Irritants in the Air

As was mentioned earlier, babies with CLD are very susceptible to respiratory illness and have a tendency to develop serious lower respiratory infections. It is important to protect your baby with CLD from exposure to germs as much as possible by keeping him away from crowds and sick people in the early months of his life. In addition, he should be protected from smoke of any kind, including smoke from cigarettes, cigars, pipes, or fireplaces, and other irritants which can cause asthma-like symptoms. If someone must smoke, ask them to do it outdoors; even if they smoke in a different room it will eventually reach your baby. Dry air heat in the winter can also be irritating and you may need to add moisture to the air with a humidifier. Babies recovering from CLD should not be exposed to kerosene heaters or the fumes from fresh paint. If you were planning to paint, try to finish a few weeks before your baby comes home from the hospital. Dust, pet hair, feathers, and other common allergens do not usually pose particular problems to children with CLD unless they develop allergies to them.

Possible Complications

In addition to their susceptibility to respiratory illnesses, babies with CLD also face an increased risk for the following conditions.

Bronchospasm or Reactive Airway Disease. When babies with CLD develop respiratory or other illnesses or are exposed to irritants like cigarette smoke, they may show symptoms of bronchospasm (also known as reactive airway disease). Similar to asthma, bronchospasm causes wheezing, coughing, and labored breathing, and occurs as the breathing passages in the chest and lungs become irritated and swollen. This tendency usually fades as your baby recovers and most children no longer develop bronchospasms by the time they are three years old.

Rehospitalization. In their first year or two, over half of the babies who have CLD will need to go back into the hospital, primarily because of a serious respiratory illness. Many of these illnesses occur in the winter months when RSV and other respiratory viruses are common.

Feeding Problems and Slow Growth. Because babies recovering from CLD need extra calories but can be difficult to feed, many grow slowly and end up on the small side. Some babies will show a spurt in growth as their CLD fades, and others will continue on "their own growth curve," i.e., showing steady growth but at a slower than normal rate.

High Blood Pressure. Some of the effects of CLD and some medications used in its treatment can cause your baby's blood pressure to be higher than normal. Babies with CLD should have their blood pressure checked at their well-baby checkups.

As Your Child Grows

Children with chronic lung disease usually outgrow their disease by about two to three years, and show minimal signs of respiratory trouble after that time, although some continue to experience episodes of asthma or reactive airway disease. Their chest X-rays may continue to show scarring and other evidence of damage from the CLD, however, so it is good to keep a copy of old films for comparison.

Many children with CLD recover completely with no lasting problems. However, children with CLD are at higher risk for long-term delays in development. The reasons for this are not completely understood at this point, but probably include a number of things that tend to go along with respiratory distress syndrome and CLD. These include fluctuations in oxygen saturation levels and other coexisting complications such as brain bleeds or PVL, and lack of adequate nutritional intake.

Necrotizing Enterocolitis (NEC)

Most babies who developed NEC in the hospital have recovered from the disease and are able to feed orally again before they come home. Although they remain at higher risk for some problems, most will grow and develop normally. However, a few of the babies who had severe cases of NEC will continue to have special needs for a few months or even longer after discharge. If your baby needs special care at home, such as intravenous or tube

---

feedings, or an ostomy, make sure you understand his care and have practiced enough to feel comfortable and competent before he is discharged.

Possible Complications

There are a number of possible complications that can occur after NEC, including problems with the intestine itself, and, for some babies, difficulty consuming and digesting adequate nutrition. The most common problems include the following.

Strictures. Strictures are the most common complication of NEC, occurring in 10 to 35 percent of surviving babies. They are sections of the intestine that have become narrowed as a result of NEC, and can cause bleeding or an obstruction (blockage). Most strictures are found within two to eight weeks after the acute phase of NEC, but it is possible for one to show up as much as six months later. If strictures cause problems such as an obstruction, they may need to be repaired surgically.

Bowel Obstruction. This is an extremely serious complication that needs a doctor's care or emergency treatment immediately. Symptoms of a bowel obstruction include irritability with crampy pain, swelling of the abdomen, severe constipation, and vomiting.

Short Bowel Syndrome (also known as Short Gut). Short bowel syndrome occurs when a significant portion of the intestine (at least 50 percent) has been surgically removed to treat a severe case of NEC. Because the intestine is so much shorter than it should be, the digestion and absorption of nutrients is significantly disrupted. The intestine gradually adapts to its shortened length and by the time a child is about two years old, digestion is usually close to normal. But until then, most babies and children with short gut will need extra nutritional support, usually in the form of intravenous total parenteral nutrition (TPN). These children are at increased risk for weight loss (or slow gain), diarrhea, anemia and other problems of digestion and nutrient absorption.

By the time they go home, most babies with short bowel syndrome will be taking at least some formula orally (usually an elemental formula such as Pregestimil or Nutramigen) and may be fed by tube or TPN at night. They may also get additional calories from sources like MCT oil or Polycose, and usually need vitamins at twice the normal dosage. Very few infants continue to have trouble with short bowel syndrome after they have turned two, but about half continue to have trouble with certain foods even after they have recovered. The most common of these are milk, corn, tomatoes, orange juice, apples, peaches, raisins, grapes, peas and chocolate.

Ostomies. An ostomy is created when a portion of the intestine is removed and the end of the intestine is brought to the surface of the abdomen in order to rest the remaining portion of the gut. An ostomy created in the small intestine is called an ileostomy; in the large intestine, a colostomy. When an ostomy is created to help treat NEC, it is usually a temporary situation, and is often closed (the two ends of the intestines reconnected) before a baby is discharged from the hospital. However, there are a few babies who come home with ostomies. If your baby will have an ostomy for a while, be sure to practice all his care in the hospital so you are familiar with it and comfortable performing it. It is important to be able to recognize the signs of intestinal illness because a baby with an ostomy can become seriously dehydrated very easily.

As Your Child Grows

Babies with milder cases of NEC who have recovered before discharge, and who are on full oral feedings and growing well, usually continue to grow and develop without any major long-term effects. However, a significant proportion of NEC survivors remain small for their ages, falling between the 3rd and 10th percentiles on growth charts.

The babies at greatest risk for growth problems and developmental delays are those who suffered from the severest cases of NEC, whether or not they had surgery. Of these, it is reported that between 43 and 75 percent will experience developmental delays. There are multiple reasons for this impact, not all of which are fully understood. Experts theorize that because NEC is a catastrophic illness that causes many stresses and complications for the infant, it increases the risks of other complications that can affect the brain, including intraventricular bleeds, shock, infection, and dips in oxygen levels in the blood. In addition, NEC makes it difficult for a baby to take in adequate nutrition during a time of rapid brain growth and development, which may lead to long-term problems and delays. With improvements in the treatment of NEC and increased knowledge of nutrition, some of these long-term effects on growth and development may be lessened in the future.

Babies with NEC are also at greater risk for being rehospitalized during the first year at home because of continuing medical problems and increased susceptibility to illness. Some babies who needed surgery will be slow to turn over, sit, and crawl because the surgery weakens the stomach muscles. As these muscles heal and gain strength, the delays will disappear and they will catch up in their development.

Hydrocephalus and Shunt Care

Hydrocephalus is not a disease but is a condition that sometimes develops after a more serious brain bleed (grades III or IV) when the flow of cerebrospinal fluid (CSF) through the ventricles in the brain is disrupted. Hydrocephalus can occur for other reasons, as well, but intraventricular bleeds are the most common cause among preemies. The ventricles are fluid-filled spaces within the brain that are normally connected with spaces around the brain and spinal cord. The body is constantly creating cerebrospinal fluid; when the ventricles become blocked or the CSF cannot be reabsorbed properly, the ventricles swell with the excess fluid and press on the surrounding brain tissue. If the swelling becomes too great or continues for too long, it can cause permanent brain damage.

With preemies, this swelling is often a temporary condition that goes away on its own or can be treated with medication or by draining the excess fluid with a series of spinal taps. However, some children need to have an artificial drainage system known as a shunt surgically implanted in order to allow the excess cerebrospinal fluid to flow out of the brain and into another area of the body where it can be reabsorbed. The shunt is a soft, flexible plastic tube which is inserted into the ventricle inside the brain, run beneath the surface of the skin and usually into the abdominal space. This is the most common type of shunt and is known as a ventriculoperitoneal shunt (VP shunt). Shunts can also be run to other parts of the

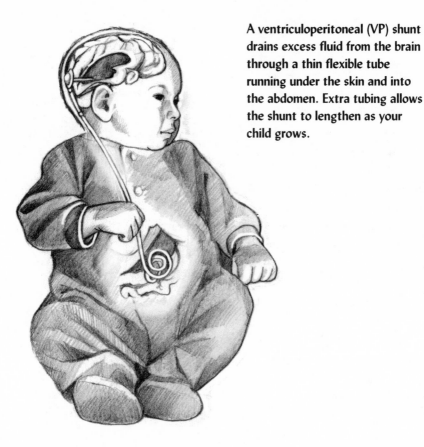

A ventriculoperitoneal (VP) shunt drains excess fluid from the brain through a thin flexible tube running under the skin and into the abdomen. Extra tubing allows the shunt to lengthen as your child grows.

body such as the heart, but this is less common. If your child needs a shunt to treat his hydrocephalus, the surgery will usually occur while he is still in the hospital. However, some babies will need to have a shunt placed later in their infancies or childhood.

If your child has a shunt:

- be sure you know what type of shunt he has;
- write down the name and model to keep with your medical records;
- have your doctor show you a sample of the shunt, and explain its component parts and how it operates;
- make sure you know whether the shunt has an on/off control valve that could be accidentally turned off, stopping the flow of CSF through the shunt.

Possible Complications

Shunts are usually fairly trouble-free and, although they do not cure hydrocephalus, they do a good job of controlling it. However, shunts can malfunction periodically, with the result that pressure builds up in your child's head again. This is a serious situation that must be cared for quickly by the neurologist or neurosurgeon who treats your child. Malfunctions are usually caused by the following.

Obstruction of the Shunt. The shunt can become partially or completely blocked by tissue, blood, or bacteria so that the flow of CSF is hindered or stopped. Depending upon the site and extent of the blockage, some or all of the shunt may need to be replaced surgically.

Infection. Infections in a shunt are caused by bacteria within your child's own body, not becaue he was exposed to illness. Most shunt infections occur within a month after surgery, but can occur as much as six months later. Shunt infections are usually treated with antibiotics and with the replacement of the shunt.

Shunt Revisions. Although not really a complication, your child's shunt may need to be lengthened or changed as he grows. Some children need to have a number of revisions made during their childhoods, but, in general, parents are told to expect that their child will need two or more revisions to adjust the shunt for his growth.

Signs and Symptoms of Increased Pressure in the Head. Because untreated hypdrocepahlus can damage the brain, it is important to recognize the signs of increased pressure (known as intracranial pressure or ICP) in your child's brain, or of an infection that could indicate that a shunt is malfunctioning. That way your child can be treated as quickly as possible, lessening the chances of serious damage.

In an infant, you may see the following:

- increased head size and bulging fontanel (the soft spot on the top of the head);
- veins in the scalp that are very visible or swollen;
- redness or swelling along the shunt line;

- changes in behavior: increased sleepiness or irritability;
- signs of illness: vomiting or fever;
- seizures; or
- frequent downward deviations of the eyes (known as sunsetting).

In a toddler or older child, you see many of the same symptoms that indicate illness or increased pressure in the head: fever, vomiting, irritability, sleepiness, seizures, redness along the shunt. An older child may also complain of a headache and you may notice that he has problems with his vision, more trouble with coordination or balance, difficulty waking up or staying awake, and declining academic abilities.

As Your Child Grows

Because the diagnosis and treatment of hydrocephalus have improved over the years, many children with this condition grow up with normal intelligence and physical development. However, children with hydrocephalus often develop a little more slowly and may have some physical problems or need special education services later in life. Your own child's development will depend upon many things, including other complications or brain damage that may have occurred along with the hydrocephalus. Your child will probably be followed closely and his development monitored throughout infancy and childhood. If he does show developmental problems, the more quickly they are recognized and responded to, the faster he will be able to progress and the better he will do overall.

Cerebral Palsy

Cerebral palsy (CP) is a name given to disorders of posture, movement, and muscle coordination caused by damage to a child's brain that usually occurs before, during, or shortly after birth. Being told that your child has CP is usually a very difficult and upsetting moment for a parent, although some parents are also relieved to finally have a name put to their vague worries or sense that something was not right with their child.

CP is an umbrella term that covers a vast array of disorders, ranging

Aided by a walker, this 2-year-old is mobile and happy.

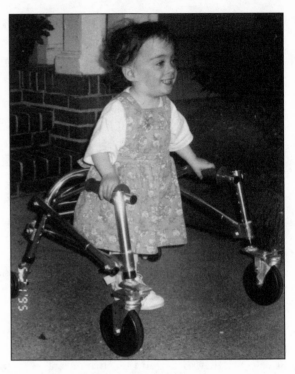

from mild muscle weakness to disabling conditions. When the diagnosis is made, usually when your child is about 12 to 18 months old, you usually do not know the extent to which your child will be affected nor the impact that it will have on your lives as a family. CP is defined as a non-progressive disorder because it does not get worse over time. However, this definition is somewhat confusing because as the brain grows and matures, the signs and symptoms of CP change even though the brain damage that causes it does not.

There are a number of different kinds of CP, but the most common type found among premature infants is the spastic type in which damage to the motor nerves in the brain causes muscle tightness and difficulty in moving normally. This is often coupled with decreased strength in the muscles of the trunk of the body including the chest, abdomen, and back. The spasticity can affect the muscles in various parts of the body, and is given different names depending on the location of the problem. The most common type found among preemies is spastic diplegia, in which the legs are affected more than the arms. Other common types are hemiplegia, in which only one side of the body is affected and the arms are usually affected more than the legs; and quadriplegia, in which arms, legs, head, and trunk are affected, and there are often problems with oral motor function as well.

Most cases of CP fall into the mild or moderate range. In mild cases, the muscle weakness or tightness that is present does not hinder the child very much. In moderate cases, the effects of CP are more noticeable, but with the use of assistive devices the impact is lessened. When a child is severely affected he is greatly hampered by the CP, and the use of assistive devices, while helpful, cannot completely overcome the disabilty.

Possible Complications

Cerebral palsy primarily affects the muscles and movement, but is associated with a number of other problems, as well.

Hearing Problems. Many children with CP have problems with recurring ear infections or an accumulation of fluid in the middle ear without an infection, both of which can cause temporary hearing loss. These problems may occur more frequently because of trouble with oral motor skills or because they may be spending more time lying down or in a reclining position.

Vision Problems. Strabismus (crossed eyes) occurs in as many as half of children with spastic CP. Problems with myopia (near-sightedness) are also more common.

Feeding and Growth Problems. Many children have feeding problems and gain weight slowly. There may be specific problems with oral motor abilities that make it difficult to suck, chew, or swallow effectively. In other cases, the effort involved in maintaining a sitting position interferes with the ability or interest in eating. This kind of problem often improves if some type of adaptive, supportive chair can be used. Problems with fine motor coordination in the hands can interfere with self-feeding, and the extra calories that some children with CP burn not only tires them out, but also makes it difficult to take in enough food to maintain their weight and growth.

Problems with Joints. Because the tightened muscles of CP can cause stress on joints, dislocations occur more frequently. In the case of spastic diplegia, hip dislocations are the most common. Sometimes tendons (such as the Achilles tendon in the heel) become shortened causing limitation in the range of motion of a joint. Braces, orthotics, and sometimes surgery can help to relieve or prevent some of these orthopedic problems.

Constipation. Constipation is another common problem among children with CP. Adding Karo syrup to formula, and increasing the number of fresh fruit and vegetables in the diet to provide bulk may help, but stool softeners or mild laxatives (such as Maltsupex or Senokot) are sometimes necessary. Always get the advice of your pediatrician or other specialist before trying to treat a problem like constipation.

Developmental Delays and Learning Disabilities. Problems with posture and movement can interfere with a child's ability to accomplish certain developmental tasks. Many children are helped by adaptive devices— chairs, special pencils, adapted utensils for feeding, braces, crutches and walkers—that help them work around their disabilities. Children with CP may also have specific learning disabilities that show up as they reach school age.

Mental Retardation. It can be very difficult to test children's cognitive abilities accurately when they have physical disabilities, so the numbers of children with CP who have below average intelligence has always been difficult to estimate. However, the incidence of mental retardation appears to be much higher among children with CP than in the general population, but many individuals have normal and above normal mental abilities.

Treatment

Cerebral palsy is not a disease that can be treated and cured. It is, instead, a disorder that can affect not just movement but many other aspects of development and growth as well. Therefore, the most successful approach to caring for a child with CP is a multidisciplinary one, in which his medical, physical, developmental, and academic needs can be met in a coordinated way.

Some of the most important aspects of your child's care may be the following:

Medical Care. Your pediatrician will provide your child's well-child care as well as diagnose any special medical problems that your child may have (see below). He or she may refer you to other specialists, depending upon the nature of your child's problems and treatment needs.

Physical Therapy. Because of the impact that CP has on movement and posture, most children with CP work closely with a physical therapist, particularly when they are young. The physical therapist can help a child learn how to move, and help to prevent some of the complications of tight muscles and spastic movements. They can also figure out what type of adaptive or assistive devices can best help your child.

Adaptive or Assistive Devices. Depending upon the types of physical problems your child has, there are a number of adaptations and devices that can help improve his posture, his ability to sit and move independently, and his ability to perform many skills on his own.

Orthotics. Some children gain a great deal of mobility with the use of special orthotics and braces. Lighter, molded plastic orthotics are available now that slip into shoes and under clothes to provide support in a way that is more comfortable for the child and less obvious to others.

Early Intervention Services. While your child is under the age of three, your local early intervention program should be able to provide you with a wide range of services. Early intervention programs emphasize the role of the family in caring for a child with disabilities and will work with and support you as you learn how to provide the care that your child needs.

School-Based Programs. After your child turns three, special education and supportive services become the responsibility of your local public school system, and many children with CP will qualify for these services. These may include special education services, as well as physical and occupational therapy. Depending upon your child's specific needs and problems, you may also need to see a neurologist, an orthopedic specialist, an otolaryngologist (ear, nose, and throat doctor), a pediatric nutritionist, an eating specialist who may be a speech pathologist or occupational therapist, a social worker, or psychologist.

Unfortunately, dealing with multiple providers and specialists can be a complicated situation for a parent to handle. Depending upon the type of health insurance you have, your primary care provider (pediatrician) may act as the central coordinator for the other specialists involved, you may be referred to a special clinic at a teaching hospital, or you may act as the central coordinator yourself. While your child is under three, you should be able to get services through your local early intervention program, and after three, through your local public school system, as mentioned above.

As Your Child Grows

The services that are available for children with cerebral palsy today ensure that most will grow and develop to the best of their abilities, and even among those with more serious cases, many will be able to attain the skills and physical capabilities to live independent lives. Children with mild CP may need little or no extra help as they grow, but you may find that they need to be steered into noncompetitive sports activities if their physical abilities begin to lag behind those of their peers.

However, being the parent of a child with moderate to severe CP is a very tiring and time-consuming job. As one parent described it, "I feel like I am an extension of my daughter." Learning to balance your own needs, your child's needs, and the needs of other family members can be a difficult task. Other children in a family can become resentful of the extra time and attention that is needed by the child with special needs. If you have other children, try to spend some one-on-one time with them on a regular basis in order to avoid this as much as possible. Use babysitters or respite care workers to get some relief for yourself and to be able to spend some regular time alone with your spouse.

Helping your child learn to become as independent as possible can also be emotionally challenging. The job of parenting changes as children grow, and all parents must begin to stand back and allow their children to do more things on their own. If your child has disabilities and many tasks are very hard for him, taking this step back can be difficult. As your child grows and you confront many of these issues, it can be helpful to talk with parents of both disabled and nondisabled children. Talking with a social worker or psychologist may also help to give you ideas on ways to handle some of the developmental hurdles and special problems that face children with disabilities and their families.

Special Situations

Coping with Multiple Medical Problems

Many babies with ongoing medical and developmental problems tend to have not just one but a number of interconnecting problems. For example, a baby recovering from CLD will need special attention paid to his respiratory problems but may also have problems with feeding, weight gain, and irritability. In addition, his physical development may be delayed and he may get sick more often. As the parent of such a baby, you will probably be seeing not only your regular pediatrician, but also a pulmonary specialist, a physical or occupational therapist, and possibly a speech pathologist and/or nutritionist to work on weight gain and feeding issues. And somewhere in there, you are also trying to be a regular parent, not only caring for your child but trying to have time to play with and enjoy him as well.

As one parent said of this situation:

"I feel like I'm kind of the general contractor for my child's life. He has all these different issues going on, and each specialist we see tells me something different, some of which makes sense and some of which doesn't. They each see a little slice of the pie, and I'm the only one who sees the whole thing. So many times I've wished there was someone I could turn to who could kind of guide me through this maze and help me make sense of it all, but so far that person has been me."

Another parent summed it up succinctly by saying, "My daughter is ten months old now and I still haven't had time just to enjoy her."

Having a child with ongoing or multiple medical needs is very difficult; it is tiring, time-consuming, confusing, and stressful. It can also be very frustrating; your child's progress may be uneven, new problems may appear, and you may feel caught in a sort of limbo, unable to get a clear sense of what to expect in the future. This happens not because your child's caregivers are unwilling to help you or are keeping things from you, but more often because they also cannot predict what may happen. Each premature baby is unique, premature babies are a relatively new group, and it is difficult to predict the ultimate outcome for any particular baby.

As a parent, however, there are a number of things you can try that may help you cope with this situation.

- Try to focus on the positive. Even though your child's progress may be uneven, try to look at it over time and identify things that have improved or gotten easier. You may want to keep a simple journal so you can look back and see how far you've come.
- Look at your child's strengths and appealing characteristics as well as his needs and problems. Appreciate all the things he can do, and don't just focus on what he can't.
- If possible, take time to enjoy your child every day, even if it is just for a few minutes. This doesn't have to involve anything special; it might just mean holding him quietly or sitting beside him watching him sleep.
- Try not to fall into the trap of seeing yourself as your child's live-in therapist. Your main job as his parent, and the one that feels the most natural and satisfying, is to love and support your child. You may need to help him with physical therapy periodically, but don't let those needs dominate your interactions with him.
- Remember that you know your own child better than anyone else does. You may need to balance some of the things that various specialists tell you with your own judgment as to your child's problems and needs.
- Be sure to get a break from caring for your child on a regular basis by trading off with your partner or finding a reliable sitter or family member. The more complicated your child's needs, the harder it can be to leave him. But you will have more energy, resilience, and an increased ability to cope if you allow yourself to get away periodically.

Dealing with Multiple Medical Providers

Children who have chronic medical problems or developmental disabilities usually are cared for by a number of different medical specialists in addition to their pediatrician or family physician. You will be at the center of this team of specialists; not only must you keep track of multiple appointments, you must try to understand what each specialist is telling you, and act as your child's advocate. Some of the following strategies may help you manage this complicated situation.

- Keep a list of your child's doctors and appointments. Include the doctor's name, the type of specialist he is, how often you should see him, the date of your last appointment and of your next scheduled visit.
- Try to get the most out of your appointments by preparing in advance. When seeing a new specialist, find out as much as you can about the doctor's specialty, why you are seeing him, and what type of services he may provide for your child. Bring with you a list of questions, and write down the answers if you need to.
- Specialists often use technical language and their own jargon. If you don't understand what the doctor is saying, ask for another explanation. Keep asking questions until you understand. If you have trouble doing this, your pediatrician should be able to provide further explanations to you at a later time.
- Specialists usually send a letter reporting their findings to your pediatrician. You may want to ask for copies of these letters and any relevant test results or evaluations to keep with your own records.

The medical providers and therapists with whom you and your child will be working are obviously an important source of help and information. But parents of children with similar problems are another valuable resource for information, support, and understanding. Parents of children with complex needs quickly become sophisticated consumers of medical care, and may be able to help you find your way more easily through the maze of medical providers and educational programs. You may meet other parents through your child's early intervention program, hospital clinics, school, and parent support and advocacy groups.

CHAPTER 12

Looking to the Future

𝄢

WHEN YOUR BABY IS BORN early, it is natural to worry about what the future might hold. But as this book has tried to show, you have good reason to feel confident about your baby's prospects. The outlook for preemies has never been better than it is right now, and the art and science of neonatology is continuing to improve. Although the recovery period is long and rocky for many babies, most recover from their early births without major problems.

However, the survival of large numbers of babies, including micro-preemies born at 750 grams (1 pounds 11 ounces) or less, is a fairly new phenomenon. Follow-up research on these children continues to explore

An older "preemie"

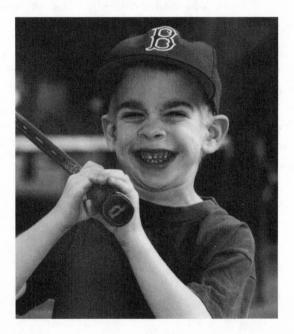

the long-term effects of prematurity. Among the many findings, two stand out. The first is that preemies as a group seem to be at higher risk for problems of attention, learning, and coordination as they grow older. These more subtle problems will be discussed below.

Secondly, prematurity, although an important factor, is only one of many possible influences that will shape your child's development and health. The environment in which she grows, the care she receives after she leaves the hospital, her personality, and other intangibles all play important roles in determining how well your child does.

There are many aspects of preemiehood that have not—and probably cannot—be identified in formal research projects. While the studies can investigate specific problems and outcomes, they have a harder time exploring the impact that prematurity has on the lives of the children themselves and on their families. This is the kind of knowledge that lies in the hearts and minds of the parents of preemies. At the end of this chapter, you will find stories from veteran parents on the challenges and joys of parenting children born prematurely.

The Preschool Years and Beyond: What the Research Shows

Over the last two decades, research has tried to uncover the long-term effects of prematurity. Preemies have been looked at in terms of their behavior, intelligence and cognitive abilities, physical growth and development, health, school achievement, and quality of life. Unfortunately, or fortunately, many of these studies offer conflicting results and inconsistent findings.

There are a few things that are clear, however:

- Major developmental problems almost always become evident within the first two years of life. If your baby has reached the age of three or so without any major problems, you can feel fairly confident that she will continue to grow and develop well.
- As a group, preemies appear to be at higher risk for subtle problems in learning, attention, and visual-motor skills.
- These problems may not show up until your child reaches school age

when academic and social demands increase and become more complex.

- Babies born at extremely low birthweights (under 1,000 grams or 2 pounds 3 ounces) are at the highest risk for these problems.
- A baby's home environment and family play a very large role in how well she does.

The More Subtle Problems of Prematurity

The most common problems reported in the follow-up research on preemie development are described below. The reasons that preemies seem to be at increased risk for these types of problems of attention, learning, and coordination are not understood at this point, and research is ongoing. Keep in mind that these problems are not unique to preemies; in any school population, many full-term children will struggle with the same challenges.

Physical Clumsiness

Many preemies seem to be less physically able or coordinated than their peers. In early childhood, physical abilities, including both large and small motor skills, develop unevenly. This uneven development continues through the preschool years, and clumsiness or lack of coordination in a preschooler is not usually a reason for concern.

But by school age (six or seven years old), physical skills among children begin to even out. A child who is less coordinated or agile may begin having more trouble keeping up with her peers physically. She may be noticeably less adept at certain skills such as running, jumping, riding a bike, throwing or catching a ball.

Clumsiness may occur among preemies for a number of different reasons:

- **Problems with motor planning.** Children who have trouble with motor planning know what they want to do but have trouble figuring out how to do it. They may have trouble performing a specific activity or it may take them longer than others to get the hang of it.
- **A generally lower level of coordination.** Some children are simply less coordinated than others, for no apparent reason.

• **Mild cerebral palsy.** Some children who have very mild cases of cerebral palsy may not be identified until later in childhood. Mild CP may show up as muscle weakness or a lack of coordination.

If your child appears to be less coordinated or physically able than her peers, discuss it with your pediatrician and perhaps a physical therapist, especially if your child becomes frustrated or upset with her lack of physical skills. It may help your child to participate in noncompetitive sports, and activities or exercises to build muscle strength and coordination. One mother whose son had motor planning problems took him to a variety of different playgrounds so that he could practice climbing and moving around different structures. He never realized that there was a therapeutic reason for these trips. Make sure that your child knows that physical abilities are only one aspect of herself and that she has many other strengths and abilities.

Slightly Decreased IQ Scores

The IQ test is one of the primary measurements of cognitive development used with children. Many factors, including socioeconomic status and parental educational levels, affect a child's IQ. But even when these factors are taken into account, preemies—as a group—do significantly less well on these intelligence tests than do normal birthweight children. Most preemies still score within the normal range (IQ of 85 or above), but a larger proportion score in the range of borderline (IQ of 70 to 84) and below normal (IQ less than 70) intelligence. Among full-term babies, approximately 14 percent have a borderline IQ and 2 percent are below normal. Among preemies, those percentages are 24 percent and 6 percent, respectively.

It is important to remember that these statistics are for groups of preemies, and can't be used to predict the level of your own child's intelligence. In addition, a child's IQ can change a bit over time. Early intervention and other educational programs, as well as a stimulating home environment, can have significant positive effects on a particular child's cognitive abilities.

Specific Learning Problems

According to the research, preemies are one and a half to four times more likely to have learning disabilities than are normal birthweight children.

In one study, about 33 percent of all preemies had school problems, as indicated by repeating a grade or being in special education. Among full-term children, only 14 percent were having similar problems. The smallest preemies, those under 1,000 grams (2 pounds 3 ounces) at birth, have even higher rates of learning problems.

The types of problems that preemies typically have fall into specific areas: mathematical skills; fine motor skills—problems with handwriting, drawing, coordination; visual-motor processing—difficulty copying patterns or putting puzzles together; and attention. A few studies reported problems in reading and language abilities, but the research on this is inconclusive.

The fact that more preemies repeat a grade or receive special education services in school may also reflect the close monitoring that many of our children receive. Parents of preemies learn early on to become good advocates for their children. As their children reach school age, they may be on the lookout for subtle problems in development or learning style. If something comes up, they know how to be assertive, and to ask for and get the services their children need.

Problems with Attention, Distractibility, and Impulsiveness

The findings of research on attention deficit disorder (ADD) and attention deficit hyperactivity disorder (ADHD) among preemies are inconsistent. Estimates of the number of children with these problems range from seven to almost 50 percent. The higher percentages are reported among the extremely low birthweight babies, those who weighed less than 1,000 grams (2 pounds 3 ounces) at birth.

Whether or not a child is officially diagnosed as having ADD or ADHD, many preemies seem to have problems with short attention spans, distractibility, and impulsiveness. These tendencies may be related to earlier problems with state regulation and the general sensitivity and disorganization of preemies' nervous systems. Certain medical complications such as PVL may also increase a child's chances of having attention problems.

If your child has difficulty focusing or maintaining her attention, there are things you can do to help. Children with serious attention problems may be helped by medication, but most ADD-like children also seem to function better with structure and predictability. Passive activities like watching TV don't help your child develop her attention span. Instead, building things, drawing, working on a project with others, circle time, and playing with other children all help build your child's ability to concentrate for extended periods. Many parents also commented that discipline is a difficult issue with these intense, active children. "Being yelled at just seems to gear Taylor up. It's almost as if he loves being yelled at; it doesn't stop him at all," said the mother of such a child. You may find that time-outs that give your child a chance to calm down, or rewarding your child for good behavior, are more effective than punishing her for bad behavior.

New Research on Adolescent Former Preemies

Until a recent study done in Canada by Saroj Saigal and her colleagues, there has been little research on the impacts of prematurity into the teenage years. Dr. Saigal investigated the experiences of a group of teenagers between the ages of 12 and 16 years who weighed less than 1,000 grams (2 pounds 3 ounces) at birth. This study differed from many in that it asked the teenagers themselves to rate their health and quality of life, and then compared their answers with those of a comparison group of similar teens who were born full-term.

The results were surprising. As a group, the former preemies had more complex health problems and disabilities including cerebral palsy, blindness, and deafness, than the comparison group. Yet when asked to rate their own health and the quality of their lives, a similar proportion of participants in both the preemie group (71 percent) and comparison group (73 percent) rated their health-related quality of life as being 0.95 or better (the scale ran from zero to one, or death to perfect health). The major difference between the two groups was that within the preemie group, a small but important number of teens with significant disabilities rated their quality of life as being much lower than that reported by any teens in the comparison group.

This research is interesting for a number of reasons, particularly because it shows how difficult it is to measure accurately the impact of prematurity. Clearly, a significant number of the former preemies who participated in the study had ongoing problems related to their early births. And yet, most were satisfied with their health and the quality of their lives. Where researchers using objective measurements would see problems, these former preemies judged themselves as being little different from anyone else their own age.

Reading and Interpreting the Research: Is It Relevant to Your Child?

Most of the research on preemie development is published in medical, pediatric, and nursing journals. You may be able to get access to these journals through a local hospital or medical school library. However, when you read the studies on the long-term impacts of prematurity, keep in mind several things that may affect how relevant the study findings are to your own child.

The Time Period of the Study. The care of preemies continues to improve, and as NICU practices change, the rates of complications and long-term effects among surviving babies also change. The findings from studies conducted before or during the early to mid-1980s may no longer accurately reflect the experience of more recently born babies. In particular, be careful of studies conducted before artificial surfactant and antenatal steroids (steroid injections given to mothers before the birth of their preemies) were used routinely.

Types of Complications Experienced by Babies in the Study. Sometimes the statistics in a study look discouraging, but when you dig a little deeper into the data, you may find that the poorer outcomes are limited to a few children with specific disabilities or severe illness. The results for healthy preemies may be much more encouraging.

How the Impacts of Prematurity Are Defined and Measured. There is little agreement in the literature about how best to measure the effects of prematurity, and how to assess their impact on the lives of preemies and their families. Definitions and measurement tools vary greatly among studies, making it difficult to compare findings across studies.

The Socioeconomic Status of the Study Population. Prematurity occurs more frequently among mothers living in poverty, and poverty is another risk factor for poor outcomes among all children, full-term as well as pree-mie. In addition, preemies seem particularly vulnerable to the negative effects of poverty. If the study population is skewed toward a lower socio-economic group, the outcomes may look particularly bad.

The Size of the Study Group. Research has shown that practice patterns vary among NICUs, and that these variations result in different rates of complications among surviving children. Larger studies that combine data from several hospitals or include all prematurely born children from a par-ticular region are able to smooth out these differences. However, these large studies are expensive to conduct and data collection can be difficult, particularly if the study period is a long one. Many of the published studies on preemies are fairly small or cover a relatively short span of time. The findings from these smaller studies may not be generalizable to the whole population of preemies.

The Voices of Experience

Much of this book has been devoted to exploring the ways in which being born prematurely changes not only your baby's beginning in life but some of the ways she grows and develops as well. For many babies, these differ-ences are temporary; for others, prematurity has a more lasting impact. But there is one place where prematurity always leaves a permanent mark, and that is on you as a parent. Simply put, being the parent of a preemie is a very different experience from being the parent of a full-term baby. Even parents whose babies were only a few weeks early and those whose chil-dren sailed relatively easily through prematurity find that they never for-get their child's early start in life.

Prematurity obviously brings challenges and anxieties to the role of parenting. But it also brings some unexpected silver linings. As you watch your child grow, you may find that you take less for granted, and that you appreciate all that she is accomplishing more fully. With my own son, I felt that I had been given a window that allowed me to watch the changes in him as he grew, and to see things I would never have otherwise seen. I was much more aware of the wonder and complexity of his development than I had been with my two full-term children.

To meet and cope with the crisis of your child's early birth and any subsequent problems also gives you a strength and confidence that you may not have had before, or may not have realized you had. It opens your eyes to a world few people know about, and helps you to gain a broader, more compassionate perspective. Although none of us would have chosen to have our babies born early, the experience allows you to see the strength and resilience of your child or children, of yourself, and of other babies and parents. It is hard not to be changed by that experience.

In closing this book, I want to share the stories of some of the many parents of preemies who have been kind enough to answer my questions and write or tell me about their children and themselves.

From the mother of a 26-weeker:

"As far as ever forgetting your child's beginnings, I don't think any of us will ever do that. Calling it 'less than ideal' is an understatement for sure. I am sometimes amazed that when I am talking to someone about my son's history, it still has the power to make me relive those emotions and really feel the way I did when I went through them the first time. Sometimes I have no trouble in talking about it but other times, it's like something sneaks up on you and you actually feel those same feelings again. I guess it is part of the ongoing grieving process we all go through. It's really like a roller coaster. You think you are coping and accepting and dealing with everything and then WHAM!!!! You are dissolving into tears and hurting for your child all over again. I just want new preemie parents to understand this is 'normal' and something we all go through over and over."

From the mother of a son born at 25 weeks gestation:

"I worked part time after Joey's birth so I could take my maternity leave when he came home. At four months, he had to have surgery for ROP which left him with one totally detached retina and one attached but with a fold through the macula so he has partial, very near-sighted vision in one eye only. When my maternity leave was over, I was a basket case sending him to day care for someone else to care for all day. Although there was no lack of love on his caregiver's part, I knew he was not getting the extra stimulation he needed to reach normal milestones because he couldn't see to imitate other kids or adults.

"I ended up quitting my job when Joey was 18 months old. Within three to four weeks after I was home with him full-time, he was walking and progressing at a tremendous rate and I believe that is why he is doing so well today. At age six, Joey is extremely mobile without a cane and it is deceptive as to how low his vision is. I have never regretted quitting my job, even though it has been seriously difficult financially.

"A week or so ago, Joey's vision teacher called me asking if I would be willing to talk about my son to a high school English class that was studying Helen Keller's life. On Friday, I went to the classsroom and talked to the kids about Joey's preemie experience, his blindness, and his present-day life in the first grade.

"It was a wonderful experience. I took in pictures of him at 1 pound 11 1/2 ounces and took along the little preemie hat from the NICU and a few other preemie mementos I have saved. When he was one, I made a card with rubber stamps including actual photocopies of his little foot-prints at two weeks of age and then stamped his one-year-old foot to show his amazing growth during the year. The kids and teacher were absolutely fascinated with the whole thing.

"I took questions from the kids and they came up with some really good ones. The only one that choked me up was when one girl asked if "after going through all this stuff, did I regret having my son?" My answer, of course, was absolutely not! If I could change the pain and struggle he went through as a preemie, yes, I would change that. But I have never regretted having him for one minute!"

From the mother of an almost teenage daughter, born at 28 weeks:
"My daughter Anna was a 28-weeker and is now twelve years old. She has mild CP. When Anna was two years old, I was told by a pediatric orthopedist that she would walk with difficulty and never be athletically inclined. I took her to another orthopedist who took a conservative approach to the whole issue and wouldn't make predictions. When she was young, Anna had physical therapy sessions weekly as well as nightly stretching exercises at home. At age three, she was fitted for bilateral AFOs (ankle foot orthotics to help support her ankles and feet) and she had a heel cord lengthening surgery at age seven.

"Anna has always been determined to try and succeed. I cannot put into words my feelings when she was nine and she showed me how she could ride her bike without training wheels. Or the pride I felt when she won a blue ribbon in basketball. In the summer of '98 we were told that she no longer needed to wear her AFOs. We celebrated by having some of her friends over for cake. Family and friends sent cards of congratulations. At the end of the evening we took the braces and cards, and placed them in a box and put them away.

"As I watch her now doing what every other preteen does, I am in awe of her. There are few who notice the slight turn of her left foot, or the way she stands with her shoulders slightly back. These are the things that remind me of the NICU so long ago. We have been through so much together, I am proud to be her mom."

From the mother of a daughter born at 23 weeks:

"Julia, my preemie, is a former 23-weeker, weighing in at 1 pound 7 ounces at birth. Today, at nearly four, she seems to have very few problems related to her prematurity. Her one big problem is her slow weight gain, but she is gaining. It's just taking her a while to catch up.

"I watch Julia a lot, and I worry all the time. She just surprises me constantly. Her preschool is a Head Start program, and they have a program for children with delays and without. Julia did not have any delays at all. In fact, she tested at age five in some areas when she was only three years old. Except for trouble reaching things like doorknobs and sinks and light switches, she is not failing any tests.

"She does seem to get banged up a lot but I don't know if it's from her prematurity or because she is a child. She has a wonderful grasp of things in life, too. She will ask questions (such as why did the policeman come to our house) and our answers (because someone hit our car with their car and broke it and drove away) do not generate blank looks or complacency but more questions that are valid and on topic. These are the times that I marvel at her. Any time she shows that she will be OK and able to successfully compete in this world with full-term children, I am excited and thrilled all over again.

"Her birthday is in April but should have been in August. So in August, we celebrate her 'second birthday' which her father and I consider to be her 'real' one. We don't shower her with gifts again, but we do have a cake and ice cream and lots of reminiscing.

"One more thing that has changed in our lives is that our faith in God has strengthened."

From the mother of two preemies, on the lasting impact of prematurity:
"It has finally dawned on me what the difference is between discussing my children with other parents of premature children, and with my friends [with full-term children]. When I tell people that Sam and Andrew are premature children they think, 'Oh, so they were born prematurely, and now they are normal children.' No! Parents of preemies understand that our children are premature children and that is what they are—they do not stop being premature children when they reach a certain age. Nothing can ever change the fact that they did not do the whole 40-week gestation bit, and that because of that they are forever going to be different from who they would have been if their birth had been different.

"We will always be premature parents. Would we have been different as parents if the birth had been different? I don't know. I never had the chance to find out. But when my boys are 16 years old, I will still classify myself as the mother of a premature child. I know that when and if my boys ever get married, I will be there with tears in my eyes remembering them in the NICU. That will stay with me forever."

From the mother of two sons born prematurely, one at 33 weeks and one at 26 weeks:
"My older son Greg was born at 33 weeks. It is amazing how things become relative; when Greg was born I considered him to be a miracle (I still do, but in different ways). Greg weighed 5 pounds and was basically a feeder-grower. He had no major problems, only needed to be in the NICU for one day, and then in the special nursery for another week until he could drink on his own. Today Greg is seven, and is doing very well at school. He's a wonderful child but he does suffer from chronic asthma.

"With Doug, my waters broke at 24 weeks and he was born by emergency C-section two weeks later. He was born with strep and pneumonia, weighed 2 pounds 3 ounces, and his Apgar scores were 0 and 1. I honestly cannot remember all the medical details surrounding his NICU stay. I know he had five blood transfusions, had two sets of chest tubes (he still has major scars from those), had a brain bleed, was on oxygen for his full stay in the NICU (3¹/₂ months). He suffered from numerous apnea episodes, and had to go back to the NICU after being home for a week after he had a serious apnea episode at home.

"For the first two years of his life, Doug was in the hospital more than he was at home. He was uncommunicative, tactile defensive, and very angry at me—I think because of all the desertions for hospital stays. His temper was terrible.

"At around the age of two years, he turned around. As soon as his speech became understandable and I stopped having to take him to the hospital so often, he developed the nature he has now. At five, he has a wonderful vocabulary, is exceptionally affectionate with everyone, and has a mind of his own. I have never been able to take him for OT (occupational therapy), PT (physical therapy), speech, or any other of the normal therapies. I run my own business and my husband's job doesn't cover our basic expenses so I have to work long and hard hours. Thankfully, Doug has achieved so much despite my limited efforts."

From the mother of a daughter born at 27 weeks:
"Amy was born at 27 weeks, weighing 1 pound 12 ounces, and 13 inches long. I had a pretty normal pregnancy until four days prior to her birth, at which point I went into preterm labor which couldn't be stopped. Amy was on the ventilator for about three weeks, and oxygen for about seven weeks. She had no brain bleeds or surgeries, although she did have renal [kidney] failure in the first few weeks that got better and is now followed on an outpatient basis. She had the usual IVs, tubes, blood transfusions, etc.

"I feel different, maybe more sensitive, because of the experiences I have had with a preemie. I don't take normal baby things for granted, and I think I am much more aware of people with all kinds of disabilities, and what the impact must be like for their families. Also, I find myself (inside) less tolerant of friends and acquaintances who seem overprotective about trivial matters with their children; I have a hard time taking them seriously when they obsess over little things. I wish I could make them see what really important things are, and how lucky they are to have their full-term healthy children who are doing fine.

From the mother of a preemie and a child born full-term:
"There are very few times when I don't remember the beginning. My daughter will always be a preemie, and we will always be preemie parents. Cait was born at 31 weeks with IUGR [intrauterine growth retardation], at 1 pound 11 ounces. Her major complication was an ischemic bowel which resolved within the first week, treated with antibiotics. She came home ten weeks later weighing 3 pounds 10 ounces. Weight gain has always and continues to be an issue. She turned five in November, and last week finally hit 30 pounds. She is 42 inches tall, but her petite size is a constant reminder of where she began.

"Cait's actual birthday is still hard, as are the holidays. She was born on November 15 and was in the hospital through Thanskgiving and Christmas that year. She didn't really start to gain weight until close to Christmas. She actually hit 2 pounds on Christmas Eve. What a gift! During that time of year, I often slip into those NICU memories. We didn't actually celebrate Christmas the year she was born, things were too hectic and she was too critical. So every Christmas since then has been extra special because she is with us and healthy. One event that was especially significant was Cait's first ballet recital when she was four and a half. When my husband saw her in her costume for the first time, it brought tears to his eyes. Although he didn't say it out loud, it was obvious he was overcome with emotion at how far she had come.

"As the parent of a preemie and a full-term son, I feel I am more appreciative of my children and their accomplishments. They both amaze me for different reasons. Cait for all she has overcome and how well she is doing considering her tenuous beginning, and David in seeing how easy things are for him. At times, since David was born, we have actually been more frightened looking back at how Cait struggled with developmental tasks compared with how easily her brother masters them. We feel we have a special bond with both of them, for different reasons: Cait because she was a preemie, and David because it took us a long time and a lot of courage to try a second time.

"I constantly find myself questioning Cait's behavior in terms of prematurity. I do find myself making excuses at times. It is such a relief to hear that some behaviors are common in full-term children. At the same time, it is comforting to know that other preemies have similar issues. As a parent, we all want our child to fit in. With our preemies, even if they don't fit into normal full-term, they are not alone since they fit into normal preemie. It took me a while to accept that differentiation, but the biggest help has been sharing stories with other parents who have walked in these shoes."

From the mother of twins born at 25 weeks:
"I think not a day goes by that I don't think about the prematurity, and how things might have been different if my children had not been born so early (at 25 weeks). I feel like I got cheated not only out of a normal birth experience but out of a typical twin experience. We very seldom get to do average family-type things due to Jack's autism and behavioral challenges. Sometimes I feel like I am running three families at once: the rare one where all three of us do something together; the one where I go somewhere with Jack, usually the doctor's; and the one where I take Jenny somewhere for her special time."

From the mother of a 24-weeker, now four:
"I often wonder if I am the same parent now that I would have been had Ben had been born at term. I really don't know, and I guess I never will. What I do know is that I take nothing for granted. When Ben was a baby I was thrilled when he learned to walk and talk. Nowadays I am equally excited when he tells a funny story, or learns to write the letters of the alphabet. But it's a thrill tempered with relief, kind of like 'thank goodness, that's another milestone I can cross off the list.' I worried about him for long weeks in the NICU, and I've never been able to let the worry go.

"I often tell people that Ben sees himself as a 'regular' kid, just like all his friends. In many ways his prematurity seems to have touched him lightly. But it has affected me profoundly. I am the parent of a premature child—and I always will be.

"Still, when I look at the bright, beautiful child I have today, I have to say prematurity wasn't what I planned. It wasn't a journey I wanted to take, or enjoyed very much in the taking. But was it worth it? Yes, indeed."

From the parents of a daughter born at 30 weeks who is now almost nine:
"Almost nine years ago, Emily was born ten weeks early, weighing 3 pounds 3 ounces. At the time we were warned about all the complications

that could happen. She did have a transfusion and came home on oxygen, which she was weaned off about a month later. We were told that Emily might have problems with gross motor activities as she grew.

"Now, as she approaches her ninth birthday, she is a beautiful, healthy child. She plays basketball, softball, soccer, and does karate, and hopes to play ice hockey next year. She is the tallest in her class, and we recently received a note from school telling us that she is above the 95th percentile for height and weight. We were advised to check with our pediatrician to see if this is 'normal.' I laughed thinking back to the tiny baby she was in the beginning. She's 'normal' all right, and there is no holding her back."

And finally, a longer story from a mother of twins born at 26 weeks, one of whom has developed typically and the other of whom has been diagnosed with autism:

"My story differs dramatically from the childbirth experiences enjoyed by my friends, coworkers, and siblings. It is fairly representative of the stories shared by many parents of premature babies, however. After four years of infertility, I was overjoyed to learn I was pregnant with twins. Pregnancy reduced those years of tears to something suddenly small. I felt beautiful, happy, and blessed by the greatest fortune imaginable. I was nervous about my ability to manage two babies, but the anxiety was welcomed. Aside from normal concerns about '10 fingers and 10 toes,' I didn't worry that my children would be anything but healthy. I was taking very good care of myself and receiving top-notch medical attention. The hard part was behind me.

"With no real warning, I went into labor 14 weeks before my due date. My labor proceeded very quickly, and my sons Louis and Adam were born by cesarean section in May of 1992. They weighed 900 grams each— roughly 2 pounds—and encountered many of the problems experienced by many preemies. The boys both had bouts of pneumonia, serious infections, and painfully slow weight gain. They were both intubated for two months and classified as having moderate BPD (bronchopulmonary dysplasia). The incident of greatest concern during their three-month hospital stay was the brain hemorrhage Adam suffered. Although the bleed was not considered severe by physicians (grade II), the possibility of long-term neurological problems was a constant worry.

"My children came home from the hospital with relatively few medical problems, given the severity of their prematurity. Louis weighed just a little under 4 pounds at three months, and feeding him was an ongoing problem, but he did grow (albeit very slowly), and he did not show any signs of respiratory issues or unexpected developmental delays. Adam was bigger when he came home—a whopping 5 pounds—but his breathing pattern was immature, and he required medication and an apnea monitor for four months. Still, given the possibilities, these were not major problems.

"Because Adam had suffered the brain bleed, we watched him very closely. We noticed some disconcerting differences between him and his twin brother shortly after they came home. Adam seemed unable to tolerate eye contact. When we held him close and looked at his face, he would invariably turn his head away. When he was lying on his back or in the swing or bouncy seat, we noticed he would stare for long periods of time at bright lights that were on. We weren't terribly alarmed by this in the first months because he was just an infant, and we didn't expect his nervous system and development to be typical. Still, there were concerns.

"With time, it became clear that Louis was developing normally. By the time he was 15 months old, his development was typical for a one-year-old. Aside from his size, there were no signs of his prematurity. Adam's development, however, became increasingly delayed. But he wasn't just developing slowly; he was developing unusually. Although he was not formally diagnosed until he was four years old, I was convinced of Adam's autism when he was just an infant. He never looked at me; he simply couldn't. And as he got older, he deviated more and more from 'normal' development. No smiles, no laughs, very few cries. I think the fact that Louis was right beside him responding to me, smiling, laughing, and crying when he was hurt or needy made Adam's issues all the more painful.

"It's hard to describe the despair I felt when Adam was a toddler. I was both scared and depressed...my sorrow was palpable. When people told me how lucky I was that the boys' issues weren't greater, I'd ask them to imagine for a moment what it would feel like if their children never looked them in the eye, never sought the comfort of their arms after a bad fall.... I would think about my boys as six-year-olds not starting school together, and I would grieve the loss of their twinship. I worried that Adam would never make eye contact or understand my love for him. I feared that I would love Louis more.... I was terribly afraid that I simply did not have what it would take to give Adam a good life.

"I'm not sure exactly when my despair started to wane and hope for my family's future began to emerge. It took me a few years to work through my grief and accept the magnitude of my loss. We all expect to have healthy children. The loss of that dream is tremendous, and I needed time to grieve. At first I was preoccupied with the magnitude of this loss. Slowly, however, it became something I could wrap my arms around. It stopped preventing me from finding my way with my little boy. And something wondrous happened. As I grew more comfortable with Adam and his autism, he grew more comfortable with me. At first his glances were furtive. But over time, they grew into lingering looks, accompanied by a gorgeous smile.

"I still understand the magnitude of my family's loss, but not to the exclusion of the great gifts of Louis and Adam. I believe I have found a way to live and thrive with the unresolved mourning surrounding Adam's autism. My sons don't have the sort of bond one often hears about between twins, but they are developing a bond. Adam's communication skills are growing, and he grows more and more comfortable with the people in his life. In fact, Adam is developing real attachment to those closest to him. The things that bring him the greatest joy are not things that the rest of us always understand, but his happiness is obvious. The most wonderful development I've observed in Adam is his genuine delight at the social time shared with his brother and teenaged stepsiblings at dinner time. Adam's family surrounds him with love and acceptance, and he responds in ways that show he can be silly, engaged, and thrilled to be the center of attention.

"While I embrace Adam and cannot envision my life without him, there are certainly things about autism that break my heart. There are also things that just wear me out from time to time. Adam's lack of concern for safety is tough to manage. He requires constant vigilance, and his issues make it hard or impossible to do some things other families take for granted. There are times when I wish I could devote more energy to Louis, who by necessity takes care of himself more than most kids his age. There are times when I really need a break. If I had anticipated some of these things when Adam was an infant, I would have thought myself unable to handle them. But I do handle them. I think what makes the difficult issues manageable is the love I feel for my son. When Adam was a baby, he was more a medical crisis than he was my son. Before I had a chance to bond with him, I was afraid of him. While I still worry, I'm no longer afraid. And although I've always been concerned about Louis and the impact of autism on him, I see evidence every day of his happiness, security, self-esteem, and remarkable sensitivity. Autism has defined our family in many ways, but it hasn't robbed us of our strength and happiness.

"I still read everything I can find about autism, and I still fantasize about the possibility of a cure. I also enjoy and get a real kick out of my son! I hug him all the time, and we love each other in our own special way, and I am no longer upset that my sons are not in first grade together. I would never have chosen autism, but I wouldn't give up Adam for anything. When I'm tired or frustrated, I turn to one of the many invaluable supports I've been fortunate to establish since my children's birth. Some of the support comes from family and long-time friends; a great deal comes from the friendships that grew out of encounters with other parents of children born prematurely. These are people I am comfortable crying and laughing with, people who help me maintain perspective and a sense of humor.

"Adam has come a long way since his days in the NICU. There are many challenges that face him, but focusing on those is not productive for me. I know that there will be help for us every step of the way. I know that my own coping skills will continue to grow as our challenges change. I understand that we've always managed and thrived better than I would have thought possible."

APPENDIXES

Appendix A: Conversion Tables

WEIGHT (Pounds and Ounces to Grams)

POUNDS / OUNCES	0	1	2	3	4	5	6	7
0	—	28	57	85	113	142	170	198
1	454	482	510	539	567	595	624	652
2	907	936	964	992	1021	1049	1077	1106
3	1361	1389	1417	1446	1474	1503	1531	1559
4	1814	1843	1871	1899	1928	1956	1984	2013
5	2268	2296	2325	2353	2381	2410	2438	2466
6	2722	2750	2778	2807	2835	2863	2892	2920
7	3175	3203	3232	3260	3289	3317	3345	3374
8	3629	3657	3685	3714	3742	3770	3799	3827
9	4082	4111	4139	4167	4196	4224	4252	4281
10	4536	4564	4593	4621	4649	4678	4706	4734
11	4990	5018	5046	5075	5103	5131	5160	5188
12	5443	5471	5500	5528	5557	5585	5613	5642
13	5897	5925	5953	5982	6010	6038	6067	6095
14	6350	6379	6407	6435	6464	6492	6520	6549
15	6804	6832	6860	6889	6917	6945	6973	7002
16	7257	7286	7313	7342	7371	7399	7427	7456
17	7711	7739	7768	7796	7824	7853	7881	7909
18	8165	8192	8221	8249	8278	8306	8335	8363
19	8618	8646	8675	8703	8731	8760	8788	8816
20	9072	9100	9128	9157	9185	9213	9242	9270
21	9525	9554	9582	9610	9639	9667	9695	9724
22	9979	10007	10036	10064	10092	10120	10149	10177

VOLUME

1 cubic centimeter (cc) = 1 milliliter (ml) = 20 drops
5 cc = 5 ml = 1 teaspoon
15 cc = 15 ml = 1 tablespoon = 1/2 ounce
30 cc = 30 ml = 1 ounce

8	9	10	11	12	13	14	15
227	255	283	312	340	369	397	425
680	709	737	765	794	822	850	879
1134	1162	1191	1219	1247	1276	1304	1332
1588	1616	1644	1673	1701	1729	1758	1786
2041	2070	2098	2126	2155	2183	2211	2240
2495	2523	2551	2580	2608	2637	2665	2693
2948	2977	3005	3033	3062	3090	3118	3147
3402	3430	3459	3487	3515	3544	3572	3600
3856	3884	3912	3941	3969	3997	4026	4054
4309	4337	4366	4394	4423	4451	4479	4508
4763	4791	4819	4848	4876	4904	4933	4961
5216	5245	5273	5301	5330	5358	5386	5415
5670	5698	5727	5755	5783	5812	5840	5868
6123	6152	6180	6209	6237	6265	6294	6322
6577	6605	6634	6662	6690	6719	6747	6776
7030	7059	7087	7115	7144	7172	7201	7228
7484	7512	7541	7569	7597	7626	7654	7682
7938	7966	7994	8023	8051	8079	8108	8136
8391	8420	8448	8476	8504	8533	8561	8590
8845	8873	8902	8930	8958	8987	9015	9043
9298	9327	9355	9383	9412	9440	9469	9497
9752	9780	9809	9837	9865	9894	9922	9950
10206	10234	10262	10291	10319	10347	10376	10404

Appendix B: Growth Charts

CDC Growth Charts: United States

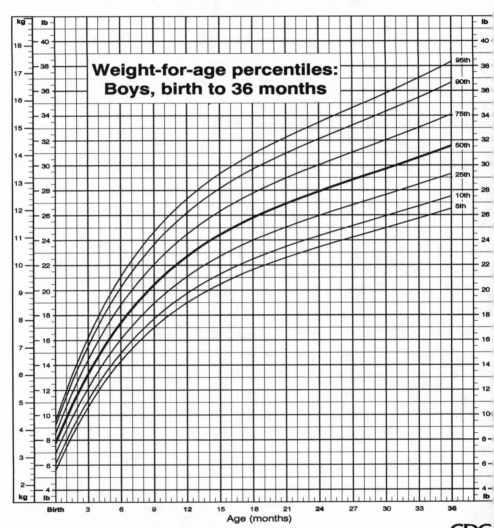

Weight-for-age percentiles: Boys, birth to 36 months

SOURCE: Developed by the National Center for Health Statistics in collaboration with the National Center for Chronic Disease Prevention and Health Promotion (2000).

CDC

CDC Growth Charts: United States

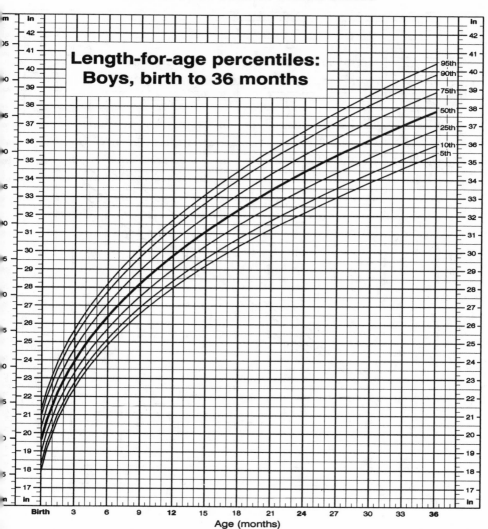

Length-for-age percentiles: Boys, birth to 36 months

Age (months)

■RCE: Developed by the National Center for Health Statistics in collaboration with
   the National Center for Chronic Disease Prevention and Health Promotion (2000).

CDC Growth Charts: United States

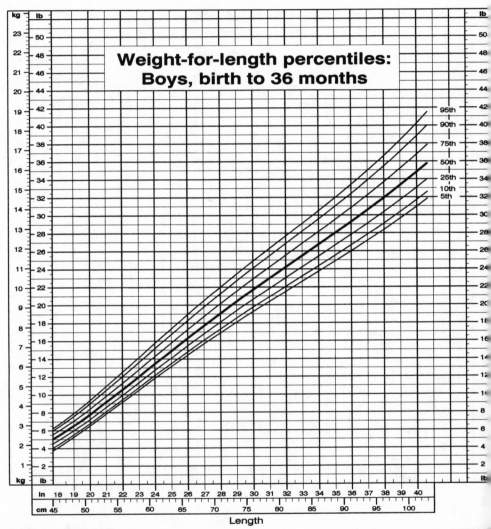

Weight-for-length percentiles:
Boys, birth to 36 months

Length

Revised and corrected June 8, 2000.

SOURCE: Developed by the National Center for Health Statistics in collaboration with
the National Center for Chronic Disease Prevention and Health Promotion (2000).

CDC Growth Charts: United States

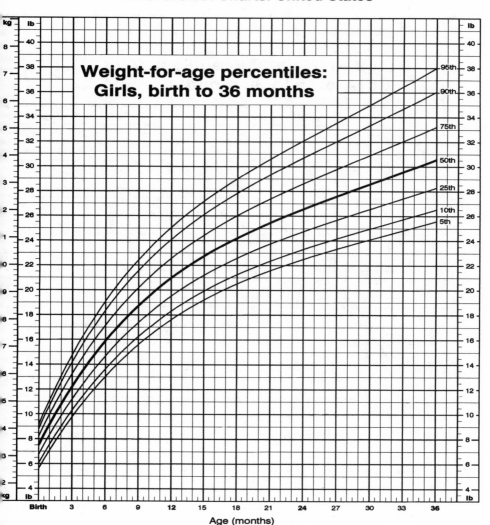

Weight-for-age percentiles: Girls, birth to 36 months

SOURCE: Developed by the National Center for Health Statistics in collaboration with the National Center for Chronic Disease Prevention and Health Promotion (2000).

CDC Growth Charts: United States

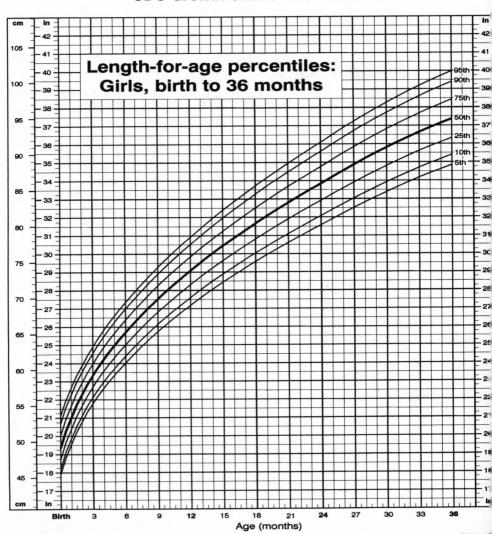

Length-for-age percentiles: Girls, birth to 36 months

SOURCE: Developed by the National Center for Health Statistics in collaboration with the National Center for Chronic Disease Prevention and Health Promotion (2000).

CDC Growth Charts: United States

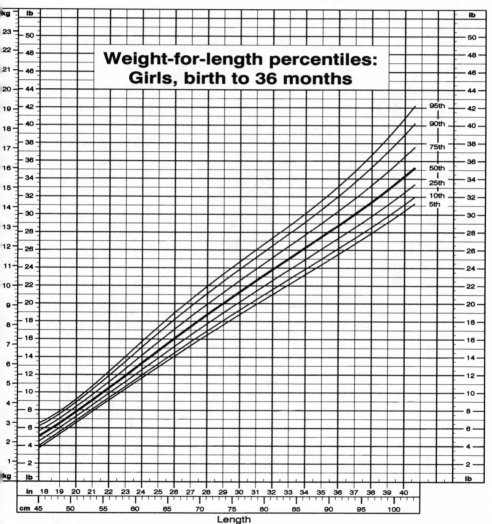

Weight-for-length percentiles: Girls, birth to 36 months

Length

Revised and corrected June 8, 2000.

SOURCE: Developed by the National Center for Health Statistics in collaboration with the National Center for Chronic Disease Prevention and Health Promotion (2000).

Appendix C: Infant CPR

Call 911 or an emergency number after starting rescue efforts.

You should start first aid if…

- The child cannot breathe at all (the chest is not moving up and down).
- The child's airway is so blocked that there's only a weak cough and a loss of color.
- The child cannot cough, talk, or make a normal voice sound.
- The child is found unconscious. (Go to CPR.)

Do not start first aid if…

- The child can breathe, cry, talk, or make a normal voice sound.
- The child has a strong cough, demonstrating that there is little or no blockage.

INFANT CHOKING (UNDER ONE YEAR OLD)

Begin the following if the infant is choking and is unable to breathe. However, if the infant is coughing, crying, or speaking, DO NOT do any of the following, but call your doctor for further advice.

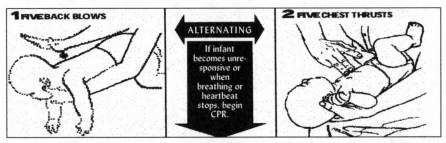

1 FIVE BACK BLOWS

ALTERNATING
If infant becomes unresponsive or when breathing or heartbeat stops, begin CPR.

2 FIVE CHEST THRUSTS

INFANT CPR (UNDER ONE YEAR OLD)

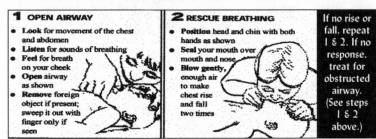

1 OPEN AIRWAY
- Look for movement of the chest and abdomen
- Listen for sounds of breathing
- Feel for breath on your cheek
- Open airway as shown
- Remove foreign object if present; sweep it out with finger only if seen

2 RESCUE BREATHING
- Position head and chin with both hands as shown
- Seal your mouth over mouth and nose
- Blow gently, enough air to make chest rise and fall two times

If no rise or fall, repeat 1 & 2. If no response, treat for obstructed airway. (See steps 1 & 2 above.)

Cardiopulmonary Resuscitation (CPR): To be used when infant is unresponsive or when breathing or heart beat stops.

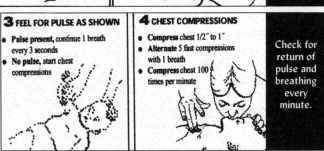

3 FEEL FOR PULSE AS SHOWN
- Pulse present, continue 1 breath every 3 seconds
- No pulse, start chest compressions

4 CHEST COMPRESSIONS
- Compress chest 1/2" to 1"
- Alternate 5 fast compressions with 1 breath
- Compress chest 100 times per minute

Check for return of pulse and breathing every minute.

CHILD CHOKING (OVER ONE YEAR OLD)

Begin the following if the child is choking and is unable to breathe. However, if the child is coughing, crying, or speaking, DO NOT do any of the following, but call you doctor for further advice.

If child become unresponsive or when breathing or heartbeat stops, begin CPR.

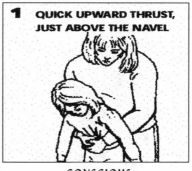

1 QUICK UPWARD THRUST, JUST ABOVE THE NAVEL

CONSCIOUS

CHILD CPR (OVER ONE YEAR OLD)

Cardiopulmonary Resuscitation (CPR): To be used when child is unresponsive or when breathing or heart beat stops.

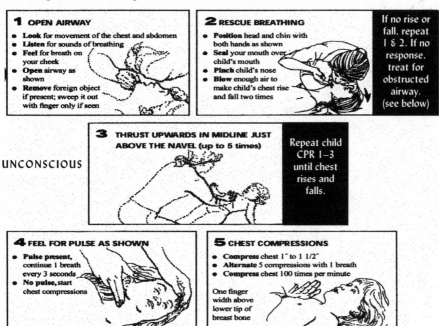

1 OPEN AIRWAY
- **Look** for movement of the chest and abdomen
- **Listen** for sounds of breathing
- **Feel** for breath on your cheek
- **Open** airway as shown
- **Remove** foreign object if present; sweep it out with finger only if seen

2 RESCUE BREATHING
- **Position** head and chin with both hands as shown
- **Seal** your mouth over child's mouth
- **Pinch** child's nose
- **Blow** enough air to make child's chest rise and fall two times

If no rise or fall, repeat 1 & 2. If no response, treat for obstructed airway. (see below)

UNCONSCIOUS

3 THRUST UPWARDS IN MIDLINE JUST ABOVE THE NAVEL (up to 5 times)

Repeat child CPR 1–3 until chest rises and falls.

4 FEEL FOR PULSE AS SHOWN
- **Pulse present,** continue 1 breath every 3 seconds
- **No pulse,** start chest compressions

5 CHEST COMPRESSIONS
- **Compress** chest 1˝ to 1 1/2˝
- **Alternate** 5 compressions with 1 breath
- **Compress** chest 100 times per minute

One finger width above lower tip of breast bone

If, at any time, an object is coughed up or the infant/child starts to breathe, call your doctor for further advice. Ask your physician for information on an approved first aid course or CPR course in your community.

Appendix D: Immunization Schedule

Recommended Childhood Immunization Schedule
United States, January – December 2000

Vaccines are listed under routinely recommended ages. [Bars] indicate range of recommended ages for immunization. Any dose not given t the recommended age should be given as a "catch-up" immunization at any subsequent visit when indicated and feasible. (Ovals) indicate vaccines to be given if previously recommended doses were missed or given earlier than the recommended minimum age.

Age ▶ / Vaccine ▼	Birth	1 mo	2 mos	4 mos	6 mos	12 mos	15 mos	18 mos	24 mos	4-6 yrs	11-12 yrs	14-16 yrs
Hepatitis B	Hep B	Hep B	Hep B		Hep B						(Hep B)	
Diphtheria, Tetanus, Pertussis			DTaP	DTaP	DTaP		DTaP	DTaP		DTaP	Td	
H. influenzae type b			Hib	Hib	Hib	Hib	Hib					
Polio			IPV	IPV	IPV	IPV	IPV	IPV		IPV		
Measles, Mumps, Rubella						MMR	MMR			MMR	(MMR)	
Varicella						Var	Var	Var			(Var)	
Hepatitis A									Hep A[B] – in selected areas			

Approved by the Advisory Committee on Immunization Practices (ACIP), the American Academy of Pediatrics (AAP), and the American Academy of Family Physicians (AAFP).

Appendix E: Resources for Parents

୫ଛ

Resources for parents of preemies are constantly increasing. One of the best new sources of information is the Internet where the number of preemie-related websites is growing exponentially. You can find websites on health and neonatology, information on specific diagnoses and disabilities, chat rooms and mailing lists, and on-line stores.

The following is, therefore, only a partial listing of all the resources currently available. I have tried to cover a broad range of parents' needs, and to select resources that can be easily located in stores or libraries, by telephone, or the Internet. Whenever possible, I have added notes on what each listed resource has to offer. Recommendations for further reading materials can also be found in the Bibliography section.

INFANT AND CHILD CARE BOOKS

American Academy of Pediatrics, Shelov, S. (ed.) *Caring for Your Baby and Young Child* (New York: Bantam Books, 1998).

Eisenberg, A., Murkoff, H.E., and Hathaway, S.E. *What to Expect the First Year* (New York: Workman Publishing, 1996).

Leach, Penelope. *Your Baby and Child: From Birth to Age 5* (New York: Alfred A. Knopf, 1997).

Sears, W. & Sears, M. *The Baby Book: Everything You Need to Know About Your Baby From Birth to Age Two* (Boston: Little, Brown & Co., 1993).

Spock, B. and Parker, S.J. *Dr. Spock's Baby and Child Care* (New York: Pocket Books, 1998).

GENERAL INFORMATION ON PREMATURITY AND RELATED ISSUES

Books for Parents

Brazy, Jane E. (ed.) *For Parents of Preemies: Answers to Commonly Asked Questions* (Madison, WI: University of Wisconsin and The Center for

Perinatal Care at Meriter Hospital, 1996). Also available over the Internet at: www.pediatrics.wisc.edu/childrenshosp/parents_of_ preemies

Davis, D. and Stein, M.T. *The Emotional Journey of Parenting Your Premature Baby: A Book of Hope and Healing* (in press) (Santa Rosa, CA: NICU Ink, 2001 [projected].

Harrison, H. *The Premature Baby Book: A Parents' Guide to Coping and Caring in the First Years* (New York: St. Martin's Press, 1983).

Hussey, B. *Understanding My Signals: Help for Parents of Premature Infants* (Palo alto, CA: VORT Corporation, 1988).

Hynan, Michael T. *The Pain of Premature Parents: A Psychological Guide for Coping* (Lanham, MD: University Press of America, Inc., 1987).

Klein, A.H. and Ganon, S.A. *Caring for Your Premature Baby: A Complete Resource for Parents* (New York: Harper Collins Publishers, Inc., 1998).

Manginello, F.P. and DiGeronimo, T.F. *Your Premature Baby: Everything You Need to Know About Childbirth, Treatment, and Parenting* (New York: John Wiley & Sons, 1998).

Smith, Timothy. *Miracle Birth Stories of Very Premature Babies: Little Thumbs Up!* (Westport, CT: Bergin & Garvey, 1999).

Tracy, A. and Maroney, D. *Your Premature Baby and Child: Helpful Answers and Advice for Parents* (New York: Berkley Publishing Group, 1999).

VandenBerg, K. A. and Hanson, M. J. *Homecoming for Babies After the Neonatal Intensive Care Nursery: A Guide for Parents in Supporting Their Baby's Early Dvelopment* (Austin, TX: PRO-ED, Inc., 1993).

Zaichkin, Jeanette. *Newborn Intensive Care: What Every Parent Needs to Know* (Petaluma, CA: NICU Ink, 1996).

Books for Children and Siblings

Lafferty, L. *Born Early: A Premature Baby's Story* (Minneapolis, MN: Fairview Press, 1998).

Murphy-Melas, E. *Watching Bradley Grow: A Story About Premature Birth* (Marietta, GA: Longstreet Press, 1996).

Pankrow, V. *No Bigger Than My Teddy Bear* (Nashville, TN: Abingdon Press, 1987). This book is currently out of print, but may be available in your local library.

Resta, Bart. *Believe in Katie Lynn* (Nashville, TN: Eggman Publishing Co., 1995).

Textbooks

Ballard, R.A. *Pediatric Care of the ICN Graduate* (Philadelphia: W.B. Saunders Co., 1988).

Bernbaum, J.C. and Hoffman-Williamson, M. *Primary Care of the Preterm Infant* (St. Louis: Mosby–Year Book, Inc., 1991).

Cloherty, J.P. and Stark, A.R. (eds). *Manual of Neonatal Care* (Philadelphia: Lippincott–Raven Publishers, 1998).

Merenstein, G.B. and Gardner, S.L. *Handbook of Neonatal Intensive Care* (St. Louis: Mosby–Year Book, Inc., 1998).

Websites for Parents

There are a growing number of websites on prematurity which can be accessed by doing a search using the word *premature* or *preemie*. I have listed a few here that offer a wide range of services, but there are many more.

Preemie-L website: www.preemie-L.org. *This website is geared toward families with premature infants and young children. There are a number of offerings: a bulletin-board–style discussion group in which messages and questions are posted for everyone to read and answer; a mailing list in which members receive and answer messages directly;* The Early Edition *on-line newspaper, and more.*

Preemie-child website: www.comeunity.com/premature. *This website is geared toward the longer-term impacts of prematurity, although it includes a lot of information on all aspects of prematurity. It also has a mailing list for parents with preemies aged four and older, in which members receive and answer messages on topics of common interest (address: www.comeunity.com/premature/preemie-child).*

The Early Edition on-line newspaper: home.vicnet.net.au/~earlyed. *A monthly newspaper from the Preemie-L website covering a range of topics around prematurity.*

Mary Searcy's Preemie Resource Page: members.aol.com/maraim/preemie.htm. *This is a comprehensive list of resources for parents of preemies.*

After the NICU: www.ixpres.com/tbangs/advice.htm. Advice from parents on various issues that arise after you bring your baby home from the hospital.

Pediatrics and Neonatology Websites

Emory Regional Perinatal Center: www.emory.edu/PEDS/NEONATOLOGY /DCP. Website of the Developmental Continuity Program, Emory Regional Perinatal Center, Atlanta, Georgia. *Contains information on common medical complications of prematurity and their implications for development, developmental milestones, and resources for parents.*

American Academy of Pediatrics: www.aap.org (website of the organization), and www.pediatrics.org (on-line *Pediatrics* journal).

Medscape Pediatrics: pediatrics.medscape.com. *Designed primarily for physicians and other health professionals, provides regular updates on research and developments in pediatrics (and other specialty areas) as well as free access to MEDLINE, the database of medical journals. Requires free one-time registration. A good place to do literature searches on various topics related to prematurity and development.*

Neonatology on the Web: www.neonatology.org. *Contains a listing of and links to many neonatology resources on the Web. This is a good place to start searching for information on specific topics.*

PREEMIE-SIZED DIAPERS

Pampers Premature Diapers
800-543-4932 Mon–Fri, 8 am–5 pm EST
800-285-6064 (in Ohio)
www.pampers.com
Many stores carry Pampers diapers and may be able to order the Premature size for you if they don't regularly carry them. Otherwise, you can order a case of Premature diapers directly using the phone numbers listed here.

Huggies Preemies Diapers (for babies up to 6 pounds)
800-447-9423 Ext. 44
800-322-0493 Ext. 44 (in Minnesota)
www.huggies.com
Huggies brand diapers are carried by many drugstores and grocery stores. If the store near you does not stock the Preemies diapers, call the company directly to order a case.

CAR SEATS

American Academy of Pediatrics. "2000 Family Shopping Guide to Car Seats: Safety and Product Information." *Pamphlet available from the AAP at 847-228-5005 or over the Internet at: www.aap.org/family/famshop.htm*

CLOTHING AND OTHER ITEMS FOR PREEMIES

Many department stores and baby stores carry clothing in preemie sizes (under five pounds). In addition, there are a growing number of sources on the Internet.

Children's Medical Ventures, Inc.
541 Main Street
South Weymouth, Massachusetts 02190
888-SOOTHIE
www.childmed.com
This company, formed in 1989 by a cooperative of 36 children's hospitals, develops and sells developmentally-supportive products for NICUs and growing babies. They offer preemie pacifiers, positioning aids, car seat inserts, and a car bed/seat designed for preemies, among many other items. This company sells both to hospitals and directly to parents.

Preemie Store...and More!
17195 Newhope Street, Suite 105
Fountain Valley, California 92708
800-O-SO-TINY (676-8469)
www.preemie.com
Offers birth announcements, books, clothing, and other items. Designed for babies as small as 1 pound through 8 pounds.

Tiny Bundles
11468 Ballybunion Square
San Diego, California 92128
858-451-9907
www.preemieclothing.com
Offers a wide array of custom-sized clothing, accessories, and books for newborn preemies, as well as older babies.

PUMPING AND BREASTFEEDING

Books

Gotsch, Gwen. *Breastfeeding Your Premature Baby* (Schaumberg, IL: La Leche League International, 1999).

Huggins, K. *The Nursing Mother's Companion, 4th Revised Edition* (Boston: Harvard Common Press, 1999).

Walker, Marsha. *Breastfeeding Your Premature or Special Care Baby: A Practical Guide for Nursing the Tiny Baby* (Weston, MA: Lactation Associates, Item # 107, 1998).

Breastfeeding Support and Education

La Leche League International
1400 North Meacham Road
Schaumburg, Illinois 60173
800-LA LECHE
847-519-7730
www.lalecheleague.org
Provides referrals to local LLLI Groups, catalog of supplies, books, and videos for nursing and pumping mothers. Also look in your local phone book under La Leche League for local phone numbers. The LLLI web site provides information on breastfeeding, access to the on-line catalog, listings of local La Leche League leaders and meetings, information on conferences, and links to other related sites.

Lactation Associates
254 Conant Road
Weston, Massachusetts 02493
781-893-3553
members.aol.com/marshalact/lactationassociates/
This organization is geared primarily toward educators and lactation professionals but publishes a number of booklets on the specific challenges of breastfeeding preemies that are appropriate for parents. Contact them for their catalog.

Lactation Professionals

The hospital where your baby was cared for may be able to refer you to a local lactation professional, or contact one of the organizations listed below for a referral. Be sure that the professional you work with has experience with preemies.

International Lactation Consultant Association (ILCA)
4101 Lake Boone Trail, Suite 201
Raleigh, North Carolina 27607
919-787-5181
www.ilca.org
Professional organization for lactation consultants. Call for referrals to certified lactation consultants in your area.

Breastfeeding National Network
(Medela, Inc.)
800-TELL-YOU (835-5968)
www.medela.com/dealers.html
Provides referrals to local lactation consultants.

Electric Breast Pump Rentals

Most mothers who will be pumping for an extended time will need to use an electric breast pump at home. Because these pumps are very expensive, most mothers rent these pumps rather than buy them. However, newer, less expensive portable models are also available that can be more easily taken to work, or if you need to travel.

The companies listed below can refer you to local rental agents; they also carry nursing and pumping supplies, and accessories. Your hospital may also be able to refer you to local suppliers.

Medela, Inc.
P.O. Box 660
4610 Prime Parkway
McHenry, Illinois 60050
800-435-8316
815-363-1166
www.medela.com

White River Concepts
924C Calle Negocio
San Clemente, California 92673
800-341-3906
949-366-8960
www.whiteriver.com

Pumping/Nursing Supplies and Equipment

There are a growing number of companies on the Internet that supply pumps and other supplies and equipment. They can usually take orders over the Internet, or they can be contacted directly by phone. A few are listed here to get you started.

Breast is Best
888-398-7987
425-485-3295
www.birthandbaby.com/Family_Resources
An on-line store that carries pumps, nursing bras, nursing aids, and more.

Lactation Innovation
888-LACTINV (522-8468)
www.lactinv.com
Carries Medela and Hollister breast pumps, as well as freezer bags, nursing pads, breast shells, nursing pillows, and other supplies.

Authentically Yours
877-799-0697 (toll free)
808-689-0697 (in Hawaii)
www.milkexpress.com
This on-line store carries Medela and Hollister pumps and replacement parts, as well as many other products.

Supplemental Nursing Devices

Supplemental nursers can be used to help build up a mother's milk supply or to make feeding easier for a baby with a weak or ineffective suck. They usually consist of a bag into which breast milk or formula is placed, and a thin, flexible tube that runs from the bag to a mother's nipple. When the baby latches on, she receives milk from both the breast and the supplemental nurser.

Supplemental Nursing System
Medela, Inc.
P.O. Box 660
McHenry, Illinois 60051
800-435-8316
www.medela.com

Lact-Aid International, Inc.
P.O. Box 1066
Athens, Tennessee 37371
423-744-9090
www.lact-aid.com

INFANT FORMULA MANUFACTURERS

If you need a special formula for your baby, check to see if your local drugstore can order it for you. If you have trouble obtaining the formula you need, contact the manufacturers directly.

Mead Johnson & Company (Enfamil, Enfamil 22, Prosobee, Lactofree, and Nutramigen)
Evansville, Indiana 47721
800-BABY-123 8 am–4:30 pm, CST
www.meadjohnson.com

Ross Laboratories (Similac, NeoSure, Isomil, Alimentum)
Consumer Relations
625 Cleveland Avenue
Columbus, Ohio 43215
800-986-8510 8:30 am–5 pm, EST
www.welcomeaddition.com

Carnation (Good Start)
800-782-7766
www.carnationbaby.com

INFANT MASSAGE

There are no books that specifically discuss massaging preemies, but the techniques described in the following books can be used with most babies by the time they come home.

McClure, V.S. *Infant Massage: A Handbook for Loving Parents* (New York: Bantam Books, 1989).

Walker, P. *Baby Massage: A Practical Guide to Massage and Movement for Babies and Infants* (New York: St. Martin's Griffin, 1996).

KANGAROO CARE

Ludington-Hoe, S. M. and Golant, S. K. *Kangaroo Care: The Best You Can Do to Help Your Preterm Infant* (New York: Bantam Books, 1993). This book is currently out of print but may be available at your local library.

Sears, W. and Sears, M. *The Baby Book: Everything You Need to Know About Your Baby From Birth to Age Two* (Boston: Little, Brown & Co., 1993). *See Chapter 14: "Babywearing: The Art and Science of Carrying Your Baby."*

ORGANIZATIONS AND SUPPORT GROUPS FOR PARENTS OF PREEMIES

Alexis Foundation for Premature Infants and Children
P.O. Box 1126
Birmingham, Minnesota 48012
877-ALEXIS-0
248-543-4169
pages.prodigy.net/thealexisfoundation/THEALEXIS1.html
An advocacy and educational organization with a mission to support parents and professionals to provide the best possible care for preemies. The foundation sponsors an annual conference for parents and professionals, and also has an on-line store that sells clothing and accessories.

National Perinatal Association
3500 E. Fletcher Avenue, Suite 205
Tampa, Florida 33613
888-971-3295
813-971-1008
www.nationalperinatal.org
Primarily an organization for professionals, the NPA works to improve perinatal care through education, research, and helping to set national priorities. Also publishes the Journal of Perinatology.

American Association for Premature Infants (AAPI)
P.O. Box 46371
Cincinnati, Ohio 45246
513-887-2888
www.aapi-online.org
The AAPI is an organization dedicated to improving the quality of health, developmental, and educational services for premature infants and their families.

Local Support Groups

In many locations, groups exist to provide support and information to families of premature infants and children. The social worker in your NICU should be able to provide you with information about groups in your area. Also refer to the listing of local groups in Mary Searcy's Preemie Resource Page *on the Internet: member.aol.com/maraim/preemie.htm. The groups are listed in the* Organizations *section of the list.*

TWINS AND HIGHER ORDER MULTIPLES

Books and Magazines

Agnew, C. L., Klein, A.H., and Ganon, J.A. *Twins! Expert Advice from Two Practicing Physicians on Pregnancy, Birth and the First Year of Life with Twins* (New York: HarperCollins, 1997).

Noble, E. *Having Twins: A Parent's Guide to Pregnancy, Birth, and Early Childhood* (New York: Houghton Mifflin Co., 1991).

Twins Magazine
5350 South Roslyn Street, Suite 400
Englewood, Colorado 80111
888-55-TWINS
303-290-8500

www.twinsmagazine.com. Twins Magazine *is published bimonthly. The website provides the table of contents of the magazine and sample articles, along with a listing of resources for parents of multiples.*

Information, Advocacy, and Support

National Organization of Mothers of Twins Clubs, Inc.
Executive Office
P.O. Box 438
Thompson Station, Tennessee 37179
877-540-0936
615-595-0936

www.nomotc.org
*Provides support, information, and educational materials for parents of twins and
higher multiples. Can link you with a local support group.*

MOST (Mothers of Supertwins)
P.O. Box 951
Brentwood, New York 11717
631-859-1110
www.mostonline.org
*National, nonprofit network that provides information, resources, and support to
parents with triplets and more.*

The Triplet Connection
P.O. Box 99571
Stockton, California 95209
209-474-0885
www.tripletconnection.org
*A national organization for expectant and new parents of triplets or higher order
multiples. Provides information, support, and networking opportunities.*

The Twin-to-Twin Transfusion Syndrome Foundation, Inc.
411 Longbeach Parkway
Bay Village, Ohio 44140
440-899-TTTS
www.tttsfoundation.org
*An international, nonprofit organization that provides support, education, and
information to families and professionals before, during, or after a case of TTTS.*

INFANT LOSS AND BEREAVEMENT

Davis, Deborah L. *Empty Cradle, Broken Heart: Surviving the Death of Your Baby*
(Golden, CO: Fulcrum Publishing, 1996).

Ilse, Sherokee. *Empty Arms: Coping with Miscarriage, Stillbirth and Infant Death*
(Maple Plain, MN: Wintergreen Press, 1990).

Sources of Books, Information, and Support

Centering Corporation
1531 North Saddle Creek Road
Omaha, Nebraska 68104
402-553-1200
www.centering.com
Publishes an extensive catalog of books, tapes, and pamphlets on loss, grief, and recovery. Includes books about and for children, as well as books about prematurity.

Wintergreen Press
3630 Eileen Street
Maple Plain, Minnesota 55359
612-476-1303
Publishes and stocks many books and videos on infant loss, grieving, and healing.

SHARE Pregnancy and Infant Loss Support, Inc.
National Office
St. Joseph Health Center
300 First Capitol Drive
St. Charles, Missouri 63301
800-821-6819
636-947-6164
www.nationalshareoffice.com
SHARE offers support and information free of charge to bereaved parents. Publishes bimonthly newsletter, and maintains listings of local support groups.

Loss in a Multiple Pregnancy

The Center for Loss in a Multiple Birth (CLIMB), Inc.
P.O. Box 1064
Palmer, Arkansas 99645
907-746-6123
www.climb-support.org
CLIMB serves parents who have lost one or more children in a multiple pregnancy. It publishes a quarterly newsletter, maintains a bibliography of information and support articles, has samples of birth and memorial announcements, and a parent contact list of other multiple birth parents who have suffered the loss of one or more of their babies.

FOR PARENTS OF CHILDREN WITH SPECIAL NEEDS

Books

Batshaw, M.L. and Perret, Y.M. *Children with Disabilities: A Medical Primer* (Baltimore: Paul H. Brookes Publishing Company, 1992).

New England SERVE. *Paying the Bills: Tips for Families on Financing Health Care for Children with Special Needs.* Available from New England SERVE, 101 Tremont Street, Suite 812, Boston, MA 02108. 617-574-9493.

Segal, M. *In Time and With Love: Caring for the Special Needs Baby* (New York: Newmarket Press, 1988).

Wolraich, M.L. *Disorders of Development & Learning: A Practical Guide to Assessment and Management* (St. Louis: Mosby-Year Book, Inc., 1996).

Resources for Advocacy, Information, and Support

Federation for Children with Special Needs
1135 Tremont Street, Suite 420
Boston, Massachusetts 02120
800-331-0688 (in Massachusetts)
617-236-7210
www.fcsn.org
The Federation is an advocacy organization for parents and parent organizations representing children with a variety of disabilities. It operates a Parent Center that offers a variety of services to parents, parent groups, and others who are concerned with children with special needs.

National Parent Network on Disabilities
1130–17th Street, NW, Suite 400
Washington, DC 20036
202-463-2299 (V/TDD)
www.npnd.org
An advocacy group based in Washington, D.C., that works to develop and implement legislation to protect and enhance the lives of children and adults with disabilities. A good source of information for parents of children with special needs or disabilities of any type.

National Information Center for Children and Youth with Disabilities (NICHCY)
P.O. Box 1492
Washington, DC 20013
800-695-0285
www.nichcy.org
NICHCY is a national information and referral center that provides information on disabilities and disability-related issues for families, educators, and other professionals. NICHCY can provide information on specific disabilities, early intervention, special education, disability organizations, and more. They offer a wide range of publications, can answer questions directly through their 800 number, and conduct searches in their library and databases. Materials also available in Spanish.

National Early Childhood Technical Assistance System (NEC-TAS)
137 East Franklin Street, Suite 500
Chapel Hill, North Carolina 27514
919-962-2001
www.nectas.unc.edu
NEC-TAS supports programs for young children with disabilities and their families covered under federal legislation (IDEA). A good source for information and publications on early intervention and special education programs.

Educational Resources Information Center Clearinghouse
on Disabilities and Gifted Education (ERIC EC)
1920 Association Drive
Reston, Virginia 20191
800-328-0272 (V/TTY)
www.ericec.org
A federally-funded center that provides access to an extensive library of publications
and information for parents and educators of children with special needs.

Exceptional Parent Magazine
Subscription Service
P.O. Box 2078
Marion, Ohio 43306
877-372-7368
On-line edition of magazine: www.eparent.com
Every year the January issue includes an extensive Resource Guide, including a listing
of state offices responsible for early intervention and special education programs, camps
and recreation programs, sources of information, products, and services.

PRO-ED
8700 Shoal Creek Blvd.
Austin, TX 78757
512-451-3246
800-897-3202
www.proedinc.com
Pro-Ed publishes and sells books and materials in the fields of psychology, special
education, and speech, language, and hearing for professionals and parents. Publishes
booklet by VandenBerg and Hanson, Homecoming for Babies After the Neonatal
Intensive Care Nursery.

VORT Corporation
P. O. Box 60132-TW
Palo Alto, CA 94306
650-322-8282
888-757-VORT (8678)
www.VORT.com
The VORT Corporation publishes and sells materials and books used for
developmental assessments and early childhood education. Includes materials for
parents of premature infants, early intervention programs, special education and
disabilities, and more. Publishes booklet by B. Hussey, Understanding My Signals:
Help for Parents of Premature Infants.

Websites of Interest

www.familyvillage.wisc.edu
The Family Village website maintains a very extensive library of information on specific disabilities, early intervention and special education programs, reading materials about and for children with disabilities, as well as a shopping mall for adaptive and assistive equipment, and much more. This website is an excellent starting point for researching information and resources on most disabilities and medical diagnoses.

www.comeunity.com
This website provides a wide range of services, information, and resources for parents adopting children or with special needs children, including preemies. Includes mailing lists that you can join to communicate with other parents in similar situations, articles on prematurity and disabilities, and reviews of books on prematurity, learning disabilities, and other specific disabilities.

www.hood.edu/seri
Special Education Resources on the Internet. Maintained by Hood College, this website is a collection of Internet-accessible information resources on disabilities in general, as well as on specific topics.

SENSORY INTEGRATION DYSFUNCTION

Kranowitz, C.S. *The Out-of-Sync Child: Recognizing and Coping with Sensory Integration Dysfunction* (New York: Skylight Press, 1998).

www.comeunity.com/disability/sensory_integration/
This website has a number of articles on SI dysfunction, a list of resources, and links to other sites.

CEREBRAL PALSY

Geralis, E. (ed.) *Children with Cerebral Palsy: A Parent's Guide* (Bethesda, MD: Woodbine House, 1991).

Leonard, J.F., Cadenhead, S.L., and Myers, M.E. *Keys to Parenting a Child with Cerebral Palsy* (Hauppauge, NY: Barron's Educational Series, Inc., 1997).

Miller, F. and Bachrach, S.J. *Cerebral Palsy: A Complete Guide for Caregiving* (Baltimore, MD: Johns Hopkins University Press, 1998).

United Cerebral Palsy (UCP)
1660 L Street, NW, Suite 700
Washington, DC 20036

800-USA-5-UCP
202-776-0406
TTY: 202-973-7197
www.ucpa.org
UCP is an advocacy and educational organization. Its website contains information
and facts about CP as well as an extensive list of resources, and a new marketplace.

www.familyvillage.wisc.edu
Under the Library heading at this website, there is an entry on CP that contains
information, resources, and links to other websites.

CHRONIC LUNG DISEASE
(BRONCHOPULMONARY DYSPLASIA)

www.cheo.on.ca/bpd/
This website from Children's Hospital of Eastern Ontario (CHEO) contains
comprehensive information about BPD, its symptoms, and treatment, including
information about nutrition and BPD.

www.lungusa.org
The website of the American Lung Association contains a brief overview of BPD and
links to other sites (800-LUNG-USA).

RETINOPATHY OF PREMATURITY

Understanding Retinopathy of Prematurity. Booklet from IRIS Medical
Instruments, Inc., Mountain View, CA, 1991 (650-962-8100).
These booklets are sold primarily to doctors and are not generally sold directly to
parents. Your child's eye doctor or an infant follow-up clinic may have copies.

www.konnections.com/eyedoc/ropstart.html
A website maintained by Ophthalmology Associates, Ogden, Utah. Gives a good
overview, with pictures, of ROP, its treatment, and possible complications.

PERIVENTRICULAR LEUKOMALACIA (PVL)

www.ucpa.org
The home page of the website of the United Cerebral Palsy Association (UCPA) has a
category called Research. Under Research, there is an entry, "Risk Factors, Causes
and Prevention of Periventricular Leukomalacia," which reviews a study published
in the journal Developmental Medicine and Child Neurology. (To go directly to
this entry: www.ucpa.org/html/research/riskfa.html)

HYDROCEPHALUS

About Hydrocephalus: A Book for Parents. Booklet from the Departments of
    Neurological Surgery and Pediatrics of the University of California, San
    Francisco, 1986. Available from the Hydrocephalus Association (see
    below).

Toporek, C. and Robinson, K. *Hydrocephalus: A Guide for Patients, Families, and
    Friends* (Sebastopol, CA: O'Reilly & Associates, Inc., 1999).

www.familyvillage.wisc.edu
On the home page of this website, click on Library. *Under the* Library *heading is an
entry for hydrocephalus that contains a very comprehensive array of information,
resources, and links to other sites.*

Hydrocephalus Association (HA)
870 Market Street, Suite 705
San Francisco, California 94102
415-732-7040
www.hydroassoc.org
*Provides support, education, and advocacy for families and professionals. Has local
chapters, and can link you with other parents. Publishes a quarterly newsletter,*
Hydrocephalus Newsletter, *and a resource list of literature they have available.
Provides the booklet* About Hydrocephalus *to new parents.*

Hydrocephalus Foundation, Inc. (HyFI)
910 Rear Broadway
Saugus, Massachusetts 01906
781-942-1161
www.hydrocephalus.org
Provides support, educational resources, and networking opportunities to families.

SUDDEN INFANT DEATH SYNDROME (SIDS)

Back to Sleep Campaign
P.O. Box 29111
Washington, DC 20040
800-505-CRIB
www.nihcd.nih.gov/sids/sids.htm
*Sponsored by the American Academy of Pediatrics, the U.S. Public Health Service,
SIDS Alliance, and Association of SIDS and Infant Mortality Programs. Will send
brochures and videos on SIDS and sleeping position in English or Spanish.*

SIDS Network, Inc.
P.O. Box 520
Ledyard, Connecticut 06339
www.sids-network.org
The website contains extensive information on SIDS, including topics such as SIDS and vaccinations, apnea, and sleep. Also contains information on the latest government statistics and links with many other sites.

Sudden Infant Death Syndrome Alliance
1314 Bedford Avenue, Suite 210
Baltimore, Maryland 21208
800-221-7437
410-653-8226
www.sidsalliance.org
A national nonprofit organization dedicated to the support of SIDS families, education, and research. Provides up-to-date information on SIDS research and other topics.

Glossary

As and Bs: an abbreviation used for spells of **apnea** and **bradycardia**.

ABR: see **auditory brainstem response**.

ADD: see **attention deficit disorder**.

ADHD: see **attention deficit disorder with hyperactivity**.

adjusted age: see **corrected age**.

AGA: see **appropriate for gestational age**.

air leak: occurs when one or more of the air sacs in the lungs tear and air escapes from the lung into surrounding tissues. See **pneumothorax.**

alveoli: tiny air sacs in the lungs where the exchange of gases occurs, i.e., oxygen enters and carbon dioxide leaves the bloodstream.

amblyopia (lazy eye): a condition in which one eye is much weaker than the other; over time, the brain begins to ignore the visual information from the weaker eye, leading to blindness in that one eye. Treated by patching the stronger eye to encourage development of the weaker eye.

anemia: a condition in which the number of red blood cells, the component of the blood that carries oxygen, falls below normal; a very common condition among newborns, including preemies.

antibodies: substances in the blood that attack and kill germs and other foreign substances in the body; provide important disease-fighting capabilities.

antibiotic: a medicine that kills or slows the growth of bacteria in the body; used to fight infections.

Apgar score: a scoring system (ranging between 0 and 10) used to assess a newborn's condition, usually at one minute and five minutes after birth. Five attributes are judged—heart rate, breathing, color, muscle tone, and reflexes—and each given a 0, 1, or 2. Preemies often have low Apgar scores.

apnea: a pause in breathing that lasts for 15 to 20 seconds, or a pause of any length that is accompanied by a slowing of the heart rate and a change in skin color to bluish or pale.

appropriate for gestational age (AGA): a term describing a baby who at birth weighs between the 10th and 90th percentiles for his gestational age.

attending physician: the physician who is in charge of the nursery at any given time, and responsible for overseeing your baby's medical care. In a NICU, the attending physician is a neonatologist. Attending physicians usually change every month.

attention deficit disorder (ADD): a neurologic syndrome marked by excessive distractibility and impulsive behavior.

attention deficit disorder with hyperactivity (ADHD): ADD coupled with a need to be in constant motion.

auditory brainstem response (ABR): a hearing test commonly used with young babies in which the brain's response to sounds is measured by recording changes in brain waves.

bagging: a common term for manually pumping air into a baby's lungs; a soft mask is placed over the baby's mouth and nose, and an attached bag is gently squeezed.

betamethasone: a type of steroid drug given by injection to a mother before her baby's birth to help speed the development of the baby's lungs.

biliblanket: a plastic blanket containing fiber-optic bililights; another method of providing phototherapy to babies to treat jaundice.

bililights: white, green, or blue lights which help break down excess bilirubin in a baby's blood to treat or prevent jaundice. See **phototherapy**.

bilirubin: a yellowish substance contained within red blood cells, and released into the blood stream when the red blood cells break down. Bilirubin is normally processed in the liver and excreted in the stool. Because preemies' immature systems cannot process bilirubin very efficiently, levels can build up in the blood and cause jaundice. See **hyperbilirubinemia**.

blood culture: a blood test to determine the presence of and type of germ causing an infection.

blood gas: a blood test to measure the levels of oxygen, carbon dioxide, and acidity in the blood.

blow-by oxygen: method of providing a little extra oxygen for a baby during a tiring activity like feeding; a gentle stream of oxygenated air is provided from a tube or mask placed near her face.

Board-certified: a term for a doctor who has completed advanced training and passed a medical board examination in a specialty area (such as neonatology).

BPD: see **bronchopulmonary dysplasia**, and **chronic lung disease (CLD)**.

bradycardia: a slowing down of the heart rate below normal; in a preemie or other newborn, a heart rate below 100 beats per minute. Bradycardia often accompanies a spell of apnea, but may also occur in response to stress, during handling or feeding, or for other reasons.

brain bleed: common term for bleeding or hemorrhage in the brain. See **intraventricular hemorrhage (IVH)**.

bronchioles: small airways in the lungs. Bronchioles are like the smaller branches of a tree, connecting the larger branches (the bronchial tubes) that enter the lungs from the trachea (windpipe), and leading to the alveoli.

bronchiolitis: an inflammation or infection of the bronchioles.

bronchopulmonary dysplasia (BPD): a type of chronic lung disease seen primarily in premature babies caused by damage from respirators and exposure to supplemental oxygen. See **chronic lung disease (CLD)**.

bronchospasm: a narrowing of the larger airways in the lungs caused by contractions of the muscles around the airways.

brown fat: a particular kind of fat that infants and small children have that is important because it can be quickly used to produce body heat. Preemies have little brown fat until they weigh over about four pounds.

button gastrostomy: a short gastrostomy tube that extends just above the skin; a longer feeding tube can be attached when needed, and, when not in use, it can be covered by a plastic flap so that it is not very noticeable under clothing.

capillaries: tiny blood vessels that lie close to the surface of the skin.

carbon dioxide (CO_2): a gas that is formed as a waste product of metabolism in the body, carried by the blood to the lungs where it is exhaled.

cardiologist: a doctor specializing in the diagnosis and treatment of heart problems.

cardiopulmonary resuscitation (CPR): a method of supporting or reviving a person whose breathing and/or heart has stopped or slowed abnormally.

CAT scan (computerized axial tomography): a diagnostic imaging technique that uses a computerized x-ray machine to construct cross-sectional pictures of internal body structures. Sometimes used to diagnose bleeding in the brain or excess fluid in the brain (hydrocephalus).

catheter: a small flexible plastic tube through which fluids are given to or drained from the body.

central line: an IV line inserted into a vein, usually in the arm, and threaded from there into a larger vein in the body close to the heart. Used to deliver medicines or nutritional solutions that would irritate small veins.

central nervous system (CNS): refers to the brain and spinal cord.

cerebral palsy (CP): a general name given to a wide range of disorders of posture, movement, and muscle coordination caused by damage to the brain shortly before, during, or after birth.

cerebrospinal fluid (CSF): clear fluid produced in the ventricles of the brain; circulates around the brain and spinal cord.

chest PT: chest physical therapy. Usually consists of gentle tapping on the chest to help loosen and remove secretions in the lungs.

chest tube: used to treat an air leak or collapsed lung; a small tube is inserted into the space between the collapsed lung and chest wall to suction out air and allow the lung to re-expand.

CHF: see **congestive heart failure**.

chronic lung disease (CLD): refers to damage to the lungs caused by the ventilators and supplemental oxygen used to treat respiratory distress syndrome in premature babies. The lungs develop areas of bleeding and scarring, and the airways become narrower and rigid. Infants are diagnosed with CLD when they still need oxygen at 36 weeks gestational age, and if certain changes are seen in their lungs on X-rays. See also **bronchopulmonary dysplasia (BPD)**.

chronological age: refers to a baby's actual age, i.e., the number of weeks or months since his birth. Compare with **corrected age**.

circumcision: the removal of the foreskin covering the tip of the penis.

CNS: see **central nervous system.**

colostomy: a surgical procedure in which a portion of the colon (a section of the large intestine) is brought to the surface of the abdomen.

colostrum: early breastmilk produced in the last part of pregnancy and the first days after delivery. Colostrum is thick and yellowish, easily digested, and rich in protein and disease-fighting substances.

congestive heart failure (CHF): a condition in which the heart does not beat effectively; can be caused by structural problems in the heart or by a number of other medical problems.

continuing care nursery: see **special care nursery.**

continuous positive airway pressure: see **CPAP.**

corrected age: the age your baby would be if he had been born on his due date. During the first two to three years of life, your baby's corrected age is a more accurate indicator of what to expect in development and behavior. Compare with **chronological age.**

CP: see **cerebral palsy.**

CPAP (continuous positive airway pressure): a type of artificial ventilation in which a constant, gentle stream of air is blown into the lungs to help keep the airways and alveoli open, making breathing easier for the baby. CPAP is usually delivered through nasal prongs or endotracheal tube.

CPR: see **cardiopulmonary resuscitation.**

CSF: see **cerebrospinal fluid.**

CT scan: see **CAT scan.**

cutdown: a surgical procedure in which a small incision is made to place an IV line into a larger vein. Cutdowns can often be done right at a baby's bedside in the nursery.

deductible: refers to the amount you must pay before your health insurance company begins to cover the costs of medical care.

DPT: refers to immunizations given to infants and young children to protect against diphtheria, pertussis (whooping cough), and tetanus.

de-satting: in the language of the NICU, refers to a drop below normal in the level of oxygen in a baby's blood. See **desaturation, oxygen.**

desaturation, oxygen (de-satting): when the oxygen level (oxygen saturation) in the blood drops below a certain point.

discharge summary: a written report summarizing a baby's history in the hospital, including any complications he has experienced, treatments received, and medical needs after discharge.

diuretic: a medication that stimulates the body to produce more urine; used to help get rid of excess fluid.

ductus arteriosus: before birth, a short blood vessel that connects the pulmonary artery directly to the aorta so that most blood being pumped from the heart bypasses the lungs and goes directly out to the body. The ductus usually closes soon after birth, sending blood into the lungs to pick up oxygen before circulating through the body. See **patent ductus arteriosus (PDA).**

early intervention program: a program that offers a range of services to infants and toddlers under age three who have or are at risk for problems with development. EI programs receive funding from federal and state governments as well as health insurance companies, and provide services to eligible families free of charge.

ECG: see **electrocardiogram**.

echocardiogram (echo): an ultrasound examination of the heart, usually done at a baby's bedside in the nursery without disturbing him.

edema: puffiness or swelling caused when excess fluid accumulates in the body.

EEG: see **electroencephalogram**.

EKG: see **electrocardiogram**.

electrocardiogram (ECG or EKG): a test in which the electrical activity of the heart is recorded in order to assess how well it is functioning.

electroencephalogram (EEG): a test in which the electrical activity of the brain is recorded.

endotracheal (ET) tube: a plastic tube inserted through the nose or mouth and into a baby's windpipe (trachea). Used to give babies extra oxygen or to help babies breathe using CPAP or a ventilator.

ENT: ear, nose, and throat doctor. See **otolaryngologist**.

erythrocyte: see **red blood cell**.

ET tube: see **endotracheal tube**.

exchange transfusion: a kind of blood transfusion in which a small amount of blood is withdrawn and simultaneously replaced with an equal volume of donor blood; a method of quickly lowering high levels of bilirubin.

extremely low birthweight (ELBW): refers to a baby born weighing less than 1,000 grams (2 pounds 3 ounces). Sometimes called micro-preemies.

extubate: to remove an endotracheal tube.

feeder-growers: a common term for babies in intermediate (Level II) care. These are babies whose health has stabilized sufficiently that they no longer need intensive care, but still need special support and medical care while they continue to grow and develop.

feeding tube: see **gavage feeding**.

fellow: in a teaching hospital, a neonatology fellow is a physician who has finished his training to become a pediatrician, and is currently in training to become a neonatologist.

fine motor skills: refers to skills involving small muscles, such as those in the hand and fingers.

flaring: refers to the nostrils being opened widely during each breath in; an indication of breathing problems or respiratory distress.

fontanel: the soft spot on the top of a baby's skull where the bones of the skull have not yet grown together.

g-tube: see **gastrostomy tube**.

gastrostomy: a surgical opening through the abdominal wall into the stomach.

gastrostomy tube: a feeding tube that is used to deliver nutritional solutions directly into the stomach. Used when the esophagus is blocked or injured, or to provide extra nutrition to babies who are having severe or long-term feeding difficulties.

gavage feeding: tube feeding. A small soft plastic tube is inserted through the nose or mouth and directly into the stomach; used to feed babies who do not yet have the oral skills to feed by bottle or breast.

gestational age: a baby's age in weeks, measured from the beginning of the mother's last menstrual period before pregnancy. Using this system, a full-term pregnancy averages 40 weeks.

gram (g, gr): a unit of weight in the metric system, commonly used in hospitals; 28 grams equals one ounce.

gross motor skills: refers to abilities involving large muscles and movement, such as sitting, walking, running, throwing a ball, etc.

heel stick: a method of obtaining a small sample of blood from a baby by pricking her heel.

hematocrit: a blood test to measure the percentage of red blood cells in the blood.

hemoglobin: an iron-containing substance in red blood cells that carries oxygen. Also a blood test that measures the level of hemoglobin in the blood.

hepatitis: a disease that causes inflammation of the liver. There are different types (A, B, C) that are caused by different viruses, and transmitted by different means.

hernia: a condition in which a portion of the small intestine pushes through weak muscles in the abdominal wall. The two most common among preemies are an inguinal hernia, where the intestine pushes through into the groin area or scrotum, and an umbilical hernia, where the intestine pushes through a weak spot around the bellybutton, causing a soft swelling.

HMD: see **hyaline membrane disease or respiratory distress syndrome**.

hyaline membrane disease (HMD): an outdated term for respiratory distress syndrome; no longer in common usage.

hydrocephalus: an abnormal accumulation of cerebrospinal fluid in the ventricles of the brain, causing swelling within the brain and possible brain damage due to pressure on surrounding tissue.

hyperalimentation (hyperal): see **total parenteral nutrition**.

hyperbilirubinemia: higher than normal levels of bilirubin in the blood; common among preemies during the first weeks of life. See **jaundice** and **bilirubin**.

iatrogenic: an injury or disease caused by medical treatment.

ICN: intensive care nursery. See **neonatal intensive care unit**.

ICP: see **intracranial pressure**.

IFSP: see **Individualized Family Service Plan**.

ileostomy: a surgically created opening in the small intestine that brings the end of the intestine to the surface of the abdomen.

immunization: a vaccination that stimulates the body to produce antibodies to a particular disease, thus reducing or eliminating the person's chances of getting that disease. Preemies are immunized based on their chronologic age rather than their corrected age.

incubator: a clear plastic box with a temperature-controlled interior; used to protect and keep preemies warm.

Individualized Family Service Plan (IFSP): in early intervention programs, a document prepared jointly by parents and EI staff that specifies a child's needs and how those needs will be met, including what services she will receive, how often, from whom, and where. IFSPs are updated at regular intervals, usually every six months at a minimum.

indomethacin: a medication used to close a patent ductus arteriosus (PDA).

infection: inflammation and illness caused when germs—bacteria, viruses, or fungi—attack certain body tissues or organs.

intracranial pressure (ICP): the pressure exerted by cerebrospinal fluid (CSF) within the ventricles of the brain.

intrauterine growth retardation: a condition in which a baby grows more slowly than usual in utero, and is smaller than normal for his gestational age at birth.

intravenous line (IV): small plastic tube or needle inserted into a vein, usually in the hand, foot, or scalp, and used to deliver fluids, medicines, and nutritional solutions.

intraventricular hemorrhage (IVH): bleeding in the brain around or in the ventricles. Also called a **brain bleed**.

intubate: to insert an endotracheal (ET) tube.

Isolette: a brand of incubator, but commonly used as a term for incubator.

IUGR: see **intrauterine growth retardation**.

IV: see **intravenous line**.

j-tube: see **jejunal tube**.

jaundice: yellowish tinting to the skin and whites of the eyes caused by high levels of bilirubin in the blood.

jejunal tube: a feeding tube inserted into the portion of the small intestine known as the jejunum; used in cases of severe reflux or vomiting so that food bypasses the stomach.

kangaroo care: skin-to-skin contact; holding your baby (usually dressed only in a diaper) against your bare chest. Provides an opportunity for close contact between baby and parent. During kangarooing sessions babies appear to sleep well, maintain their body temperatures, and have steady heart and breathing rates.

kernicterus: brain damage caused by very high levels of bilirubin. A rare complication now that levels of bilirubin are monitored closely, and babies receive phototherapy early before levels can climb too high.

kilogram (kg): measure of weight in the metric system; equals 1,000 grams, or 2.2 pounds.

lanugo: soft downy hair on the body of a fetus or young preemie, particularly noticeable on the shoulders and upper back. Disappears as the baby matures.

large for gestational age (LGA): refers to a baby who is larger than normal (above the 90th percentile in weight) for his gestational age at birth.

let-down reflex: the initial flow of milk from the milk storage reservoirs within the breast down to the nipple; may be accompanied by a tingling or gripping sensation, and milk dripping or spurting from the nipples.

LGA: see **large for gestational age.**

LP: see **lumbar puncture.**

leukocyte: see **white blood cell.**

Level I nursery: a hospital nursery staffed and equipped to care for healthy mothers and newborns.

Level II nursery: a hospital nursery that can care for moderately premature infants, or those who no longer need intensive care. Also called an intermediate or special care nursery, or step-down unit.

Level III nursery: can provide intensive care for the youngest preemies, and critically ill newborns of any age; usually found in a large urban teaching hospital or regional medical center.

low birthweight (LBW): refers to any infant born weighing less than 2,500 grams, or 5 pounds 8 ounces. Babies can have low birthweights because they were born prematurely, or had problems with growth during the pregnancy.

lumbar puncture (LP, spinal tap): a procedure in which a needle is inserted between the vertebrae of the lower back, and a small amount of spinal fluid is withdrawn. May be used to get a sample of spinal fluid if an infection is suspected, or to drain excess cerebrospinal fluid.

magnetic resonance imaging (MRI): a diagnostic technique that uses a magnetic field to create pictures of organs and tissues within the body. Can create clearer images than CAT scans or ultrasounds.

maternal transport: transferring a pregnant mother before delivery from one hospital to another that can provide the appropriate level of care for both mother and baby. Usually occurs when a baby is expected to need intensive care after birth.

MCT oil: see **medium-chain triglyceride (MCT) oil**.

medium-chain triglyceride (MCT) oil: can be added to breast milk or formula to provide extra calories; easily digested by preemies' immature digestive systems.

meningitis: inflammation or infection of the meninges, membranes surrounding the brain and spinal cord. If meningitis is suspected, a lumbar puncture will usually be performed to test the spinal fluid for evidence of infection.

micro-preemie: a baby born weighing less than 750 grams (1 pound, 11 ounces).

monitor: similar to a small television, a monitor records and displays information about such things as heart rate, breathing rate, oxygen saturation levels, and body temperature.

murmur: sound made by blood flowing through the heart; some murmurs occur when there are problems with how the heart is operating, but many occur normally.

myopia: near-sightedness.

nasal cannula: soft plastic tubing that ends in two short prongs in the nostrils; used to administer supplemental oxygen and/or CPAP.

naso-gastric tube: see **NG tube**.

NBICU: newborn intensive care unit. See **neonatal intensive care unit**.

nebulizer: small machine that delivers humidified air and medications in a fine mist that is inhaled.

NEC: see **necrotizing enterocolitis**.

necrotizing enterocolitis (NEC): serious disorder of the bowel in which a portion of the bowel wall is damaged or dies.

neonatal: refers to the newborn period, from birth through the first 28 days of life.

neonatal intensive care unit (NICU): special nursery within a hospital equipped and staffed to care for very premature and sick newborns. Usually located in a teaching hospital or regional medical center. Also known as a Level III nursery, newborn intensive care unit (NBICU), or intensive care nursery (ICN).

neonatal nurse practitioner: a registered nurse who has received advanced training, usually through a master's degree program, in the diagnosis, care, and treatment of the problems of newborns, including preemies.

neonatologist: a pediatrician who has completed advanced training and is Board certified in neonatology.

neonatology: a pediatric subspecialty that deals with the diagnosis, care, and treatment of problems of pregnancy, labor, delivery, and newborns, including preemies.

NG (naso-gastric) tube: small flexible tube inserted through the nose, down the esophagus, and into the stomach; used to feed preemies who are too young or sick to feed by mouth. See **gavage feeding**.

NICU: see **neonatal intensive care unit**.

NNP: see **neonatal nurse practitioner**.

NPO: abbreviation for the Latin words meaning "nothing by mouth." Used when a baby should not be fed or given liquids by mouth.

occupational therapist (OT): a therapist who specializes in the development of fine motor skills; with preemies, OTs also assess behavioral responses and recommend ways of handling, feeding, and positioning babies to reduce stress and promote development.

ophthalmologist: physician specializing in the diagnosis and treatment of eye problems.

OPV: oral polio vaccine. Preemies begin their OPV series at two months (chronological age), but do not usually receive this vaccine until they are discharged from the hospital.

orthopedist: physician who specializes in diagnoses and treatment of problems of bones and joints.

orthotics: splints or braces used to support joints or limbs, or to improve movement.

OT: see **occupational therapist**.

otitis media: infection of the middle ear.

ostomy: an artificial opening created surgically. See **ileostomy, colostomy, gastrostomy,** and **tracheostomy**.

otolaryngologist: a physician specializing in the diagnosis and treatment of problems of the ear, nose, and throat.

oxygen (O_2): a gas that makes up 21% of regular room air; necessary for life.

oxygen hood: plastic box or hood placed over a baby's head to provide supplemental oxygen.

palate: the roof of the mouth.

patent: medical term meaning "open."

patent ductus arteriosus (PDA): a condition in which the ductus arteriosus, part of the fetal circulatory system, remains open and functional after birth rather than closing as it should. See **ductus arteriosus**.

PDA: see **patent ductus arteriosus**.

pediatric intensive care unit (PICU): a unit in the hospital that cares for critically ill infants and children admitted to the hospital after the newborn period (i.e., after the first 28 days of life).

PEG tube: see **percutaneous endoscopic gastrostomy tube**.

percutaneous endoscopic gastrostomy tube (PEG tube): a gastrostomy tube that is inserted without surgery; the tube is threaded down the esophagus into the stomach guided by an endoscope (a flexible tube with a lighted end), and then brought to the surface of the skin through a small incision.

perinatal: before, during, and after birth; usually includes the period of time from about week 20 of a pregnancy to one month after delivery.

perinatologist: an obstetrician who specializes in diagnosing and treating problems of pregnant women, fetuses, and newborns.

periodic breathing: irregular breathing pattern; breathing interrupted by pauses of up to 10 to 20 seconds. Common among all newborns, and especially among preemies.

periventricular leukomalacia (PVL): damage to the white matter of the brain caused by infection or insufficient blood flow.

phototherapy: light therapy; method of lowering high levels of bilirubin in newborns by exposing their skin to bright lights. See **bililights, hyperbilirubinemia,** and **jaundice**.

physical therapist (PT): a therapist who specializes in problems in coordination and in development of large motor skills.

PIE: see **pulmonary interstitial emphysema**.

pneumogram (sleep study): a test monitoring a baby's breathing and heart rate, oxygen saturation levels, and sometimes episodes of reflux during sleep to diagnose the reasons for any irregularities in breathing patterns. Sometimes called a pneumocardiogram.

pneumomediastinum: an air leak into the center of the chest.

pneumonia: inflammation or infection in the lungs.

pneumothorax: a condition that occurs when air escapes from the lung through a hole or tear, and becomes trapped between the lung and chest wall. The trapped air exerts pressure on the lung, causing it to collapse. Also known as an **air leak**.

Polycose: a brand name of a powdered form of easily digested sugars, added to breastmilk or formula to increase calories.

premature infant: a baby born before the end of the 37th week of pregnancy.

projectile vomiting: refers to forceful vomiting, usually by an infant.

pulmonary: having to do with the lungs.

pulmonary edema: an accumulation of fluid in the lungs.

pulmonary interstitial emphysema (PIE): a condition that occurs when air leaks from the air sacs into surrounding tissue in the lungs.

pulse oximeter: a small light sensor that measures the oxygen levels in the blood; usually attached to a finger or toe.

radiant warmer: a small open bed with heating elements above it. Often used right after delivery or for very sick newborns, it allows the staff to have easy access to care for the baby while keeping her warm. Also called a **warming table**.

RBC: see **red blood cell**.

RDS: see **respiratory distress syndrome**.

red blood cell (RBC, erythrocyte): the component of the blood that carries oxygen.

resident: a doctor who has completed medical school and is in training in a particular area of medicine. Most residents in the NICU are pediatric residents, i.e., they are in training to become pediatricians.

residual: food remaining in the stomach from a previous feeding at the time of the next feeding. Large residuals indicate feeding or digestion problems.

respirator: see **ventilator**.

respiratory distress syndrome (RDS): respiratory trouble that many preemies develop because their lungs are immature at birth. RDS is caused by a lack of surfactant within the lungs, a substance that keeps the air sacs from collapsing and sticking together.

respiratory syncytial virus (RSV): a common virus that causes respiratory infections; among newborns and babies with respiratory problems, can cause a serious lower respiratory infection (bronchiolitis and pneumonia).

RSV: see **respiratory syncytial virus.**

reticulocyte: an immature red blood cell; the presence of reticulocytes in the blood indicates the body is producing red blood cells.

retina: the light-sensitive lining of the back of the eye; responsible for sending visual images to the brain.

retinopathy of prematurity (ROP): an eye disease of prematurity; caused when the normal growth of blood vessels in the retina is disrupted. ROP often resolves with no treatment and no lasting damage to the eye, but if severe, can lead to scarring, retinal detachment, and blindness.

retractions: refers to a drawing in of the chest between the ribs and at the collarbone with each breath taken; an indication of breathing problems or respiratory distress.

ROP: see **retinopathy of prematurity.**

rounds: daily visits to each baby by the medical care team to discuss problems, progress, and plans for care.

scalp IV: a small IV placed in a vein in an infant's scalp.

seizure: abnormal electrical activity in the brain, usually causes involuntary muscle movements.

sensorineural hearing loss: hearing loss caused by damage to the inner ear or to the nerves that carry sound to the brain.

sensory integration dysfunction (SI dysfunction): abnormal or inefficient processing of sensory information by the brain, leading to oversensitivity or undersensitivity to stimuli such as sound, touch, light, and movement.

sensory system: body system composed of organs that allow you to see, hear, taste, feel, and smell.

sepsis: a general infection throughout the body.

septicemia: an infection in the blood.

serous otitis: accumulation of thick fluid in the middle ear.

SGA: see **small for gestational age.**

short bowel syndrome: occurs when a significant portion of the intestine (at least 50 percent) has been surgically removed; disrupts digestion and the absorption of water and nutrients. Also known as **short gut.**

short gut: see **short bowel syndrome.**

shunt: a thin tube used to drain excess fluid from one area of the body to another, such as a ventriculoperitoneal shunt used to treat hydrocephalus by allowing excess fluid to drain from the ventricles in the brain to the abdomen (peritoneum). Also, an abnormal connection between two areas of the body, such as a patent ductus arteriosus, which causes a right-to-left or left-to-right shunt of the blood flow.

SIDS: see **sudden infant death syndrome**.

SI dysfunction: see **sensory integration dysfunction**.

sleep study: see **pneumogram**.

small for gestational age (SGA): newborn whose weight is abnormally low (usually below the 10th percentile) for his gestational age.

spastic diplegia: a form of CP marked by increased muscle tone causing stiff, awkward movements; affects the legs more than the arms. The most common form of CP among premature babies.

special care nursery: a nursery equipped and staffed to care for moderately premature babies, recovering preemies, or any newborns who need extra care after birth. Also known as a Level II nursery, step-down unit, or continuing care nursery.

spinal tap: see **lumbar puncture**.

step-down unit: see **special care nursery**.

steroid: a medication that reduces inflammation and swelling.

streptococcus, Group B: a type of bacteria sometimes found in the vagina which can cause pneumonia in newborns.

strabismus: a condition in which the eyes do not work together in a coordinated way; eyes may either turn in or turn out.

sudden infant death syndrome (SIDS): the sudden unexplained death of a sleeping infant who is less than a year old.

sunsetting: refers to a downward gazing of the eyes; can be a symptom of increased intracranial pressure.

surfactant: a soap-like substance found in mature lungs that keeps the sides of the air sacs in the lungs from sticking together and collapsing. Artificial forms of surfactant are now available to help babies until they begin to produce surfactant naturally.

TCM: see **transcutaneous monitor**.

theophylline: a stimulant that is used to treat apnea.

tocolytic drugs: drugs used to slow or stop premature labor contractions, such as Terbutaline.

total parenteral nutrition (TPN): intravenous solution that contains all the nutritional elements a baby needs—proteins, fats, sugar, minerals, vitamins. Used when a baby cannot take in food orally for an extended time. Also known as **hyperalimentation**.

TPN: see **total parenteral nutrition**.

trachea: windpipe; tube that connects the throat to the bronchial tubes in the lungs.

tracheostomy: a surgical opening made into the windpipe (trachea), made to allow air to enter lungs if throat is obstructed. A breathing tube can be inserted through a tracheostomy.

transcutaneous monitor (TCM): a small device placed against an infant's skin to measure oxygen levels in the blood.

tube feeding: see **gavage feeding**.

ultrasound: a diagnostic technique that uses sound waves to create a picture of internal organs in the body. Painless and noninvasive, ultrasound tests can usually be performed at a baby's bedside in the nursery.

umbilical catheter: small, flexible plastic tube inserted into one of the blood vessels of the bellybutton (umbilicus) and used to deliver medication and fluid, take blood samples, and monitor blood pressure. Often used soon after birth.

under the lights: a term referring to phototherapy, or being under bilirubin lights to treat jaundice.

ventilator: a machine that breathes for a baby, or assists her breathing. Also known as a respirator.

ventricle: a small hollow chamber. The two lower chambers of the heart are called ventricles, and there are ventricles deep within the brain that produce cerebrospinal fluid and provide a cushioning system for the brain.

very low birthweight (VLBW): any infant who weighs less than 1,500 grams (3 pounds 5 ounces) at birth.

vital signs: the basic signs of life—heart rate, body temperature, breathing (respiration) rate, and blood pressure.

VLBW: see **very low birthweight**.

warming table: see **radiant warmer**.

white blood cell (WBC): component of the blood that helps to fight infection.

X-ray: diagnostic technique that uses electromagnetic waves to create an image of internal body structures.

Bibliography

℘

INTRODUCTION

Statistics on Prematurity

Ventura, S.J., et al. "Final Data for 1997." *National Vital Statistics Reports* 47(18): National Center for Health Statistics, Hyattsville, Maryland, 1999.

The reports containing these statistics are usually available in the government documents room of large public libraries, or can be accessed over the Internet at www.cec.gov/nchswww/. There is a two-year lag in reporting, so, for example, the statistics for 1998 were available in spring 2000.

CHAPTERS 1 AND 2: FIRST QUESTIONS and LEARNING YOUR WAY AROUND THE NICU

Survival and Disability Rates

Grogaard, J.B., et al. "Increased Survival Rate in Very Low Birth Weight Infants (1500 grams or less): No Association with Increased Incidence of Handicaps." *Journal of Pediatrics* 117(1), 1990.

McCormick, M.C. "Has the Prevalence of Handicapped Infants Increased with Improved Survival of the Very Low Birth Weight Infant?" *Clinics in Perinatology* 20(1), 1993.

General Information on Prematurity and the Care of Preemies

Brazy, Jane E. (ed.) *For Parents of Preemies: Answers to Commonly Asked Questions* (Madison: University of Wisconsin and The Center for Perinatal Care at Meriter Hospital, 1996). Also available over the Internet at: www.pediatrics.wisc.edu/childrenhosp/parents_of_preemies.

Cloherty, J.P. and Stark, A.R. (eds). *Manual of Neonatal Care* (Philadelphia: Lippincott-Raven Publishers, 1998).

Harrison, H. "Special Article: The Principles of Family-Centered Neonatal Care." *Pediatrics* 92(5), 1993.

Koh, T.H.H.G. and Jarvis, C. "Promoting Effective Communication in NICU by Audiotaping Parents-Neonatologist Conversations." *International Journal of Clinical Practice* 52(1): 1998. Excerpts from this article are also available in the keynote address "Promoting Partnership with Parents" from the Annual Conference of the Alexis Foundation and Preemie-L, Chicago, IL, 1999, at www.preemie-L.org/chicago8.htm

Merenstein, G.B. and Gardner, S.L. *Handbook of Neonatal Intensive Care* (St. Louis: Mosby-Year Book, Inc., 1998).

U.S. Congress, Office of Technology Assessment, "Neonatal Intensive Care for Low Birthweight Infants: Costs and Effectiveness" (Health Technology Case Study 38), OTA-HCS-38 (Washington, DC: U.S. Congress, Office of Technology Assessment, December 1987).

Zaichkin, Jeanette. *Newborn Intensive Care: What Every Parent Needs to Know* (Petaluma, CA: NICU Ink, 1996).

CHAPTER 3: PARENTING IN THE HOSPITAL

Traditional Holding and Kangaroo Care

Bosque, E.M., et al. "Physiologic Measures of Kangaroo Versus Incubator Care in a Tertiary-Level Nursery." *Journal of Obstetric, Gynecologic, and Neonatal Nursing* 24(3), 1995.

Legault, M. And Goulet, C. "Comparison of Kangaroo and Traditional Methods of Removing Preterm Infants from Incubators." *Journal of Obstetric, Gynecologic, and Neonatal Nursing* 24(6), 1995.

Ludington-Hoe, S.M. and Golant, S.K. *Kangaroo Care: The Best You Can Do to Help Your Preterm Infant* (New York: Bantam Books, 1993).

Infant Massage

Field, T. "Massage Therapy for Infants and Children." *Developmental and Behavioral Pediatrics* 16(2), 1995.

McClure, V. S. *Infant Massage: A Handbook for Loving Parents* (New York: Bantam Books, 1989).

Scafidi, F., et al. "Massage Stimulates Growth in Preterm Infants: A Replication." *Infant Behavior and Development* 13, 1990.

Walker, P. *Baby Massage: A Practical Guide to Massage and Movement for Babies and Infants* (New York: St. Martin's Press, 1996).

Comfort and Individualized Care

Als, H. and Gibes, R. *Newborn Individualized Developmental Care and Assessment Program (NIDCAP): Training Guide* (Boston: Children's Hospital, 1986).

Als, H., et al. "Individualized Developmental Care for the Very Low-Birth-Weight Preterm Infant: Medical and Neurofunctional Effects." *Journal of the American Medical Association* 272(11), 1994.

Buehler, D.M., et al. "Effectiveness of Individualized Developmental Care for Low-Risk Preterm Infants: Behavioral and Electrophysiologic Evidence." *Pediatrics* 96(5), 1995.

Cole, J.G., et al. "Changing the NICU Environment: The Boston City Hospital Model." *Neonatal Network* 9(2), 1990.

Gorski, Peter. "Developmental Intervention During Neonatal Hospitalization: Critiquing the State of the Science." *Pediatric Clinics of North America* 38(6), 1991.

Hussey, B. *Understanding My Signals: Help for Parents of Premature Infants* (Palo Alto, California: VORT Corporation, 1988).

Lawhon, Gretchen. "Management of Stress in Premature Infants." In Angelini, D.J., et al. (eds.) *Perinatal/Neonatal Nursing: A Clinical Handbook* (Boston: Blackwell Scientific Publications, 1986).

Merenstein, G.B. "Individualized Developmental Care: An Emerging New Standard for Neonatal Intensive Care Units?" (Editorial) *Journal of the American Medical Association* 272(11), 1994.

VandenBerg, K.A. "Basic Principles of Developmental Caregiving." *Neonatal Network* 16(7), 1997.

Oral Feeding and Breastfeeding Premature Infants

Gotsch, Gwen. *Breastfeeding Your Premature Baby* (Schaumberg, Illinois: La Leche League International, 1999).

Gross, S.J., et al. "Nutritional Composition of Milk Produced by Mothers Delivering Preterm." *Journal of Pediatrics* 96, 1980.

Lau, C., et al. "Oral Feeding in Low Birth Weight Infants." *The Journal of Pediatrics* 130(4), 1997.

Lucas, A. and Cole, T.J. "Breast Milk and Neonatal Necrotising Enterocolitis." *Lancet* 336(Dec.22/29), 1990.

Meier, P. and Anderson, G. "Responses of Small Preterm Infants to Bottle and Breast Feeding." *MCN: American Journal of Maternal-Child Nursing* 12, 1987.

Meier, P., et al. "The Accuracy of Test-Weighing for Preterm Infants." *Journal of Pediatric Gastroenterology and Nutrition* 10, 1990.

Meier, P., Brown, L.P., and Hurst, N.M. "Breastfeeding the Preterm Infant." In Riordan, J. and Auerbach, K.G. (eds.), *Breastfeeding and Human Lactation*, 2nd *Edition* (Sudbury, Massachusetts: Jones & Bartlett, 1998).

Nyqvist, K.H., et al. "Supporting a Preterm Infant's Behaviour During Breastfeeding: A Case Report." *Journal of Human Lactation* 12(3), 1996.

Walker, Marsha. *Breastfeeding Your Premature or Special Care Baby: A Practical Guide for Nursing the Tiny Baby* (Weston, Massachusetts: Lactation Associates, Item # 107, 1998).

Ziemer, M.M. and George, C. "Breastfeeding the Low-Birthweight Infant." *Neonatal Network* 9(4), 1990.

Emotional Reactions to Premature Birth

Affleck, G., et al. "Mothers, Fathers, and the Crisis of Newborn Intensive Care." *Infant Mental Health Journal* 11(1), 1990.

Castellano, C. "Parenting a Premature Baby." *Mothering*, Fall, 1988.

Davis, D. and Stein, M.T. *The Emotional Journey of Parenting Your Premature Baby: A Book of Hope and Healing* (in press) (Santa Rosa, CA: NICU Ink, 2001 [projected]).

Hynan, Michael T. *The Pain of Premature Parents: A Psychological Guide for Coping* (Lanham, MD: University Press of America, Inc., 1987).

Miles, M.S., et al. "Sources of Support Reported by Mothers and Fathers of Infants Hospitalized in a Neonatal Intensive Care Unit." *Neonatal Network* 15(3), 1996.

Miles, M.S. and Holditch-Davis, D. "Parenting the Prematurely Born Child: Pathways of Influence." *Seminars in Perinatology* 21(3), 1997.

Financing Care for Premature Infants

SSI for Premature Infants. Regional SSA Public Information Bulletin, No. 05-94, Boston Region, January, 1994.

Medicaid (Title XIX) and *State Child Health Insurance Programs (SCHIP) (Title XXI)*. Further information can be obtained from your state Medicaid or medical assistance office, or, at the federal level, from the Health Care Financing Administration of the Department of Health and Human Services. Their Internet website is: www.hcfa.gov/

CHAPTER 4: COPING WITH MEDICAL COMPLICATIONS

General References on Medical Complications

See references listed above for Chapters 1 and 2.

Apnea of Prematurity

Miller, M.J. and Martin, R.J. "Apnea of Prematurity." *Clinics in Perinatology* 19(4), 1992.

Perlman, J.M. and Volpe, J.J. "Episodes of Apnea and Bradycardia in the Preterm Newborn: Impact on Cerebral Circulation." *Pediatrics* 76(3), 1985.

Jaundice (Hyperbilirubinemia)

Although each hospital nursery has its own protocols determining when treatment for hyperbilirubinemia should begin, typical guidelines are the following:

For babies

- under 1,000 grams, phototherapy begins within 24 hours, and an exchange transfusion occurs at levels of 10-12 mg/dl;

- between 1,000 and 1,500 grams, phototherapy begins at bilirubin levels of 7 to 9 mg/dl, and exchange transfusion at 12 to 15 mg/dl;

- between 1,500 to 2,000 grams, phototherapy begins at levels of 10 to 12 mg/dl, and exchange transfusion at 15 to 18 mg/dl;

- between 2,000 and 2,500 grams, phototherapy begins at 13 to 15 mg/dl, and exchange transfusion at 18 to 20 mg/dl;

From *Manual of Neonatal Care*, Cloherty, J.P. and Stark, A.R. (eds.), (Philadelphia: Lippincott-Raven Publishers, 1998).

Blood Transfusions

Blood Transfusions: Knowing Your Options. Pamphlet from Pall Biomedical Products Company, East Hills, New York.

Respiratory Distress Syndrome and Chronic Lung Disease

American Lung Association Fact Sheets, "Respiratory Distress Syndrome" and "Bronchopulmonary Dysplasia," American Lung Association, 1-800-LUNG-USA.

Hanson, J. (ed.) *Parent Guide to Bronchopulmonary Dysplasia (BPD)* . Booklet from the American Lung Association of New Mexico and The Pediatric Pulmonary Program at the University of New Mexico, 1992.

Jobe, A.H. "Pulmonary Surfactant Therapy." *New England Journal of Medicine* 328(12), 1993.

Jobe, A.H., et al. "Beneficial Effects of the Combined Use of Prenatal Corticosteroids and Postnatal Surfactant on Preterm Infants." *American Journal of Obstetrics and Gynecology* 168(2), 193.

Northway, W.H., et al. "Late Pulmonary Sequelae of Bronchopulmonary Dysplasia." *New England Journal of Medicine* 323(26), 1990.

Schwartz, R.M., et al. "Effect of Surfactant on Morbidity, Mortality, and Resource Use in Newborn Infants weighing 500 to 1500 g." *New England Journal of Medicine* 330(21), 1994.

Air Leak (Pneumothorax)

Wyatt, T.H. "Pneumothorax in the Neonate." *Journal of Obstetric, Gynecologic, and Neonatal Nursing* 24(3), 1995.

Retinopathy of Prematurity

Page, J.M., et al. "Ocular Sequelae in Premature Infants." *Pediatrics* 92(6), 1993.

Phelps, D.L. "Retinopathy of Prematurity." *Pediatric Ophthalmology* 40(4), 1993.

Understanding Retinopathy of Prematurity. Booklet from IRIS Medical Instruments, Inc., Mountain View, California, 1991.

Necrotizing Enterocolitis (NEC)

Stoll, B.J. and Kliegman, R.M.(eds.) "Necrotizing Enterocolitis." *Clinics in Perinatology* 21(2), 1994.

Walsh, M.C., et al. "Severity of Necrotizing Enterocolitis: Influence in Outcome at Two Years of Age." *Pediatrics* 84(5), 1989.

Intraventricular Hemorrhage (IVH) and Periventricular Leukomalacia (PVL)

Dammann, O. and Leviton, A. "Maternal Intrauterine Infection, Cytokines, and Brain Damage in the Preterm Newborn." *Pediatric Research* 42(1), 1997.

Dammann, O. and Leviton, A. "Infection Remote from the Brain, Neonatal White Matter Damage, and Cerebral Palsy in the Preterm Infant." *Seminars in Pediatric Neurology* 5(3), 1998.

Philip, A.G.S., et al. "Intraventricular Hemorrhage in Preterm Infants: Declining Incidence in the 1980s." *Pediatrics* 84(5), 1989.

Rogers, B., et al. "Cystic Periventricular Leukomalacia and Type of Cerebral Palsy in Preterm Infants." *Journal of Pediatrics* 125(1), 1994.

Roth, S.C., et al. "Relation Between Ultrasound Appearance of the Brain of Very Preterm Infants and Neurodevelopmental Impairment at Eight Years." *Developmental Medicine and Child Neurology* 35, 1993.

Verma, U., et al. "Obstetric Antecedents of Intraventricular Hemorrhage and Periventricular Leukomalacia in the Low-birth-weight Neonate." *American Journal of Obstetrics and Gynecology* 176(2), 1997.

Volpe, J.J. *Neurology of the Newborn, Third Edition* (Philadelphia: W.B. Saunders Co.)

Volpe, J.J. "Brain Injury in the Premature Infant: Overview of Clinical Aspects, Neuropathology, and Pathogenesis." *Seminars in Pediatric Neurology* 5(3), 1998.

Volpe, J.J. "Cognitive Deficits in Premature Infants." Editorial, *New England Journal of Medicine* 325(4), 1991.

Volpe, J.J. "Neurologic Outcome of Prematurity." *Archives of Neurology* 55(3), 1998.

Infant Loss

Davis, Deborah L. *Empty Cradle, Broken Heart: Surviving the Death of Your Baby* (Golden, Colorado: Fulcrum Publishing, 1996).

Ilse, Sherokee. *Empty Arms: Coping with Miscarriage, Stillbirth and Infant Death* (Maple Plain, Minnesota: Wintergreen Press, 1990).

Kavanaugh, K. "Parents' Experience Surrounding the Death of a Newborn Whose Birth is at the Margin of Viability." *Journal of Obstetric, Gynecologic, and Neonatal Nursing* 26(1), 1997.

Wall, S.N. and Partridge, J.C. "Death in the Intensive Care Nursery: Physician Practice of Withdrawing and Withholding Life Support." *Pediatrics* 99(1), 1997.

CHAPTER 5: MAKING PROGRESS TOWARD HOME

Circumcision

American Academy of Pediatrics, Task Force on Circumcision, "Circumcision Policy Statement." *Pediatrics* 103(3), 1999. Available at www.aap.org/policy/re9850.html

American Academy of Pediatrics. "Circumcision: Information for Parents." Pamphlet available from the AAP, Elk Grove, Illinois (800-433-9016) or at www.aap.org/family/circ.html

Car Seats

American Academy of Pediatrics. "2000 Family Shopping Guide to Car Seats: Safety and Product Information." Pamphlet available from the AAP or over the Internet at: www.aap.org/family/famshop.htm

Bass, J.L., et al. "Monitoring Premature Infants in Car Seats: Implementing the American Academy of Pediatrics Policy in a Community Hospital." *Pediatrics* 91(6), 1993.

Bull, M.J. and Stroup, K.B. "Premature Infants in Car Seats." *Pediatrics* 75(2), 1985.

American Academy of Pediatrics, Committee on Accident and Poison Prevention. "Safe Transportation of Newborns Discharged from the Hospital." *Pediatrics* 86(3), 1990.

American Academy of Pediatrics, Committee on Injury and Poison Prevention and Committee on Fetus and Newborn. "Safe Transportation of Premature and Low Birth Weight Infants." *Pediatrics* 97(5), 1996.

Discharge Guidelines

Committee on Fetus and Newborn, American Academy of Pediatrics. "Hospital Discharge of the High-Risk Neonate — Proposed Guidelines." *Pediatrics* 102(2), 1998.

CHAPTERS 6 AND 7: AS YOUR BABY SETTLES IN and CARING FOR YOUR BABY AT HOME

Adjusting to Home

Ballard, R.A. *Pediatric Care of the ICN Graduate* (Philadelphia: W.B. Saunders Co., 1988).

Bernbaum, J.C. and Hoffman-Williamson, M. *Primary Care of the Preterm Infant* (St. Louis: Mosby-Year Book, 1991).

Blackburn, S. "Problems of Preterm Infants After Discharge." *Journal of Obstetric, Gynecologic, and Neonatal Nursing* 24(1), 1995.

Gorski, P.A. "Fostering Family Development after Preterm Hospitalization." In Ballard, R.A. *Pediatric Care of the ICN Graduate* (Philadelphia: W.B. Saunders Co., 1988).

Kenner, C. And Lott, J. "Parent Transition After Discharge from the NICU." *Neonatal Network* 9(2), 1990.

VandenBerg, K.A. and Hanson, M.J. *Homecoming for Babies After the Neonatal*

Intensive Care Nursery: A Guide for Professionals in Supporting Families and Their Infants' Early Development (Austin, Texas: PRO-ED, Inc., 1993).

VandenBerg, K.A. and Hanson, M.J. *Homecoming for Babies After the Neonatal Intensive Care Nursery: A Guide for Parents in Supporting Their Baby's Early Development* (Austin, Texas: PRO-ED, Inc., 1993).

Sleep Position and Sudden Infant Death Syndrome (SIDS)

American Academy of Pediatrics, Task Force on Infant Positioning and SIDS. "Positioning and Sudden Infant Death Syndrome (SIDS): Update." *Pediatrics* 98(6), 1996.

Hoffman, H.J. and Hillman, L.S. "Epidemiology of the Sudden Infant Death Syndrome: Maternal, Neonatal, and Postnatal Risk Factors." *Clinics in Perinatology* 19(4), 1992.

Hunt, C.E. and Shannon, D.C. "Sudden Infant Death Syndrome and Sleeping Position." *Pediatrics* 90(1, Part 1), 1992.

Lockridge, T. "Now I Lay Me Down to Sleep: SIDS and Infant Sleep Positions." *Neonatal Network* 16(7), 1997.

Willinge, M., et al. "Defining the Sudden Infant Death Syndrome (SIDS): Deliberations of an Expert Panel Convened by the National Institute of Child Health and Human Development." *Pediatric Pathology* 11(5), 1991.

General Information on Baby Care

American Academy of Pediatrics, Shelov, S. (ed.) *Caring for Your Baby and Young Child* (New York: Bantam Books, 1994).

Eisenberg, A., Murkoff, H.E., and Hathaway, S.E. *What to Expect the First Year* (New York: Workman Publishing, 1996).

Leach, Penelope. *Your Baby and Child: From Birth to Age Five* (New York: Alfred A. Knopf, 1997).

Ludington-Hoe, S.M. and Golant, S.K. *Kangaroo Care: The Best You Can Do to Help Your Preterm Infant* (New York: Bantam Books, 1993).

Sears, W. and Sears, M. *The Baby Book: Everything You Need to Know About Your Baby From Birth to Age Two* (Boston: Little, Brown & Co., 1993).

Spock, B. and Parker, S.J. *Dr. Spock's Baby and Child Care* (New York: Pocket Books, 1998).

American Academy of Pediatrics and American Academy of Dermatology. "Fun in the Sun: Keep Your Baby Safe. Guidelines for Parents." Pamphlet available from the AAP, Elk Grove, Illinois.

Immunization of Preemies

American Academy of Pediatrics, Committee on Infectious Diseases. "Recommended Childhood Immunization Schedule—United States, January–December 2000." *Pediatrics* 105(1), 2000.

American Academy of Pediatrics, Committee on Infectious Diseases. "Update on Timing of Hepatitis B Vaccination for Premature Infants and for Children with Lapsed Immunization." *Pediatrics* 94(3), 1994.

Khalak, R., et al. "Three-Year Follow-up of Vaccine Response in Extremely Preterm Infants." *Pediatrics* 101(4), 1998.

LaMar, K. "Implementing an Immunization Program in the Neonatal Intensive Care Unit." *Neonatal Network* 16(3), 1997.

Respiratory Syncytial Virus (RSV)

American Academy of Pediatrics, Committee on Infectious Diseases. "Respiratory Syncytial Virus Immune Globulin Intravenous: Indications for Use." *Pediatrics* 99(4), 1997.

American Academy of Pediatrics, Committee on Infectious Diseases. "Prevention of Respiratory Syncytial Virus Infections: Indications for use of Palivizumab and Update on the Use of RSV-IGIV." *Pediatrics* 102(5), 1998.

American Academy of Pediatrics, Impact-RSV Study Group. "Palivizumab, a Humanized Respiratory Syncytial Virus Monoclonal Antibody, Reduces Hospitalization from Respiratory Syncytial Virus Infection in High-risk Infants." *Pediatrics* 102(3), 1998.

Lehr, M.V. and Simoes, E.A.F. "A Weapon Against RSV for Children at Risk." *Contemporary Pediatrics* 15(2), 1998.

Maycock, D.E. and Redding, G. "Recommended Guidelines for Use of Synagis and Respigam in Infants and Children." Website from Children's Hospital and Regional Medical Center, Seattle, Washington (http://neonatal.peds.washington.edu/NICU-WEB/RSV_Prevention.asp).

Apnea and Home Monitoring

Miller, M.J. and Martin, R.J. "Apnea of Prematurity." *Clinics in Perinatology* 19(4), 1992.

National Institutes of Health Consensus Development Conference Statement. "Infantile Apnea and Home Monitoring." In Ballard, R.A. (ed.), *Pediatric Care of the ICN Graduate* (Philadelphia: W.B. Saunders Co., 1988).

Whitaker, S. "The Art and Science of Home Infant Apnea Monitoring in the 1990s." *Journal of Obstetric, Gynecologic, and Neonatal Nursing* 24(1), 1995.

CHAPTER 8: FEEDING YOUR BABY AT HOME

General Feeding Information

Also see references under Oral Feeding and Breastfeeding in Chapters 2 and 3, and Adjusting to Home and General Information on Baby Care in Chapters 6 and 7.

Lasky, Vicki. *Feed Me! I'm Yours* (NewYork: Meadowbrook Press, 1994).

Satter, Ellyn. *Child of Mine: Feeding with Love and Good Sense* (Palo Alto, California: Bull Publishing Co., 1991).

Satter, Ellyn. *How to Get Your Kid to Eat...But Not Too Much: From Birth to Adolescence* (Palo Alto, California: Bull Publishing Co., 1987).

Breastfeeding at Home

Huggins, K. *The Nursing Mother's Companion* (Boston: The Harvard Common Press, 1999).

Hill, P.D., et al., "Breastfeeding Patterns of Low-Birth-Weight Infants After Hospital Discharge." *Journal of Obstetric, Gynecologic, and Neonatal Nursing* 26(2), 1997.

Kavanaugh, K., et al., "Getting Enough: Mothers' Concerns About Breastfeeding a Preterm Infant After Discharge." *Journal of Obstetric, Gynecologic, and Neonatal Nursing* 24(1), 1995.

Kavanaugh, K., et al., "The Rewards Outweigh the Efforts: Breastfeeding Outcomes for Mothers of Preterm Infants." *Journal of Human Lactation* 13(1), 1997.

Kurakawa, J. "Finger-feeding a Preemie." *Midwifery Today* 29, 1994.

Mead, L.J., et al., "Breastfeeding Success with Preterm Quadruplets." *Journal of Obstetric, Gynecologic, and Neonatal Nursing* 21(3), 1992.

Meier, P., et al. "A New Scale for In-Home Test-Weighing for Mothers of Preterm and High Risk Infants." *Journal of Human Lactation* 10(3), 1994.

Feeding Challenges and Reflux

American Pseudo-obstruction and Hirschsprung's Disease Society. "Gastroesophageal Reflux." From website: www.tiac.net/users/aphs /reflux.htm

Babbitt, R.L., et al. "Behvioral Assessment and Treatment of Pediatric Feeding Disorders." *Developmental and Behavioral Pediatrics* 15(4), 1994.

Singer, L.T., et al. "Feeding Interactions in Infants with Very Low Birth Weight and Bronchopulmonary Dysplasia." *Developmental and Behavioral Pediatrics* 17(2), 1996.

Colic

Balon, A.J. "Management of Infantile Colic." *American Family Physician* 55(1), 1997.

Lehtonen, L.A. and Rautava, P.T. "Infantile Colic: Natural History and Treatment." *Current Problems in Pediatrics* 26, 1996.

Treem, W.R. "Infant Colic: A Pediatric Gastroenterologist's Perspective." *Pediatric Clinics of North America* 41(5), 1994.

CHAPTER 9: FROM INFANCY TO AGE THREE

Also see references under General Information on Prematurity and the Care of Preemies in Chapters 1 and 2, and under School-age Outcome Studies in Chapter 12.

Research on Preemie Development in the First Years

Bartlett, D. And Piper, M.C. "Neuromotor Development of Preterm Infants Through the First Year of Life: Implications for Physical and Occupational Therapists." *Physical and Occupational Therapy in Pediatrics* 12(4), 1993.

Bernbaum, J. and Hoffman-Williamson, M. "Following the NICU Graduate." *Contemporary Pediatrics* 3(June), 1986.

Blackburn, S. "Problems of Preterm Infants after Discharge." *Journal of Obstetric, Gynecologic, and Neonatal Nursing* 24(1), 1995.

Blackman, J.A. "Neonatal Intensive Care: Is It Worth It? Developmental Sequelae of Very Low Birthweight." *Pediatric Clinics of North America* 38(6), 1991.

Dubowitz, L. "Neurological Assessment." In Ballard, R. (ed.), *Pediatric Care of the ICN Graduate* (Philadelphia: W.B. Saunders Co., 1988).

Hack, M., et al. "Outcomes of Extremely Low Birth Weight Infants." *Pediatrics* 98(5), 1996.

Hulseman, M.L. and Norman, L.A. "The Neonatal ICU Graduate: Part I. Common Problems." *American Family Physician* 45(3), 1992.

Msall, M.E., et al. "Risk Factors for Major Neurodevelopmental Impairments and Need for Special Education Resources in Extremely Premature Infants." *Journal of Pediatrics* 119(4), 1991.

Oehler, J.M., et al. "Behavioral Characteristics of Very-Low-Birth-Weight Infants of Varying Biologic Risk at 6, 15, and 24 Months of Age." *Journal of Obstetric, Gynecologic, and Neonatal Nursing* 25(3), 1996.

Siegel, M.D. "Advances in Neonatology: View from a Practicing Physician." *Pediatric Clinics of North America* 40(5), 1993.

Thom, V.A. "Physical Therapy: Follow-up of the Special-Care Infant." In Ballard, R. (ed.), *Pediatric Care of the ICN Graduate* (Philadelphia: W.B. Saunders Co., 1988).

Grogaard, J.B., et al. "Increased Survival Rate in Very Low Birth Weight Infants (1,500 grams or less): No Association with Increased Incidence of Handicaps." *Journal of Pediatrics* 117(1), 1990.

Scottish Low Birthweight Study Group. "The Scottish Low Birthweight Study: I. Survival, Growth, Neuromotor and Sensory Impairment." *Archives of Disease in Childhood* 67, 1992.

Growth

Casey, P.H., et al. "Growth Status and Growth Rates of a Varied Sample of Low Birth Weight, Preterm Infants: A Longitudinal Cohort from Birth to Three Years of Age." *Journal of Pediatrics* 119(4), 1991.

Hack, M., et al. "Catch-up Growth During Childhood Among Very Low-Birth-Weight Children." *Archives of Pediatric and Adolescent Medicine* 150, 1996.

Hirata, T. And Bosque, E. "When They Grow Up: The Growth of Extremely Low Birth Weight (≤ 1000 gm) Infants at Adolescence." *Journal of Pediatrics* 132(6), 1998.

Kitchen, W.H., et al. "Very Low Birth Weight and Growth to Age Eight Years: I. Weight and Height."*American Journal of Diseases of Children* 146(1), 1992.

Ross, G., et al. "Growth Achievement of Very Low Birth Weight Premature Children at School Age." *Journal of Pediatrics* 117(2), 1990.

Sensory Integration Problems

Kranowitz, C.S. *The Out-of-Sync Child: Recognizing and Coping with Sensory Integration Dysfunction* (New York: Perigee Book, 1998).

Common Health Concerns

Cunningham, C.K., et al. "Rehospitalization for Respiratory Illness in Infants of Less Than 32 Weeks' Gestation." *Pediatrics* 88(3), 1991.

Doyle, L., et al. "Audiologic Assessment of Extremely Low Birth Weight Infants: A preliminary report." *Pediatrics* 90(5), 1992.

Dusick, A. "Medical Outcomes in Preterm Infants." *Seminars in Perinatology* 21(3), 1997.

Furman, L., et al. "Hospitalization as a Measure of Morbidity Among Very Low Birth Weight Infants with Chronic Lung Disease." *Journal of Pediatrics* 128(4), 1996.

Hack, M., et al. "Health of Very Low Birth Weight Children During Their First Eight Years." *Journal of Pediatrics* 122(6), 1993.

Kitchen, W.H., et al. "Respiratory Health and Lung Function in Eight-Year-Old Children of Very Low Birth Weight: A Cohort Study." *Pediatrics* 89(6), 1992.

Kitchen, W.H., et al. "Health and Hospital Readmissions of Very-Low-Birth-Weight and Normal Birth-Weight Children." *American Journal of Diseases of Children* 144, 1990.

McCormick, M.C., et al. "Hospitalization of Very Low Birth Weight Children at School Age." *Journal of Pediatrics* 122(3), 1993.

Emotional Challenges

Miles, M.S., et al. "Maternal Concerns About Parenting Prematurely Born Children." *MCN: American Journal of Maternal-Child Nursing* 23(2), 1998.

Seow, W.K. "Effects of Preterm Birth on Oral Growth and Development." *Australian Dental Journal* 42 (2), 1997.

CHAPTER 10: GETTING THE MOST OUT OF EARLY INTERVENTION AND SCHOOL-BASED PROGRAMS

Information about Early Intervention Programs

Ad Hoc Part H Work Group. "Helping Our Nation's Infants and Toddlers with Disabilities and Their Families: A Briefing Paper on Part H of the Individuals with Disabilities Education Act (IDEA) 1986-1995." Preliminary Report. Submitted to the Federal Interagency Coordinating Council, April 20-21, 1995 (Chapel Hill, North Carolina: National Early Childhood Technical Assistance System [NEC-TAS], 1995).

Hurth, J.L. and Goff, P.E. *Assuring the Family's Role on the Early Intervention Team: Explaining Rights and Safeguards* (Chapel Hill, North Carolina: National Early Childhood Technical Assistance System [NEC-TAS], 1998).

Massachusetts Department of Public Health, Early Intervention Services, Boston. Various pamphlets and booklets, including *Welcome to Early Intervention in Massachusetts: Your Guide to Early Intervention Programs throughout the Commonwealth; Welcome to the Individualized Family Service Plan;* and *Is Your Baby Blooming? If Not, Early Intervention Can Help.*

National Early Childhood Technical Assistance System (NEC-TAS) and the Office of Special Education Programs (OSEP) of the U.S. Department of Education. *Part H Updates, 2nd Edition: Updates on Selected Aspects of the Program for Infants and Toddlers with Disabilities (Part H) of the Individuals with Disabilities Education Act (IDEA)* (Chapel Hill, North Carolina: NEC-TAS, 1998).

Trohanis, P. "Progress in Providing Services to Young Children with Special Needs and Their Families: An Overview to and Update on Implementing the Individuals with Disabilities Education Act (IDEA)." *NEC-TAS Notes*, Number 7, 1995.

Shackelford, J. "State and Jurisdictional Eligibility Definitions for Infants and Toddlers with Disabilities Under IDEA." *NEC-TAS Notes*, Number 5, Revised, 1998.

In the section on the *Individualized Family Service Plan (IFSP)* in this chapter, the list of possible topics is based on materials developed by the Anne Sullivan Center Early Intervention Program, Lowell, Massachusetts, from several assessment tools. They are used here with the permission of the Director.

Effectiveness of Early Intervention

Bennett, F.C. and Guralnick, M.J. "Effectiveness of Developmental Intervention in the First Five Years of Life." *Pediatric Clinics of North America* 38(6), 1991.

Bennett, F.C. and Scott, D.T. "Long-Term Perspective on Premature Infant Outcome and Contemporary Intervention Issues." *Seminars in Perinatology* 21(3), 1997.

Brooks-Gunn, J., et al. "Enhancing the Cognitive Outcomes of Low Birth Weight, Premature Infants: For Whom is the Intervention Most Effective?" *Pediatrics* 89(6), 1992.

Brooks-Gunn, J., et al. "Effects of Early Intervention on Cognitive Function of Low Birth Weight Preterm Infants." *Journal of Pediatrics* 120(3), 1992.

McCarton, C.M., et al. "Results at Age Eight Years of Early Intervention for Low-Birth-Weight Premature Infants: The Infant Health and Development Program." *Journal of the American Medical Association* 277(2), 1997.

McCormick, M.C., et al. "Early Educational Intervention for Very Low Birth Weight Infants: Results from the Infant Health and Development Program." *Journal of Pediatrics* 123(4), 1993.

McCormick, M.C., et al. "The Health and Developmental Status of Very Low-Birth-Weight Children at School Age." *Journal of the American Medical Association*, 267(16), 1992.

Transition to Special Education Programs

Danaher, J. "Preschool Special Education Eligibility Classifications and Criteria." NEC-TAS Notes, Number 6, Revised, 1995.

FACTS/LRE (Family and Child Transitions into Least Restrictive Environments) Information Series.

Booklet #2: *Entering a New Preschool: How Service Providers and Families Can*

Ease the Transitions of Children Turning Three Who Have Special Needs (1994)

Booklet # 4: *Planning Your Child's Transition to Preschool: A Step-by-Step Guide for Families* (1995)

(University of Illinois at Urbana-Champaign, Champaign, Illinois: FACTS/LRE

Hausslein, Evelyn. *Turning Three: Moving from Early Intervention to Preschool — A Handbook for Parents* (Boston: The Federation for Children with Special Needs, 1995).

Massachusetts Department of Education, Division of Special Education. *A Parent's Guide to Special Education Regulations*, 1992.

CHAPTER 11: CARING FOR A CHILD WITH SPECIAL MEDICAL OR DEVELOPMENTAL NEEDS

Also see the references in Chapter 4.

General Overviews of Medical and Developmental Outcomes

Ballard, R.A. *Pediatric Care of the ICN Graduate* (Philadelphia: W.B. Saunders Co., 1988).

Batshaw, M.L. and Perret, Y.M. *Children with Disabilities: A Medical Primer* (Baltimore: Paul H. Brookes Publishing Company, 1992).

Bernbaum, J.C. and Hoffman-Williamson, M. *Primary Care of the Preterm Infant* (St. Louis: Mosby-Year Book, Inc., 1991).

Dusick, A. "Medical Outcomes in Preterm Infants." *Seminars in Perinatology* 21(3), 1997.

Wolraich, M.L., *Disorders of Development & Learning: A Practical Guide to Assessment and Management* (St. Louis: Mosby-Year Book, Inc., 1996).

Chronic Lung Disease

Giacoia, G.P., et al. "Follow-up of School-age Children with Bronchopulmonary Dysplasia." *Journal of Pediatrics* 130(3), 1997.

Robertson, C.M.T., et al. "Eight-Year School Performance, Neurodevelopmental, and Growth Outcome of Neonates with Bronchopulmonary Dysplasia: A Comparative Study." *Pediatrics* 89(3), 1992.

Vohr, B.R., et al. "Neurodevelopmental and Medical Status of Low-Birthweight Survivors of Bronchopulmonary Dysplasia at 10 to 12 Years of Age." *Developmental Medicine and Child Neurology* 33, 1991.

Walsh, M.C., et al. "Severity of Necrotizing Enterocolitis: Influence on Outcome at Two Years of Age." *Pediatrics* 84(5) 1989.

Hydrocephalus

About Hydrocephalus: A Book for Parents. Booklet from the Departments of Neurological Surgery and Pediatrics of the University of California, San Francisco, 1986.

Toporek, C. and Robinson, K. *Hydrocephalus: A Guide for Patients, Families and Friends.* Sebastopol, California: O'Reilly & Associates, Inc., 1999.

Cerebral Palsy

Blackman, J.A. "Disorders of Motor Development: Cerebral Palsy." In Wolraich, M.L., *Disorders of Development & Learning: A Practical Guide to Assessment and Management* (St. Louis: Mosby-Year Book, Inc., 1996).

Geralis, E. (ed.) *Children with Cerebral Palsy: A Parents' Guide* (Bethesda, Maryland: Woodbine House, 1991).

Leonard, J.F., Cadenhead, S.L., and Myers, M.E. *Keys to Parenting a Child with Cerebral Palsy* (Hauppauge, NY: Barron's Educational Series, Inc., 1997).

Coping with Complex Medical or Developmental Problems

Capper, L. *That's My Child: Strategies for Parents of Children with Disabilities* (Washington, D.C.: Child and Family Press, Child Welfare League of America, Inc., 1996).

Segal, Marilyn. *In Time and With Love: Caring for the Special Needs Baby* (New York: Newmarket Press, 1988).

CHAPTER 12: LOOKING TO THE FUTURE

School-age Outcome Studies

Chapieski, M.L. and Evankovich, K.D. "Behavioral Effects of Prematurity." *Seminars in Perinatology* 21(3), 1997.

Hack, M.B., et al. "School-Age Outcomes in Children with Birth Weights under 750 g." *New England Journal of Medicine* 331(12), 1994.

Hack, M., et al. "Long-Term Developmental Outcomes of Low Birth Weight Infants. *The Future of Children* 5(1), 1995.

Hille, E.T.M., et al. "School Performance at Nine Years of Age in Very Premature and Very Low Birth Weight Infants: Perinatal Risk Factors and Predictors at Five Years of Age." *Journal of Pediatrics* 125(3), 1994.

Klebanov, P.K., et al. "School Achievement and Failure in Very Low Birth Weight Children." *Developmental and Behavioral Pediatrics* 15(4), 1994.

Leonard, C.H. and Piecuch, R.E. "School Age Outcome in Low Birth Weight Preterm Infants." *Seminars in Perinatology* 21(3), 1997.

Leonard, C.H., et al. "Effect of Medical and Social Risk Factors on Outcome of Prematurity and Very Low Birth Weight." *Journal of Pediatrics* 116(4), 1990.

McCormick, M.C. "Has the Prevalence of Handicapped Infants Increased with Improved Survival of the Very Low Birth Weight Infant?" *Clinics in Perinatology* 20(1), 1993.

Piecuch, R.E., et al. "Outcome of Extremely Low Birth Weight Infants (500 to 999 Grams) Over a 12-Year Period." *Pediatrics* 100(4), 1997.

Resnick, M.B., et al. "Educational Outcome of Neonatal Intensive Care Graduates." *Pediatrics* 89(3), 1992.

Ross, G., et al. "Social Competence and Behavior Problems in Premature Children at School Age." *Pediatrics* 86(3), 1990.

Ross, G., et al. "Educational Status and School-Related Abilities of Very Low Birth Weight Premature Children." *Pediatrics* 88(6), 1991.

Saigal, S., et al. "Self-perceived Health Status and Health-Related Quality of Life of Extremely Low-Birth-Weight Infants at Adolescence." *Journal of the American Medical Association* 276(6), 1996.

Scottish Low Birthweight Study Group. "The Scottish Low Birthweight Study: II. Language Attainment, Cognitive Status, and Behavioural Problems." *Archives of Disease in Childhood* 67, 1992.

Skuse, D. "Survival After Being Born Too Soon, But at What Cost?" (Editorial comment on study by Wolke and Meyer) *The Lancet* 354 (July 31), 1999.

Taylor, H.G., Hack, M., et al. "Achievement in Children with Birth Weights Less Than 750 Grams with Normal Cognitive Abilities: Evidence for Specific Learning Disabilities." *Journal of Pediatric Psychology* 20(6), 1995.

Tyson, J.E. and Broyles, R.S. "Progress in Assessing the Long-term Outcome of Extremely Low-Birth-Weight Infants." *Journal of the American Medical Association* 276(6), 1996.

Vohr, B., et al. "Effects of Intraventricular Hemorrhage and Socioeconomic Status on Perceptual, Cognitive, and Neurologic Status of Low Birth Weight Infants at Five Years of Age." *Journal of Pediatrics* 121(2), 1992.

Vohr, B.R. and Msall, M.E. "Neuropsychological and Functional Outcomes of Very Low Birth Weight Infants." *Seminars in Perinatology* 21(3), 1997.

Waber, D.P. and McCormick, M.C. "Late Neuropsychological Outcomes in

Preterm Infants of Normal IQ: Selective Vulnerability of the Visual System." *Journal of Pediatric Psychology* 20(6), 1995.

Wolke, D. and Meyer, R. "Cognitive Status, Language Attainment, and Prereading Skills of Six-Year-Old Very Preterm Children and Their Peers: the Bavarian Longitudinal Study." *Developmental Medicine & Child Neurology* 41, 1999.

Acknowledgments

This book began many years ago as an idea that wouldn't go away, and it is my great pleasure to acknowledge the many people—both professionals and parents—who helped to turn that idea into a reality. First, I would like to thank my agent, Kit Ward, who guided me through the process of putting together a book proposal, provided valuable feedback on ideas and drafts, and supported my efforts throughout this project with warmth and good humor. I am grateful to Bruce Shaw at The Harvard Common Press for taking a chance on an unknown writer, to editors Dan Rosenberg and Debra Hudak for their patience and skill, and to the rest of the staff who have helped to produce this book. It has been nothing but a pleasure to work with you all. Thanks also to editor Adrienne Lieberman for streamlining my prose and ridding it of an enormous number of unnecessary words, and to Gail Pool and the members of the Radcliffe Seminars writing class for their help in shaping the book in its early stages.

I am indebted to a long list of individuals who work with preemies for generously sharing their time, knowledge, and experience, and greatly enhancing my understanding of the many issues facing preemies and their parents. I would like to single out a few of these for special thanks.

At the very top of this list is Linda Van Marter, MD, MPH, neonatologist of Children's Hospital in Boston, who cared for Philip and his parents with great kindness and skill during our early days in the NICU, and who was the first professional with whom I discussed my idea of writing a book for parents of preemies. Linda has been an invaluable source of information and support throughout this project. She has discussed with me the many aspects of prematurity and its impact on babies and parents, has shared her vast library of research articles, patiently answered my many questions, and provided feedback on drafts. Writing this book would have been much more difficult without her help. I would also like to thank Marie McCormick, MD, ScD, Chairman of the Department of Maternal and Child Health of the Harvard School of Public Health, who reviewed with me the research on long-term outcomes for preemies, commented on drafts, and clarified many aspects of the research that I found confusing. I am grateful, as well, to Jane Stewart, MD, Co-Director of the Infant Follow-up Clinic of Children's Hospital, Boston, for her help, particularly with the chapter on medical complications, and for providing an Introduction to the book. And for his behind-the-scenes impact on the book, I would like to thank our pediatrician, Dan Epstein, MD. His advice when we first brought Philip home from the hospital woke me up to the ongoing differences between preemies and full-term infants, and, over the years, he has continued to provide good health care, answers to questions on a vast range of topics, and good cheer.

Many other professionals who work with preemies provided valuable information on various aspects of preemies and preemie development, and I thank everyone with whom I met over the past five years. In particular, I would like to acknowledge the contributions of the following individuals: Maureen Hack, MB, ChB, Director of High Risk Follow-up, Neonatal Unit of Rainbow Babies and Children's Hospital, Cleveland, Ohio, for her early interest in this project and comments on the book proposal and book outline; Betty Vohr, MD, of Women and Infant's Hospital, Providence, R.I., for a discussion on issues in preemie development; Linda Zaccagnini, RNC, MS, NNP, of Beth Israel-Deaconess Medical Center, Boston, for a review of common problems and routine care for preemies in the hospital; Caryn Doumas, RN, and Carol Shockley, RN, staff nurses and primary caregivers in the NICU at Brigham and Women's Hospital, Boston, for advice on ways in which parents can be involved in caring for their babies; and Steven Ringer, MD, Director of Newborn Medicine, Brigham and Women's Hospital, Boston, for reviewing the proposal and final draft of the book, and for his interest and support. And for answering numerous questions about services provided by social workers in hospital nurseries, I thank Tamara May, MSW, LICSW, at Brigham and Women's Hospital, Boston.

Cathy Chapman, MD, of Children's Hospital, Boston, neurologist and neighbor, provided a crash course in neurology and brain anatomy while sitting at my kitchen table one morning. Alan Leviton, MD, Olaf Dammon, MD, and David Bellinger, PhD, of the Neuroepidemiology Unit of Children's Hospital, Boston, spent several hours with me explaining white matter damage in preemies, its possible causes and effects, and current research efforts. Janice Ware, PhD, formerly Director of Pediatric Psychology, and Jane Holmes-Bernstein, PhD, Director of the Neuropsychology Program at Children's Hospital, Boston, reviewed common issues in cognitive development in preemies.

For information on breast-feeding preemies, I would like to thank Michelle Weisberg, RN, IBCLC, lactation specialist at Brigham and Women's Hospital, Dot Norcross of Lactation Care, Newton, MA, and Marsha Walker of Lactation Associates, Weston, Massachusetts. Thanks to Arden Hill, MS, CCC-SLP, and Kara Fletcher, MS, CCC-SLP, speech pathologists and coordinators of the Swallowing Disorders Program at Children's Hospital, for their informative seminar on growth, eating disorders and their treatment, and to Arden, who answered many questions in a follow-up telephone conversation. Nancy Terres, PhD, RNC, of the Graduate Nursing Program, MGH Institute of Health Professions, provided a great deal of useful information on feeding disorders and their treatment, as well. Dan Shannon, MD, Unit Chief, Pediatric Pulmonary and Cystic Fibrosis Unit, Massachusetts General Hospital, reviewed and commented on sections of the book on SIDS and sleep position. Guidance on issues of small and large motor development were provided by occupational therapist Cindy Sutton, OTR, formerly of Massachusetts General Hospital, and Joanne Sweeney, PT, and Jill Lewis, PT, physical therapists at Riverside Early Intervention Program, Needham and Dedham, Massachusetts.

I would like to thank the directors of several early intervention programs who provided background information on EI, access to staff members who work with preemies, and referrals to preemie parents: Margaret Mahoney of the Anne Sullivan Center, Lowell, Massachusetts; Tom Maloney, former director of the Riverside Early Intervention Program, Needham, Massachusetts; and Lorraine Sanak, Waltham-Weston EI Program, Waltham, Massachusetts. Thanks to Laura Aldrich, current director of Riverside EI Program for providing a sample IFSP and photograph of an EI session. I would also like to thank Pat McLean, RN, for sharing her broad knowledge of preemies from her work at the Richie McFarlane EI Center in Stratham, New Hampshire.

Evelyn Hausslein, formerly Director of Early Intervention for the Federation for Children with Special Needs, Boston, and Karen Algus, parent advocate, helped with background information and resources on special education, and the transition from early intervention to school-based programs. And Eileen Sullivan, Early Childhood Coordinator for the Newton Public Schools, Newton, Massachusetts, generously reviewed with me the contents of a typical IEP form.

This book would not have been complete without the details of life with preemies that I learned from the many parents I interviewed. I am grateful to them all for sharing their experiences and their children with me, and thank them for helping others through their voices in this book. I would particularly like to thank Diana Zais, parent of preemie twins, who has enriched my life as a friend, and who helped this project enormously by being willing to discuss all the special ups and downs of preemie parenting. A special thanks as well to Jill Baranoski, Anne Costello, Diane Hendrigan, Iris Hardin, Dale Murphy, Donna Rassulo, and Lesley Ann Rosowski. Members of NICU:Parent Support, Inc., of Newton, Massachusetts, have provided a wonderful support network over the past eight years, and their interest in this book is greatly appreciated. I would also like to thank Allison Martin, owner of the Internet-based Preemie-Child email support group, and to all the members of the group who shared their experiences and knowledge on-line; many of their contributions are included at the end of the book under "Voices of Experience."

And finally, my friends and family have been incredibly patient and supportive through the many years it has taken to complete this book. Their continued interest and encouragement have meant a lot to me. Thanks to Linda Atkinson and my mother, Rosalie Leach, who read the manuscript with fresh eyes, and improved it with insightful comments. My gratitude also goes to Marion Vendituoli, Anne and Alun Jones, Kim Streetman, and John Wolf for their steady encouragement. And last, but not least, my love and thanks to my husband, Paul, and my children, Megan, Charlie, and Philip, each of whom contributed in their own ways to the creation of this book, and whose support was indispensable to me.

Index

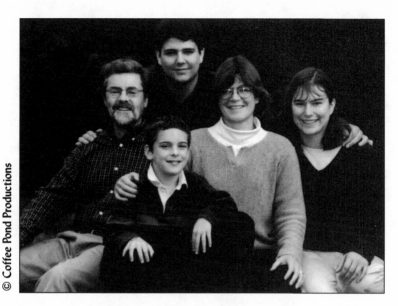

About the Author

Susan L. Madden, M.S., was inspired to write *The Preemie Parents'*
Companion after the birth of her own premature child. The book developed from her observations of the joys and challenges of helping her son
grow, and of the ways his behavior and development differed from those of
her full-term children. Drawing upon her firsthand experience as the
mother of a preemie, her academic training in public health, and her professional experience as a health and health-administration writer, Madden
devoted countless hours of research, interviews, and writing to creating a
thorough, accessible, up-to-date, and much-needed guide to successfully
and lovingly raising a healthy preemie.

A graduate of Harvard/Radcliffe College with a Master's degree in
Health Policy and Management from the Harvard School of Public
Health, Madden has long been involved in health care and has written
and spoken extensively on health-related issues. She has co-authored two
books: *A Guidebook on Geriatric Program Development in Community and*
Migrant Health Centers (published by the Government printing office) and
Methods of Controlling Ancillary Usage: A Guidebook for Hospital Admin-
istrators (published by the Massachusetts Hospital Association). Susan
Madden lives in the Boston area with her husband and three children.